D1082177

COSMOPOLITAN CONCEPTIONS

Cosmopolitan Conceptions   IVF Sojourns in Global Dubai

MARCIA C. INHORN

Duke University Press   Durham and London   2015

© 2015 Duke University Press
All rights reserved
Printed in the United States of America on acid-free paper ∞
Cover design by Natalie F. Smith; interior design by
Heather Hensley
Typeset in Chaparral Pro by Westchester Publishing Services

Library of Congress Cataloging-in-Publication Data
Inhorn, Marcia Claire, [date]
Cosmopolitan conceptions : IVF sojourns in global Dubai /
Marcia C. Inhorn.
pages cm
Includes bibliographical references and index.
ISBN 978-0-8223-5913-5 (hardcover : alk. paper)
ISBN 978-0-8223-5933-3 (pbk. : alk. paper)
ISBN 978-0-8223-7535-7 (e-book)
1. Fertilization in vitro, Human—United Arab Emirates—Dubai.
2. Medical tourism—United Arab Emirates—Dubai. I. Title.
RG135.I5834 2015
362.1981'780599095357—dc23   2015009494

Cover art: Burj Dubai (Burj Khalifa). Dubai, United Arab Emirates.
© philipus / Alamy.

CONTENTS

ILLUSTRATIONS

PROLOGUE

Rahnia's Reproductive Journey

On February 4, 2007, I met Rahnia in an in vitro fertilization (IVF) clinic called Conceive, located strategically on the border between the emirates of Dubai and Sharjah, two of the seven principalities that make up the United Arab Emirates (also known as "the UAE" or "the Emirates," terms that will be used interchangeably in this book).[1] Rahnia was a stunning half-Ethiopian, half-Eritrean Muslim woman who had fled the civil war in her divided countries,[2] becoming a teenage refugee in London. There she eventually met Ahmed, a fellow Muslim refugee from Sudan. "It was very hard to hunt down a Muslim man in the UK [United Kingdom]," Rahnia explained. "And when I met him, it was very hard to conceive, very hard. But I'm very optimistic. I see bright light at the end of the tunnel."

Rahnia agreed to share with me her story of marital infertility and duress and the tumultuous journey that had landed her in a clinic far away from home. With her three-year-old IVF daughter, Wisal, by her side, Rahnia told me this story, hoping that it would somehow "help others" in their own quests for conception. Her story is transcribed verbatim, with minor editing for clarity and definition of some key terms. (Medical terms used by Rahnia are defined in the medical glossary at the end of this book.) I have included my questions to Rahnia, although most of her story was delivered to me in English and with no prompting. I have italicized parts of Rahnia's narrative that she delivered with particular emphasis. With Rahnia's knowledge, I have changed her name (and those of her family members) to protect her identity, given the sensitivity and confidentiality of several parts of her story. However, the story itself has not been altered and is presented here in its full form, in Rahnia's own words.

In Her Own Words

Rahnia: "Well, let me tell you my story. We tried for five years, but there was no natural conception. We tried going to different doctors, using different medications. They did hormonal treatments, but they said the only option was IVF. That was in the UK, and actually, *not one doctor diagnosed the problem in the UK!* No diagnostic tests were done in the UK. This is because there is no system of private medicine in the UK. Most people use the National Health Service [NHS]. I work and I pay taxes, and so I'm entitled to use the NHS. But they did no diagnostic tests, and I was given some kind of medicine, tablets, to stimulate my eggs. I tried for years without any doctor telling me what was wrong. So I traveled to Egypt."

Marcia: "Oh, I've lived in Egypt! Why did you go to Egypt?"

Rahnia: "Well, Egypt was a coincidence, because my brother was there, and I went to visit. And at the same time, I was depressed, and so I thought I would see an obstetrician. I found a local doctor, and I explained my situation, and she said: *'You've taken all this medication without any diagnostic test?!'* So a [diagnostic] laparoscopy was done there, in Cairo, at Misr El Gadida Hospital. I couldn't find one IVF center there, and actually, I wasn't sure at that time if I was interested, because I was not sure if IVF was my best option. But, as I was growing older, maybe one option was pregnancy through IVF."

Marcia: "What did they tell you in Egypt?"

Rahnia: "This is very confidential, but I had chlamydia [a sexually transmitted infection]. It was untreated and perhaps I had it since I was a teenager. This is the reason why I am infertile. My [fallopian] tubes—there are lots of adhesions [that is, scar tissues], and they removed the adhesions. They did a good job, and we were both, my husband and I, treated for chlamydia. This chlamydia I did not know about in the UK. It was discovered in Egypt. To boost my fertility, those Egyptian doctors also gave me Clomid [a fertility drug] again.

"Because I live in the UK, and I had taken all of these medications there, I wanted a shortcut. So I went to seek IVF in the UK in 2002. But, actually, I had to pay for it. I would have tried to use the NHS, because you have one entitlement for [free] IVF if you've been infertile for several years. But you have to wait for two years [on the NHS waiting list]. So I had to make a shortcut. I said, 'Let's make the impossible possible.' I got money from family and friends to go to a private clinic. The cheapest IVF, including the cost of medications, was still about £3,000 [approximately $5,000]."

Marcia: "That's a lot of money!"

Rahnia: "When you're desperate, you do the impossible. But I was unlucky again. I had an ectopic pregnancy [a tubal pregnancy]. It was on the right-hand side. But it was not discovered by the clinic that I was pregnant."

Marcia (shocked): "Really?"

Rahnia: "The level of service there in the UK is very bad. I went for a scan [an ultrasound]. They said, 'Okay, you're pregnant but spotting. Let's give it a few days.' That same night, I fainted and was rushed to the emergency. They had missed the ectopic, and I would have lost my very life. I went back to the NHS for the emergency ectopic, and they said they didn't know how that private IVF center could have failed to treat me. I had to have my tube removed, my right tube, and the left one was damaged. I lost *so* much blood; I was given four units of blood, because it was an emergency situation. Though I *must* say that those doctors at the NHS, they saved my life."

Marcia: "What happened then?"

Rahnia: "Well, again, I was desperate. That was 2002—no, 2003. At that time, because I had the ectopic pregnancy, automatically I was put onto the [NHS] waiting list [for IVF], but they said it will be two years. Again, I was desperate. I had been trying for five to six years, and I didn't want to wait two more years. Again, I went to another [private IVF] center, which brought me luck. I had her [pointing to her three-year-old daughter, sitting by her side] through a regular IVF cycle. It was similar to the first one, the cheapest I could find. And this time, I had some frozen embryos. I had *several* frozen [IVF] cycles, a countless number.[3] There in the UK, they never count frozen embryo transfers. They only count fresh cycles. They don't acknowledge frozen cycles for some reason, maybe because they don't succeed as much."

Marcia: "Did you ever get pregnant with a frozen cycle?"

Rahnia: "I actually got a clinical pregnancy with a frozen cycle.[4] I had *so* many frozen cycles. Each time I would go for a fresh cycle, I would get eight good embryos, *very* good, *very* good. But they only allow you to use two embryos in the UK. They will only put two back [in the uterus]. If I have six frozen, and if they can only transfer two at a time, then I can try thrice. That cost, of about £500 to £600 [$850–$950], is nothing compared to a fresh cycle. I had two fresh cycles at two different clinics, and I got her [Wisal, the daughter] on the second one. After her—I did three fresh after her. And *a lot* of frozen cycles. It could be seven to eight fresh and frozen cycles overall. But I've never been successful after that one cycle. I'm still trying. I'm trying."

Marcia: "Do you feel like you need a second child?"

Rahnia: "To be honest, I'm in a better situation with my daughter. God blessed me with her. But I have fear. In case an accident or something killed her, as a mother, I have all kinds of worries. It's *terrible*. I want at least two children, whatever God gives. The joy you get from children can't be compared."

Marcia: "So you keep on trying IVF?"

Rahnia: "Yes, but, as I said, in the last cycle, it was a fresh cycle, and it cost a fortune. They did a blastocyst transfer, and it was *very* demanding. It had a lot of consequences. But I had *good eggs*—at least ten good eggs. I was blessed with very, very good eggs, and so they got actually eight or nine embryos, all very good. Obviously, they have to be kept differently in the blastocyst phase. We reached four very good embryos by day five. But according to UK law, I was only able to put back two [in the uterus]. I lost two, because they couldn't freeze them, and they were discarded. I *begged* the doctor to put at least three [embryos back into the uterus], but he said that the clinic would [have to] 'close its doors' if he did that. I understand that he has to follow the rules, but they are extremely strict."

Marcia: "It's not like that in the US, where I come from. We don't have these kinds of restrictions."

Rahnia: "I *love* the US. I actually searched to go to the US, one clinic in Virginia, but it's very expensive. They have a 'package' amount, but it's many thousands of dollars. And that clinic said they will make you pregnant or give you your money back—a refund."

Marcia: "Could you have gone?"

Rahnia: "No, not really. I am working in a job there in the UK. I work in recruitment. We recruit for casual workers in a company. And even though I like my job, my personal circumstances create stress. All the stress. It was [would have been] *really* hard for me to leave, to go to the

US. Finally, I decided to take an unpaid leave from work, an unpaid leave. They are very nice to enable me to leave."

Marcia: "So you decided to take a leave from work to travel?"

Rahnia: "Yes, because I had to journey in my life. First, to get pregnant. Then to go back from where I came, to see my family. I left sixteen years ago because of the war. I was able to come out due to the consequences of the civil war, but some are still trapped there. I thought part of the reason IVF failed so many times is my longing—my feeling of needing to go back. I said: 'Let me rest my soul before I do another IVF.' Plus, my extended family hasn't seen my daughter. So I went back. I tell you, *I'm on a journey*! That's why I came to Dubai. I intend to do IVF!

"My husband wasn't in favor of this. My husband said, 'Put the treatment off. It will drive you mad!' But I arranged to go to India, Mumbai. I found a clinic. I searched the Internet, and I found clinics in India, the US, Canada, and Italy. Before going to Africa, I had already gone to Italy. But unfortunately, the guy [doctor] I met, he was only able to do a [diagnostic] laparoscopy. He couldn't help me with IVF. It was not his field, he told me. He found water in my remaining tube that needs to be removed before I should consider IVF. Plus, Italy also restricts the number of embryos, just like the UK. If you produce lots of eggs, they can only put two to three embryos back, and the rest are destroyed. *That's blocking my way! I had to run away from there!*

"Back in the UK, I met a friend of a friend, who was pregnant with twins. I met her and, even though people don't openly talk about IVF—people are not honest about their fertility treatment—she obviously had heard rumors that I've been trying for years. She got pregnant through IVF in this center [Conceive], but she was not willing to give me the number. So I was hunting down the number on the Internet. I found a center in El Rashid Hospital in Dubai, and I e-mailed a few other places, and they put me off: 'You're better off in the UK. Why would you come here? You are in a better place [in the United Kingdom].' But the level of service [in the United Kingdom] might not be good. And they have restrictions, rules you have to obey.

"I went to the Internet, thinking I'll just find Conceive there. I found Conceive, but only the address. Their website was 'under construction.'"

Marcia: "Were you surprised?"

Rahnia: "It was a shock! It's such a developed country [the UAE], and yet again the website was missing. It's so surprising. When I came here and I see a nice clinic like this, and they don't even have a website! But at least I got the number [of Conceive], before I traveled back to Ethiopia, Sudan, and Eritrea with my husband. At least I could put to rest those feelings. I saw my family, and I saw for the first time how difficult their situation is. But what can I do? I can't help the whole country. So I e-mailed Dr. Pankaj [Conceive's clinical director] from Ethiopia. But there was no response. I called, and there was no response. I called the emergency number, and I'm not even—I'm not a patient, but I called the emergency number. I was told that Dr. Pankaj was in India until the new year.

"I *had* to catch him, so I came from Ethiopia straight to this clinic on New Year's Day. I *insisted* to the receptionist that I needed to see him. She said that this was his first day back and he would be very busy. But I said I *must* see him. I saw him and explained the situation. He was even astonished and said, 'Why are you here?' But no one understands what I'm going through, the rules, the restrictions in the UK. Even the fluid in my tube cannot be removed there."

Marcia: "Why not?"

Rahnia: "Because in my situation, I have my [IVF] daughter, and so I'm on the waiting list. I had my previous place on the list withdrawn because I now have a child. I want more children with my husband. But as long as you have a child from the same man, you're done. *Khalas* [finished]! I have a child, but, okay, I want one more. But in the UK, they gave me a scenario: If I have another relationship, then I could have another IVF child to 'bond' [with a new partner]. *Am I forced to divorce my husband? Leave him?* I don't blame them [the NHS]. They are doing what is fair. But minimal things, like the fluid removal—I pay taxes. I work. I should be entitled to that."

Marcia: "So you came here to Conceive."

Rahnia: "So, in early January, Dr. Pankaj actually discovered fluid in the tube on the left—what do you call it?"

Marcia: "Hydrosalpinx?

Rahnia: "Yes, hydrosalpinx. Can you write it down? [I wrote it down for her on her interview consent form.] So he said that we should remove that and then proceed with IVF. My husband was here with me, because we'd come from Ethiopia. But they were fully booked here, and so they couldn't do it right away. He said I should go back home and then he would book the [operating] theater for February. So it never occurred to me that he meant for me to have the laparoscopy to remove the fluid [in the United Kingdom] way back in January.

"Today is February 4. I came all the way back from London, and I haven't had the fluid removed. But he *won't* turn me down. When he scanned me, the water is not there. It's a good sign *or* a bad sign, because the water could come back. He told me, 'It's a gamble.'"

Marcia: "So are you willing to try IVF here, even if it's a gamble?"

Rahnia: "Yes, sadly. Well, I'm trying to be optimistic. Now, I'm just starting Gonal F [a hormonal medication]. I just want to try a cycle [of IVF]. Obviously, here, there are not restrictions on how many embryos you can put back."

Marcia: "Here, they normally put back three, and they do freeze [excess embryos]."

Rahnia: "India was the best, actually. In India, they do put in four embryos. If there is a multiple pregnancy [three or more fetuses], they do 'reduce' [through a form of selective abortion]. So I'm 'holding onto' India. But I went back to London in early January, and then I just came back here on January 30."

Marcia: "Do you have a place to stay?"

Rahnia: "No, I'm actually staying in a hotel, using my credit card, and *it is expensive*! But I've been traveling like this, just because of the fear I have. I know my situation is better than a childless couple. But I daydream. I have a fear of something happening to her [Wisal]."

Marcia: "Does your husband want more children?"

Rahnia: "Oh, yes. My husband—I *do* think he wants more children. Of course, he wanted more than the one daughter we have. And society itself. I consider myself to be 'invisibly disabled.' *It is a disability, and it cannot be discussed openly.* You're isolated in your own world. I *hate* where I come from [East Africa]. That's not a nice thing to say, but I *hate* the people I associate with. They just get pregnant easily, quickly, and they wouldn't see a problem with it. I'll just give you an example. My friend, we started at the same time. I had my daughter, and she had her son. And now she's on her fourth. For her, just like a 'click,' and she's pregnant.

"The society bullies you."

Marcia: "Verbally?"

Rahnia: "No, not verbally. But people say: 'What are you trying to *be*? Are you trying to be westernized? A westernized woman? *You are an African!*' Usually, the people I meet, would they understand that I've got a fertility problem? *No, they won't!* You can't really openly have a conversation with friends."

Marcia: "And your family?"

Rahnia: "My in-laws, they put pressure on him, obviously, and I have to deal with him. Our people just put you down. It's really too much for a human being to handle. I don't blame anyone. I was just born unlucky in terms of being infertile, and I know, deep down, I *will* have another child. I *do* believe. *I strongly believe that I will have another child.*"

Marcia: "But it sounds like you're under a lot of pressure right now."

Rahnia: "I think, yes, the whole world surrounding me is looking at me. 'What's she doing? Is this [pregnancy] going to happen to her?' I just pray that God will bless me, then everyone will be quiet. *They will find a different target! Someone else to focus on!* But it's not easy, being *far* away from your country. We say we are 'settled' [in the United Kingdom]. We try to integrate, become educated, work. But your own society criticizes you for who you are. And to be honest, they are telling him: '*Leave this woman. She's infertile! Find another one!' All* of them—the Sudanese, Ethiopians, Eritreans. All the ethnic minorities from Africa have got this attitude. Even from the Middle East as well!"

Marcia: "But aren't you protected a little bit by being in the UK?"

Rahnia: "To a certain extent. But I've been married for ten years, and if I were back in Sudan, there would be no stopping him. *He would definitely have a few wives and endless children!* The whole family, everyone would get a name[sake]! So, yes, it's protective in a way to be in the UK. To be honest, my confidence is *not* down because of this problem. Sometimes I stand up to him. 'I am *not* the one with the problem!' Sometimes in arguments—he said, 'If I don't love you, I wouldn't go through all this.' I told him, 'If you think you are doing me a favor, it's not a favor! I have ovaries. I have eggs. Only my tubes are the problem. I can get a sperm donor for £250 [$400]. But we are married. We are an entity. It's a 'package' when you're married. *If you had had a fertility problem, I would have done the same for you!'*

"So, in a way, you see, I can lift my head when I'm in the UK. In the UK, they *don't* care if you have a child. A child is like a commodity; it's like a mortgage. They start their families at the age of thirty-five, and I totally agree with that attitude. But, because [of] where I come from, it's a culture clash. I'm in the middle of this, and I pay two prices. All this criticism."

Marcia: "What about your family? Do they try to protect you?"

Rahnia: "My family? Well, they're all right. But it's better talking to a stranger than to my family. They listen. They do have sympathy. But they are not up to my expectations in terms of support. I still get the feeling that they're holding back. And, obviously, none of them do have any problem. *No one is infertile in my family*, or not that I know of, really. I've lived outside for such a long time, that my home is in the UK. I do feel it's my home, but society is trying to make you feel . . . UK society tries to make you feel like 'You don't belong here.'"

Marcia: "So you're caught between two worlds."

Rahnia: "It is like that. There are two problems. I can't really talk about the political situation in my own society, and integrating into the UK is difficult. I must say, however, that I love UK people, the British. I really admire them. I like them. *I just feel I owe them something, because they rescued me when I was a refugee.* They rescued me from war and rape and all these kinds of things in Eritrea, in Africa. They saved me, and they educated me to work. I owe them my whole life. I'm so grateful, and also my husband came as a refugee from Sudan."

Marcia: "And as a refugee, you're entitled to a number of benefits, right?"

Rahnia: "As I said, regardless of where you come from, as long as you pay the national tax, you're entitled to get medical care. There is no segregation in medicine, which is good. But here [in the UAE], it's citizens of the country only [who receive subsidized care]."

Marcia: "Did you know that before you came here?"

Rahnia: "Well, I got onto the Internet, and oh my God! *The minute you type in the word 'infertility,' you just open 'India'!* There are different ways to search on Google, and still you get India, which is really interesting, very interesting. Dubai is still backward. It's not on the Internet. But I'm here now, and my husband, he's back in the UK. He will be coming here, maybe February 11, that day. Dr. Pankaj says, 'We'll tell you the specific day when your husband should be here.'

"This time, he [her husband] was very pleased when he saw Dr. Pankaj. The first thing Dr. Pankaj identified was water in my tube, and he actually said that this is the reason why I've had *so many failed IVFs!* It's due to the water, which 'poisons the embryo.' This satisfied my husband. Deep down, he thought that something is wrong with my tube or my ovaries, or whatever. Dr. Pankaj said I've got water in my tube, and he said he just needs to remove or clip my tube prior to the IVF. *My husband was overjoyed, because this is the treatment!* He said it's water in the tube, and it makes sense. He only had to make one [ultrasound] scan, and it gave all the context for my failed IVFs. We expected in the

UK to find out what is wrong, but no one ever mentioned this in the UK. It cost me a fortune to track down, to find just a simple reason. So it all came down to a problem I have, like a simple problem. He said, 'You've got a problem, and first you have to solve the problem.'"

Marcia: "You said you've spent a fortune. Is it costing you a lot to be here?"

Rahnia: "Right now, the two of us are in Dubai in a hotel, and I'm using credit cards. I'm hoping it's only two weeks; I don't want to stay more than two weeks, because it costs me a fortune. Every day here is 250 dirhams [$70], minimum. It's more expensive than rent, than a mortgage in the UK."

Marcia: "Back in the UK, would you call yourself middle class?"

Rahnia: *"No! We're lower class in the UK.* So this is really difficult for us. It's extremely difficult, to have all these expenses, having to use credit cards and go into debt. I would say so far, just to estimate all the previous treatments 'til now, I've spent £17,000 [$27,000]. *That is a lot of money, to put myself into debt!* But for this, it's important. So what can you do? I have to try. I just pray and ask my God to make this treatment be the last one. Please bless me with a child—or twins or triplets! I don't mind."

Marcia: "Does your husband want a son?"

Rahnia: "Yes, there is some pressure, but they never spell it out. But you can see it. But to me, really, it's not about a girl or a boy. It's just having a healthy child and to have a sibling for my daughter. That is my main concern. *It would matter to my husband to have a son.* But if our daughter has a sibling, it will calm him down.

"I just feel that my marriage is on the edge of the hill. *If there is one tip, it will just*—it is on the edge right now. We are having a hard time. It's a marriage problem. He *is* getting pressure. I can understand. But all this medicine I'm taking. I'm injecting myself. Then the husband, the discrimination, the expense, and the waiting. I just wish I had married a Western man. It wouldn't be a problem then."

Marcia: "Did you ever consider that?"

Rahnia: "I wouldn't mind being with a Western man. If it would have clicked, I wouldn't mind. But it's just a cultural issue. I wish I would have ignored my culture. When I married, I needed to believe I was being sensible. But should all of your culture and society interfere with your marriage? In Western society, no, they can't, or at least less so.

It's just the comfort between you and him. So infertility is less likely to be a problem.

"But his mother, she's Egyptian."

Marcia: "Oh, really?"

Rahnia: "Yes, she migrated to Sudan years ago. They are all Turkish-Egyptians, living in Khartoum. My husband left as a refugee to [go to] the UK. Some of his family are in the UK, but mostly in Sudan. *But the telephone is enough to create misery in your marriage!* They're always calling. I hate their attitude. The minute they call, [they ask,] 'Is there anything on the way?' I had to ignore them. But the first year of marriage, I would talk to them. The last four years, until I had her [Wisal], *I ignored any phone calls,* so that I wouldn't have to speak to them. It hurt. *It hurt endlessly.*"

Marcia: "Can I ask if you would ever have considered egg donation as a way to help with your expenses, even though you're Muslim?"[5]

Rahnia: "I'm not opposed to donation. I actually contacted, I already contacted a few centers in the UK to help me with the cost if I would donate my eggs. I was turned down, not because of my eggs, but because of the number of failed IVFs. I would have done this without notifying my husband, *because it is just my egg, not his sperm!* It would be creating happiness, just helping another couple. *This would satisfy me.* Other women can't even ovulate; they have no eggs. Why not help them and, at the same time, help myself with the cost? Yet again, I was restricted because of the failed IVFs."

Marcia: "Did you know that egg donation is not allowed in Islam?"[6]

Rahnia: "Yes, I knew the religion was against it. *They might just slaughter me if they knew!* But I live in the UK. It's a civilized country. So they have a different attitude toward religion and life. *I'm not harming another!* I'm helping another, not hurting anyone. If adoption is allowed, right, why not donate eggs?

Marcia: "But adoption isn't allowed in Islam."

Rahnia: "*It is legal, I think. I can adopt.* You actually get a reward for adopting a child.[7] So donating eggs is like adopting a child."

Marcia: "Would you consider adopting a second child?"

Rahnia: "I *did* consider this. But my husband—I wouldn't discuss this kind of thing with my husband. But if I did, I think I would get my way. If it was a choice between donation or adoption, he definitely *would* adopt, but donation, no. But our financial situation wouldn't allow us to raise an adopted child. To donate my eggs, *he would not allow, but I would!* It will help me, and it's not about finances only. I would still be using my credit card. But it's about making another infertile couple complete. It's a gift. I was incomplete before I had my daughter, and now I feel I can help. I have to be there for others. I definitely think my eggs would help others. But it's just the restrictions—all of the laws in the UK—which are really irritating."

Marcia: "So they make no exceptions to the law in the UK?"

Rahnia: "In the UK, *they cannot allow the laws to be broken!* The clinics would refuse. One of the professors—actually, this is very interesting. When I had frozen embryos to put back, and three of them were very good, *he wanted to put them all back*. But he can't. I begged him to consider it. He said, 'There *are* three, but I can't put them all back, I can't put them back.' I see in his eyes that he wants to, but he can't because of all these restrictions. He is wanting to, but he can't."

Marcia: "We don't have these kinds of embryo transfer restrictions in America."

Rahnia: "I love America for all of these kinds of freedoms. Why not allow more embryos? Why control all of this at the government level? You just make people run away from your country, literally. *I have to run, imagine!* I have to basically run from one point to another—to Italy, to Egypt, to Dubai. And my plan was to go to Bombay."

Marcia: "Let's hope you'll stop running!"

Rahnia: "I just hope, *insha'Allah* [God willing]! I just hope that this problem disappears for good."

Marcia: "Where are you now in your cycle?"

Rahnia: "I've already gotten scanned. I've gotten an appointment, and I've had my first injection. I'll be injecting myself for the next seven days."

Marcia: "Will you stay here, or go back to the UK?"

Rahnia: "I think I should stay here. I don't know really if it's better to be here. The cost is maybe the same as if I travel to the UK and come back again. The hotel is 250 dirhams [$70] a day. The flight is £250 to £280 [$400–$440] for a round-trip flight, but my daughter is maybe £220 [$345], because of the child discount. So, together, it's £500 [$800] for me and my daughter to fly, and then my husband will come. So the sensible thing is to stay here, even if it's 250 [dirhams] a day for a hotel."

Marcia: "Where are you staying?"

Rahnia: "In Dubai, the Shams Hotel."

Marcia: "How did you find them?"

Rahnia: "Actually, I contacted a hotel by Internet, through e-mailing from Ethiopia. The Internet is very limited there, and so my booking was canceled. When I got here to the hotel, they said, 'We e-mailed you because we don't have space.'"

Marcia: "What did you do?"

Rahnia: "The taxi driver just brought me to another hotel. Luckily, *there are lots of hotels in Dubai!*"

Marcia: "Was the second hotel okay?"

Rahnia: "Well, it's okay. What can you do?"

Marcia: "How are you and your daughter managing?"

Rahnia: "We just walk around. I'm really bored. For eating, we just 'take away' every day—breakfast, lunch, and dinner."

Marcia (commenting on the remarkable poise of Rahnia's three-year-old daughter): "She's amazing. I've never seen such a well-behaved child!"

Rahnia: "She's calm. I'm grateful. God compensated me in that aspect."

Marcia: "Is your husband happy to have her?"

Rahnia: "Oh, yes! *Extremely happy. I don't think he loves anything else but her.*"

Marcia: "Do you love him?"

Rahnia (pausing): "Kind of. Yes. But I don't know what love is anymore. It was a pressurized thing when I married him. My family was looking at me as an '*African girl, lost in the West!*' I can have boyfriends, and so they pressured me a lot to marry. This guy [her husband] approached me, I and said, 'Okay,' just to shut them down. He saw me somewhere and asked me to marry him. *But I did accept!* There was no way of, like, finding another Muslim man in Britain at the time. So I went into marriage just in terms of honor to my family."

Marcia: "Had you had any other relationships?"

Rahnia: "I did have another boyfriend in the UK, because it was *very* difficult to get a Muslim man. I *can't* marry a Christian man, because it would dishonor the family. But, if the time was now, I *would* have married, regardless of the family. My old boyfriend, he had a car accident and passed away."

Marcia: "Oh . . ."

Rahnia: "Yes, it's very sad. He was a British guy, and he would definitely take me back now if he were alive."

Marcia: "Can I ask, how do you think you got chlamydia?"

Rahnia: "To be honest, I really don't know how. This is a question I couldn't answer. I was not really sleeping around. I only had one boyfriend. I never liked to go around. I really don't know. After marriage, when they discovered I had chlamydia, I sat down and talked to my husband. I know that I never deceived him in any way. *But he might have been deceptive.* I don't know. I can't know."

Marcia: "Was he upset about the chlamydia?"

Rahnia: "There were no arguments. No issues to discuss. I was honest with him that I had had a boyfriend previously. I would really like to know how I got this, to rest my soul, to rest my mind. *Because a sexually transmitted disease caused my infertility!* When I told my husband, he asked me no questions, and he accepted the treatment. He was treated also. In a way, maybe he was unfaithful, or from before marriage. I don't know. He didn't say that he was not. And there was no anger.

"I said, 'Okay, deep down, at last, we got somewhere. Even in the UK, such a simple test to detect chlamydia. Sixteen years of living there, and they never suggested it. It never occurred to them that I might have that kind of chlamydia. *Thanks to those Egyptians!* They detected it. They are the ones who treated it. I praise them, honestly."

Marcia: "Are his sperm good after the treatment?"

Rahnia: "He's absolutely fine. I just suspect he gave me chlamydia, but I don't really care. I don't know if he has affairs, *but I don't believe men! And a big issue is HIV and AIDS, oh yes!* And definitely you have to be healthy. You cannot just play around. Every time we get the results [of HIV testing], I say, 'Oh my God! This kind of gives me faith that he never cheated on me. But I was confronting him, and telling him we must get tested. At first he asked, 'How dare you?!' But we've had multiple tests, always on my initiative. I'm *very* careful, because that small infection caused all these things to happen to me, *so I'm extremely careful about HIV.*"

Marcia: "Do you use condoms with him?"

Rahnia: "Condoms? Oh, yes. Throughout our marriage, although not constantly. But when I need to, I have them. It's the only solution to keep any kind of infection away. I can only trust myself. I try to believe him, just so that I feel comfortable in my marriage. But I am the one to distrust. If my Dad cheated on my mother . . ."

Marcia: "Did he?"

Rahnia: "Yes! It happened, in Africa. And I know that it's *very easy to have an affair!* I could easily have an affair with my colleague."

Marcia: "Do you ever feel like you want to divorce him and marry a British guy?"

Rahnia: "I thought about that. Now, that will bring me back to the invisible disablement matter. The reason why? So, for example, as far as I can see, in the UK society, I might perhaps find a nice guy. But for a nice relationship to develop, to make it bond, you need to have a child."

Marcia: "Even in the UK?"

Rahnia: "Yes, I see lots of my colleagues. They have a partner for a few years. If the relationship is solid, they definitely have a child. If not, they walk away. So I am invisibly disabled. I have to stick to this marriage."

Marcia: "But what about a divorced man with children?"

Rahnia: "Yeah, but still, from my friends, what I've seen, *unless the guy definitely doesn't want more children*, most of them do, regardless of their previous marriage and children. But that's the freedom I have. The advantage I have is that I could definitely live on my own with my daughter. If you have your freedom, with no cultural issues pressing on you, you will definitely find your soul mate, I believe. I just wonder about being with someone else. *I think about it a lot, really.* But every marriage has its own issues. I think I'll be happy [in this marriage] if another child comes, but I'll also be happy if my marriage walks away. I'll be grateful if I have a child, and my confidence will be boosted. I'll live happily for the rest of my life, *insha'Allah*."

Marcia: "How will you manage with another child? Will you continue to work?"

Rahnia: "In this financial crisis, I have to work. I have to leave my daughter at day care and have other people take care of her. In the UK, you can only go to school at age five. At age four, all children go to preschool. At age three, you're entitled to a £100 grant [$160] a month for two and a half hours [of day care] per day. But because I work full time, she goes to a private nursery. I have no choice. I have to be working. It doesn't get me a lot of money, but it's peace of mind, primarily. If I stay home, I only think of cooking, and I lose my skills. I just focus on what to eat, and it's demoralizing. I made the decision when she was nine months to look for work. I found a job. Luckily, they are very nice people, but it's not big pay. All my money goes to her nursery. Every dollar goes to send her to nursery. But I do realize that I'm investing in her. I had the opportunity to withdraw her from the nursery, because I'm on unpaid leave right now, so I can take her out. But I want her to learn English well, in addition to Amharic and Arabic."

Marcia: "What does your husband do for a living?"

Rahnia: "He works retail. He's a salesperson. *Our finances are very shaky!* We only have money to live from day to day. But it's okay. At least I'm not on benefits [welfare]. *I couldn't do that!* Because I do want to work. I could be on benefits, but I want to work. I went to university and have an honors degree in computing and business. In terms of the UK, I am more educated than my husband. He was educated in Egypt, all in Arabic. I can only barely read and write Arabic, but he speaks so-so English, with an accent. It's very difficult for him, culturally. But we just have to work and pay off the debts. We're £17,000 [$27,000] in debt. It will take us a couple or three years' time to pay this off. But if this [IVF] works out, I will be able to save that money. *All this money just to have a baby!*"

Marcia: "Can I ask you, what do you think of the term 'reproductive tourism'? Could you call yourself a 'reproductive tourist'?"

Rahnia: "Reproductive tourism? The first time I have seen the word, to be honest, is when I read actually the [study] ad. I kind of understand what it means, but it doesn't describe me."

Marcia: "Why not?"

Rahnia: "Well, it actually is too light of a term to describe my disability, which is invisible. Maybe this disability is ignored, not known by others. It's never discussed. But maybe some people would like to know my suffering. I'm going around the world, and my words have never been heard by any one person besides you. Because nobody asked me. Nobody asked me why. Nobody cared. I need some level of understanding. I need to be recognized. *What I've been going through is not tourism!* I have seen some kind of fertility tourism on the Internet in Malaysia. *'While on holiday, do your IVF!'* I would definitely associate that with just another holiday. But the term 'tourism,' perhaps in my own view, doesn't actually reflect what it is. What I'm trying to do is more than tourism—*a lot more than tourism. It's desperation!* It's out of desperation that I'm doing this. *'The impossible to make possible.'* It's desperation that's really driving me from one country to another. It's desperation that drives me around the world. So the term 'traveler' would be right, *but not a tourist!* The term 'tourism' is *not good.*"

Marcia: "Do you have anyone to talk to about all this?"

Rahnia: "There *are* other people, but I don't say to them what I've done trying to get pregnant. Then it accumulates in me, with no way of letting it out. Up until this point, I couldn't say any of it—not to the right person. There was no right person until you came along."

Coda

In the days that followed, I saw Rahnia many times in Conceive's ultrasound scanning area, where I gave small treats to Wisal, including papers and pencils for drawing. Rahnia reiterated several times how much my being there had helped her to "sleep well at last," and how much I had unburdened her by listening to her entire story. Toward the end of February, Rahnia's husband, Ahmed, flew to Dubai for the semen collection necessary before the IVF procedure.

All seemed well on the day of Rahnia's egg collection, which was on a Thursday. However, when I came to the clinic on a Sunday morning, I met Ahmed, who I noted was very tall and visibly agitated. He said that something had gone terribly wrong over the weekend. Indeed, I found Rahnia in acute distress on her way to the operating room. Apparently, back at the hotel, Rahnia had developed a high fever, nausea, and diarrhea, with profound pain over her entire body. Even being touched was exquisitely painful. Ahmed had called Conceive's emergency number, and painkillers were prescribed for Rahnia. But as the infection grew worse, Dr. Pankaj advised Ahmed to take Rahnia immediately to the emergency room of the American Hospital in Dubai. Rahnia and Ahmed had no money, however. Their entire trip had been put on credit cards, and they felt that they could not risk the expense of a lengthy hospitalization.

Given their predicament, Dr. Pankaj told Ahmed to bring Rahnia immediately to the clinic, where high-dose, intravenous antibiotics were administered. Rahnia spent two days and nights in a clinic bed under intensive antibiotic therapy. Dr. Pankaj performed a diagnostic laparoscopy, only to discover a massive pelvic infection of unknown origin. Furthermore, the pelvic infection had spread into Rahnia's bloodstream, leading to a more generalized septicemic infection. Cupfuls of bloody liquid were removed from Rahnia's pelvis, in an attempt to try to discern the origin of her infection.

I kept vigil with Rahnia, as she lay in agony in the recovery room. When Dr. Pankaj came to check on her, she asked both of us, rhetorically: "Why me? What kind of sin have I done that caused all these bad things to happen? Maybe I was not good to my mother. I don't know." Dr. Pankaj said kindly, "Well, the Hindus have an answer for that. Everything bad that happens in this life is simply the working out of your karma from a previous life. You have no control over it." I added, "You have done nothing wrong. It's not your fault."

Fortunately, the intravenous antibiotics delivered at Conceive seemed to work, significantly reducing the symptoms of infection. When the infection appeared to be under control, Dr. Pankaj told Rahnia that she needed to return immediately to the United Kingdom, because she was risking her life by not being able to access emergency medical treatment in the UAE. He told me—and later Rahnia—that the "worst things happen to the nicest people."

By midweek, Rahnia was feeling much better, and I found her sitting by herself in a clinic chair. She recounted her physical ordeal in excruciating detail, and I told her that going through all of these IVFs was not worth it if it meant risking her life. She agreed that she did not want to leave her daughter an orphan. She told me that her husband had been "really there for me" during this whole episode, and that without him, she couldn't have managed this difficult month in the Emirates. I sensed that this life-threatening episode had brought them closer together. Perhaps Ahmed realized that his wife, the mother of his only child, had almost died in her attempt to conceive under cultural pressure.

I saw Rahnia on her last day at the clinic. She, Ahmed, and Wisal were scheduled to leave for London at 4:00 PM on Emirates Airlines. She told me that they had had to switch their flights many times, with extra charges being levied with each new ticket. Finally, Ahmed had argued with the airline, telling them that it was unfair to compound these charges when his wife was facing a life-threatening medical emergency. Fortunately, the airline relented.

At our final farewell, both Rahnia and I became tearful, telling each other how much we had helped each other and how special we found the other to be. She promised to e-mail me, although she admitted that getting to an Internet café was always difficult for her. She hoped that I would publish her story, so that "my words will be heard" by others.

I learned from the clinic later that week that Rahnia and her family had returned home safely. I never learned what kind of infection had nearly killed Rahnia, nor whether it was sexually transmitted in nature. Most of all, I hoped that Rahnia would become pregnant with the child that she was desperately seeking. Two weeks later, Conceive contacted Rahnia back in the United Kingdom. Sadly, her reproductive journey to and from Dubai had come to a bitter end, as her ninth attempted IVF, poisoned by an unknown infection, had failed to produce a pregnancy.

INTRODUCTION
IVF Sojourns

sojourn: 1. *n.* A temporary stay at a place.
2. *v.* Stay temporarily; reside for a time.
—*Oxford English Dictionary*

Desperation and Aspiration

Rahnia, whose story opens this book, casts herself as a "runner," a woman moving frenetically from country to country in a tortuous quest for conception. Rahnia hoped that her journey would serve as a cautionary tale for other would-be reproductive travelers. She also hoped that her story would shed light on the intense longing and despair of infertile women, who experience an "invisible disability" in a fertile world that neither appreciates nor understands their suffering.

Indeed, for many women—and men—around the world, infertility is a dire social burden. Infertility assaults an adult's personhood and gender identity. It can lead to marital duress, divorce, and abandonment. In many societies, infertility causes intense social stigma and community ostracism. The experience of infertility inspires those who can to undertake reproductive travel as a solution to their suffering and to satisfy their intense longings for children. Such desire for children underlies every reproductive quest. Rahnia and many others who travel for in vitro fertilization (IVF) describe their emotional desires for a child as "desperate"—an affective driver of reproductive mobility that cannot be underestimated.

Thus, reproductive travelers are often under considerable pressure in their attempts to conceive. Some of these pressures are economic, while others are logistical. Women may feel pressured because of their advancing ages and a "ticking" biological clock, while men may feel pressured to keep their own infertility secret. Some pressures are legal, forcing infertile couples to become law evaders. Other pressures are related to the difficult moral dilemmas surrounding IVF, including actions that may defy religious orthodoxy.

Rahnia's story is a case in point. Having fled as a refugee from the war-torn countries of Eritrea and Ethiopia, she faces cultural discrimination and multiple restrictions as she attempts to access IVF in Britain's public health care sector. Although Rahnia is grateful for subsidized medicine under the National Health Service (NHS), she faces rationed access to IVF, long waiting lists, and embryo transfer restrictions that force her to bypass the NHS system altogether. Having fled the NHS, Rahnia encounters a poorly regulated private medical sector, where her lack of quality care results in an emergency, life-threatening, ectopic pregnancy. Furthermore, IVF in the private sector is not cheap; Rahnia spends a small fortune financing eight IVF cycles in private clinics in the United Kingdom, going deeper and deeper into debt. When Rahnia decides that it is finally necessary to travel abroad for IVF services, she is out of money and out of luck, using credit cards to finance her ultimately unsuccessful journey.

It is important to note that Rahnia chooses to seek treatment in the United Arab Emirates—also known as the UAE or the Emirates, terms that will be used interchangeably in this book—because of word-of-mouth and Internet referrals, and the geographic and cultural proximity that it affords her as an East African–born Muslim woman. She decides to come to the UAE for IVF in conjunction with a trip "back home" to East Africa. There, Rahnia hopes that she can "rest her soul" from feelings of longing, which she believes are negatively affecting her IVF prognosis. Dubai, as the tourism hub of the Emirates, has made it particularly easy for East Africans like Rahnia—who have no access to IVF in their home countries—to travel for extended periods on special visitors' visas. Moreover, the UAE is located in the geographic center of many other Muslim nations, serving as a kind of hub for the Muslim diaspora. Because of the UAE's favorable location, reproductive travel can be choreographed with visits to family back home. For Muslims, the UAE also represents a zone of cultural comfort in a country that undertakes IVF according to Islamic sharia laws.

At the end of Rahnia's reproductive journey, she almost dies. Indeed, many women whose reproductive travel stories are told in this book have risked their lives in their quests for conception. Medical emergencies and catastrophes are a common occurrence in reproductive travel—belying the notion that IVF journeys are some form of leisure travel. After two near-death experiences, one in the United Kingdom and one in the Emirates, Rahnia is a vociferous critic of the term "reproductive tourism," which is used routinely in the media and scholarly literature to describe this form of travel. Although she casts herself as a kind of reproductive sojourner, her travels have never been for tourism or for any kind of pleasure. In Rahnia's case, the four hedonistic enchantments of the Emirates—sun, sand, sex, and shopping—are entirely beside the point. Thus, when she is asked if she can possibly conceive of herself as a "reproductive tourist," she is offended by this label, which makes a mockery of her "invisible disability" and her multifarious forms of embodied suffering.

Despite its unfortunate ending, Rahnia's reproductive quest is also a journey filled with hope. Moving from the United Kingdom to East Africa to the Emirates—then home to London and back again to the Emirates—is about "making the impossible possible." Rahnia's greatest hope in life, one that has kept her going for many years, is to make a second test-tube baby, thereby solidifying her marriage and providing a sibling for her daughter. Although she recognizes the great difficulties that this journey will entail, Rahnia describes herself as being "very optimistic," seeing "bright light at the end of the tunnel."

Rahnia's story bespeaks the desperate measures, considerable perils, and unfulfilled promises of IVF sojourns. But it is also a story of aspiration—of one woman's valiant struggle to conceive. The threads of both desperation and aspiration are woven throughout this text—a book that is purportedly about "reproductive tourism" but that insists on removing that term from the conceptual lexicon before we even begin.

Reproductive "Tourism"?

In the twenty-first century, infertile women and men who cross national and international borders in pursuit of conception through IVF are called "reproductive tourists." Rahnia is clearly a reproductive tourist according to the following definition: "the travelling by candidate service recipients from one institution, jurisdiction or country where treatment is not available to another institution, jurisdiction or country where they can obtain the kind of medically assisted reproduction they desire."[1]

Rahnia is one in a long line of infertile women who have traveled in search of IVF. It is fair to claim that "reproductive tourism" is as old as IVF itself. From the moment that IVF was invented, reproductive travel was undertaken, some of it under conditions of secrecy. Lesley Brown, the world's first "test-tube mother," would be considered a reproductive tourist by today's standards. She and her husband, John, traveled across southern England (from Bristol to Cambridge) to meet the inventors of IVF, Professor Robert G. Edwards and his physician partner, Dr. Patrick Steptoe. The world's first "test-tube baby," Louise Brown, was delivered on July 25, 1978, in a distant third location (Oldham Hospital, Lancashire) to avoid media scrutiny and moral condemnation concerning Louise's test-tube conception. Within weeks of her birth, long-term infertile couples were traveling from all over Europe to Bourn Hall, Cambridge, the world's first IVF clinic, to obtain the new technology of conception.

IVF was developed by Edwards and Steptoe to overcome blocked fallopian tubes, the condition from which both Rahnia and Lesley Brown suffered. IVF essentially bypasses the fallopian tubes by hormonally stimulating the ovaries to produce excess eggs, removing those eggs directly from the ovaries, mixing them with spermatozoa in a petri dish, and then transferring the fertilized embryos into a woman's uterus. (See the glossary at the back of this book for further details about IVF and other medical terms throughout the chapters.) However, it took more than thirty years for the importance of IVF to be fully recognized by the scientific community. On October 4, 2010, the Nobel Prize committee bestowed its award for physiology and medicine on Edwards, a University of Cambridge reproductive physiologist, in recognition of his development of IVF. Well into his eighties by this point and very frail, Edwards was unable to travel to Stockholm, Sweden, to accept the award. He passed away three years later, at the age of eighty-seven. Lesley Brown, the world's first IVF mother, had passed away a year earlier, at the age of sixty-four.[2] Both of these pioneers had lived just long enough to watch the world's first test-tube baby, Louise Brown, herself become pregnant (without any IVF assistance) and become a mother of a son, Cameron.

Louise Brown was the first of an estimated five million IVF children to have been born by the second decade of the new millennium.[3] This book is not about those IVF babies, but rather about their parents—the men and women like John and Lesley Brown who have had to travel to achieve an IVF conception. Little is known about the number of these IVF-seeking travelers. But increasing evidence suggests that reproductive travel is a highly significant and growing global phenomenon.

How did this kind of reproductive travel become known as reproductive tourism? It began rather simply in 1991, when two legal scholars,

Bartha M. Knoppers and Sonia LeBris, coined the term "procreative tourism" to describe the movement of IVF-seeking couples across international borders; a decade later, a prominent Belgian bioethicist, Guido Pennings, began publishing a series of influential articles on what he called "reproductive tourism."[4] Pennings focused his attention on reproductive border crossings within the European Union (EU). In particular, he was highly critical of the "patchwork" of IVF laws within the EU—a "legal mosaic" that was leading to "law evasion" among IVF-seeking couples. "Reproductive tourism" to other countries, Pennings argued, was a form of "moral pluralism in motion," or a way for infertile couples to circumvent restrictive laws in the absence of legal harmonization within the EU.

Intrigued by the topic of reproductive tourism, the media soon joined the conversation. On January 25, 2005, the *New York Times* published an article titled "Fertility Tourists Go Great Lengths to Conceive."[5] The *Wall Street Journal*, the BBC, and many other news outlets followed suit, publishing stories about American and European "fertility tourists" who had traveled to countries such as Israel, South Africa, and India to obtain low-cost, legally unrestricted IVF.[6]

But the question remained: Was "tourism" the correct term to describe this particular form of travel? A group of reproductive scholars headed by Nicky Hudson and Lorraine Culley, well-known sociologists of infertility and assisted reproduction in Britain, published a state-of-the art review of the literature on the subject.[7] Of fifty-four scholarly articles surveyed in their review, thirty-six were commentaries or "debate papers." The biggest debate by far surrounded terminology. As several commentators noted, the term tourism refers to pleasure travel and implies both financial freedom and choice of destination, as well as the luxury of being on a holiday. Thus, it may not reflect the difficult experiences of most infertile couples who seek IVF services across borders. Although some scholars insisted that tourism reflects the broader economic infrastructures that underpin the global fertility market and its link to the tourism industry,[8] most commentators argued for a more "neutral" term, decoupling this form of IVF travel from leisure.

In one of the most compelling commentaries, the legal scholar Richard Storrow questioned the use of "fertility tourism" as an appropriate synonym for reproductive travel. As he noted, tourism is a type of traveling that revolves around leisure, pleasure, and free time. Fertility tourism, on the other hand, is quite a different story: "Fertility tourism occurs when infertile individuals or couples travel abroad for the purposes of obtaining medical treatment for their infertility. Fertility tourism may also occur in the reverse, when the infertile import the third parties necessary for their fertility treatment. These definitions of fertility tourism are, on the one hand, difficult to harmonize with the idea of tourism as pleasure travel, particularly given that some infertile individuals describe their condition as devastatingly painful and their effort to relieve it as requiring enormous physical and emotional exertion."[9]

In an effort to find a better term, scholars have in recent years proposed more neutral alternatives, including "transnational reproduction," "reproductive travel," and "cross-border reproductive care," now shortened to its rather awkward acronym, CBRC.[10] Interestingly, and for no compelling conceptual reason, the last term (or its acronym) has rapidly gained the widest acceptance in the scholarly literature, judging by the sheer number of citations since 2010.[11] However, cross-border reproductive care, too, is a vexed term. "Care" may be a questionable component of the cross-border reproductive experience, given the potential for physical trauma and commercial exploitation. Some scholars have suggested that "cross-border reproductive services" may be a more accurate and neutral term.[12]

Whether reproductive travelers should be called "patients" has also been fundamentally questioned, since many reproductive travelers are not technically infertile. Single women and men wanting children, as well as gay couples hoping to become parents, are increasingly traveling abroad for assisted reproduction, often in search of gestational surrogates in resource-poor countries.[13] Within such a global market of "gay reproductive tourism" and "single mothers (and fathers) by choice," those seeking assisted reproduction services may be conceptualized as reproductive "consumers," reproductive "agents," or reproductive "opportunists."[14] Thus, the very terminology used to describe this phenomenon and the people who participate in it remains far from settled.

I have been drawn into these terminological debates, changing my position over time based on my ethnographic engagement.[15] When I first arrived in the Emirates in 2007, I was still using the popular term reproductive tourism to describe my study to potential participants. However, like Rahnia, most of the infertile couples I met at Conceive recounted difficult journeys across regional and international borders in pursuit of conception. In virtually every case, infertile couples described their preferences not to travel, if only legal, trustworthy, and affordable services were available closer to home. Furthermore, they told me bluntly that my brightly colored study ad on reproductive tourism did not resonate with their experiences. Most of them did not consider themselves to be tourists of any kind, even if they had traveled great distances. For example, a Greek woman told me, "When I was reading the ad, the word 'tourism,' for me, always refers to people traveling happily. It's almost like—'infertility' and 'tourism,' the words don't go together. I don't know. Under which heading do you put it? But I always think of traveling for happy reasons. I don't think this is tourism because it's for a medical reason. So when I was reading the [study] ad, I didn't really get what it meant."

Other men and women told me that the term tourism implies "fun," "leisure," and "holidays under the sun." Yet their own travel was undertaken out of the desperate need for a child and was highly stressful and costly. Reproductive tourism, they argued, was a cavalier and insensitive term, making a mockery of infertile people's heartbreak and suffering. For example, an infertile couple who had already tried IVF in their home countries of Sweden and Lebanon, as well as the Czech Republic, had this to say:

> **She:** To me, tourism means a vacation, and this is certainly *not* a vacation! It's not like shopping for a child. It's a terrible term. It's not like cosmetic surgery. Fine, you can go abroad for that. But that's something else. For kids, it's another story. It's a lot of searching.
> **Marcia:** What would you call yourselves?
> **She:** Reproductive searchers.
> **He:** In need of reproduction—I, N, O, R. But it will spoil your holiday. You will not have fun!
> **She:** You can't drink wine. How much fun is that?
> **He:** You can't drink wine, and you have to live with someone who is full of hormones!
> **She:** And on a sofa bed! I'm not sure what kind of tourism is that!

These kinds of comments suggest that the term reproductive tourism could not begin to reflect the stresses of infertile travelers' journeys. It misrepresented their subjective worlds of physical and emotional suffering. Furthermore, most had felt "forced" to travel abroad in order to obtain IVF services that were not readily available or optimally delivered in their home countries. In this regard, Rahnia's comments on reproductive tourism in the prologue bear repeating: "The term 'tourism,' perhaps in my own view, doesn't actually reflect what it is. What I'm trying to do is more than tourism—*a lot more than tourism. It's desperation!* It's out of desperation that I'm doing this. '*The impossible to make possible.*' It's desperation that's really driving me from one country to another. It's desperation that drives me around the world. So the term 'traveler' would be right, *but not a tourist!* The term 'tourism' is *not good.*"

I take Rahnia and her fellow reproductive travelers' critiques very seriously, and this book challenges the assertion that reproductive tourism is an appropriate term for IVF-related travel. It also calls into question many other recent claims about reproductive tourism, including that it is motivated by the search for "cut-rate" IVF bargains in vacation locales; that "reproductive tourists" are selfish consumers, making calculated choices within a free market economy; that the reproductive marketplace operates as a "baby business," with entrepreneurial IVF clinics and physicians simply out to "make a buck"; and that IVF travel is entirely "elective," undertaken to overcome a "luxury" disability of Western career couples, who have delayed their childbearing for too long. Indeed, Rahnia's story belies these many facile characterizations. Her travel to the Emirates was arduous, costly, and taxing, both physically and emotionally. In the end, she almost died—without producing the IVF baby she so desired.

Understanding the IVF sojourns of women like Rahnia demands a heightened ethnographic and ethical sensitivity, as well as new forms of theoretical conceptualization. As of this writing, there is still no resolution to the terminological debate about what to call reproductive travel. Reproductive tourism prevails in the popular media, and cross-border reproductive care has gained currency in the medical and bioethical literature. However, neither term is regularly used by those infertile couples who travel. When asked, they generally prefer the term "reproductive travel" to any other label.

In this book, I will use the term reproductive travel because it is truer to infertile people's wishes. However, because reproductive travel and reproductive travelers can become cumbersome if used repeatedly, I will use the shorthands *reprotravel* and *reprotravelers* as convenient contractions (similar to, say, *reprogenetics*, which is used to describe the merger of reproductive and genetic medicine). In this book, my interlocutors are reprotravelers, because all of them had traveled or were traveling in search of IVF. Some of this reprotravel was to the Emirates, some of it was out of the Emirates, and, as we shall see, much of it was to and from, back and forth, in and out of the UAE.

This book attempts to shed light on the IVF sojourns of these infertile reprotravelers. Why did they leave their countries of origin in search of IVF? Why did they settle on the Emirates as a location to make a test-tube baby? Rahnia's reprotravel story begins to answer some of these questions. Rahnia desperately wanted an IVF sibling for her daughter, but she could not access optimal IVF services in the United Kingdom, with its strict regulations and rationing of care. She chose to travel to the Middle East because Muslim clerics there had legitimized IVF to overcome infertility many years earlier (in 1980, in fact). Such early Islamic authorization of IVF in the Middle East has served to bolster the region's attractiveness for infertile Muslims such as Rahnia, who are living in diasporic settings. But traveling to the Emirates also made sense for Rahnia because of Dubai's easily obtainable entrance visa, available lodging, and proximity to her natal family in East Africa.

The globalization of IVF from sites of Euro-American invention to other parts of the world, such as the Muslim Middle East,[16] has led to the production of unique IVF hub sites, such as Dubai. There, IVF practitioners serve an increasingly diverse international clientele of infertile reprotravelers. This book takes readers into the "womb" of a truly cosmopolitan IVF clinic (Conceive) located in this emerging global reprohub. Although reprotravel may be as old as IVF itself, the emergence of such cosmopolitan clinics and global reprohubs is a new and unique by-product of twenty-first-century reproductive mobilities.

Reprotravel as Global Form

The existence of cosmopolitan clinics such as Conceive that attract reprotravelers from around the world suggests that the scale of twenty-first-century reproductive mobility may be significant. Still, little is known about the scope of global reprotravel, and its extent is difficult to assess. The largest empirical study to date—sponsored by the European Society for Human Reproduction and Embryology Taskforce on Cross Border Reproductive Care—involved forty-six IVF clinics in six destination countries in Europe, including Belgium, the Czech Republic, Denmark, Slovenia, Spain, and Switzerland.[17] Based on the analysis of 1,230 completed patient questionnaires, the study estimated that there was a minimum of 24,000–30,000 cross-border IVF cycles in Europe each year, involving 11,000–14,000 patients. The main reason for travel, according to the patients who responded to the survey, was "unfriendly" legislation in their home countries—such as the prohibition of certain techniques (for example, egg donation), or inaccessibility of the techniques because of patient characteristics (such as age, sexual orientation, or marital status).

Outside of Europe, only one attempt has been made to assess the extent of reprotravel on a global level.[18] As part of an international process of data collection for the International Committee Monitoring Assisted Reproductive Technologies (ICMART), clinics in eleven countries were surveyed about "outgoing" treatment cycles. The data showed that patients from these countries had undertaken approximately 5,000 cross-border IVF cycles in more than twenty-five other nations. Collectively, the fifteen "recipient" country clinics that reported data estimated that 7,000 couples traveled from nearly forty countries to receive IVF. However, the authors acknowledge that these data are incomplete and largely estimates. In general, the absence of any kind of global registry of IVF clinics and the minimal international monitoring of cross-border IVF cycles are obstacles to the collection of reliable international statistics.

Reprotravel, as a global metric, remains a twenty-first-century mystery. However, in addition to Dubai, a number of sites have clearly emerged in the past decade as reprohubs offering specialized IVF services. The first of these reprohubs is Belgium, known for its early 1990s invention of intracytoplasmic sperm injection (ICSI), a variant of IVF designed to overcome male infertility.[19] More generally, Belgium is regarded as one of the most liberal European destinations with a wide range of assisted reproduction services.[20] Spain has recently cornered the market on oocyte (egg) donation, purportedly because Spanish women are the most "altruistic" in the world.[21] Denmark, meanwhile, has become the international center for sperm donation, because of its home-grown company, Cryos Denmark, which boasts the world's largest sperm bank.[22] Yet not all reprohubs are in Europe. For example, one study from Latin America shows a thriving reprotravel sector in Argentina, Brazil, Chile, and Mexico.[23] Furthermore, Latin America has been at the international forefront in the development of two regional IVF clinic registries, which are able to track the movement of patients across the region. That said, the Argentinian IVF clinics that are most aggressively promoting "reproductive tourism packages" to foreigners remain unaffiliated with regional registries. Thus, the scope of reprotravel to and from Argentina, at least, is well beyond the official gaze of the regional monitors.

India and Thailand deserve special mention because the governments of these nations are encouraging the growth of a reprotravel industry. India is perhaps the most widely known global reprohub, with more than five hundred registered IVF clinics and many centers specializing in commercial gestational surrogacy. India has become renowned (or notorious, depending on one's vantage point) as the global hub for transplant and surrogacy "tourism," both of which rely on a steady supply of poor Indian bodies.[24] In the world of commercial gestational surrogacy, India has now earned the dubious monikers of "the world's baby factory," "the reproductive assembly line," and the place where "giving birth is outsourced."[25] Calling India the "mother destination" for commercial gestational surrogacy, sociologist Sharmila Rudrappa nonetheless suggests that commercial gestational surrogacy involves more than crass reproductive exploitation.[26] For example, sensitive ethnographic research by Rudrappa and her fellow sociologist Amrita Pande depict the reproductive decision making, material aspirations, and affective relationships sustained by some gestational surrogates with their Western commissioning couples.[27] Nonetheless, it is clear that the Indian government is promoting commercial gestational surrogacy as a new kind of "niche market" for the country, with profits projected to reach $6 billion in the second decade of the twenty-first century.[28]

Thailand, which has marketed itself as the world's premier medical tourism hub, is also developing a controversial reproductive niche. There reprotravelers can now access IVF with preimplantation genetic diagnosis (PGD), which can be used for the purposes of sex selection. The anthropologist Andrea Whittaker, who has been following the growth of IVF in Thailand, worries that the Thai promotion of PGD will create a "new sex trade" among Asian and other foreign couples, who want to make sure that they are conceiving sons, and not daughters.[29]

In both of these Asian countries, reprotravelers can stay in five-star hotels, which may be adjacent to "five-star hospitals" with their own internal IVF units.[30] Some IVF clinics appeal to infertile couples by using romantic tourist images and vacation resort inducements. Morning clinic visits may be followed by afternoon pampering in a resort's spa, with massages, gourmet food, and villas on the beach. Even with the international travel, the costs are much lower, and the success rates may not be so different from those found at home. Thus, as Storrow notes, "on the supply side of the equation, clinics that cater to fertility tourists appear to welcome the development of new markets and have undertaken to market their services so as to create a fantasy of conceiving a child during a romantic holiday."[31]

Medicine in Motion

As is clear in the cases of India and Thailand, reproductive medicine has become embedded in a much larger industry of so-called "medical tourism," which has burgeoned over the past decade and which now operates on an increasingly coordinated global scale. Five major reasons have been proffered for the growth of the medical tourism sector in countries like India and Thailand since the beginning of the current millennium.[32] The first reason is the privatization of health care. Vigorously endorsed by the World Bank since 1993, privatization has reduced states' commitment to health care, leaving many people un- or underinsured, with little if any access to health care services. Those who have been "pushed out" of home-country care may travel abroad to seek more affordable, accessible services elsewhere. The second reason is uneven access in public health care systems. Many Western European nations, as well as Canada and Australia, subsidize health care for their citizens. However, "elective" procedures such as IVF may be rationed or unavailable on a regular basis. The result is long waiting times for certain procedures, sometimes lasting several years. Those who cannot afford to wait—for example, women who are "aging out" of their fertility—may seek services abroad, where immediate access to medical services is virtually guaranteed. Third, certain procedures may be unavailable or illegal in some countries. For example, IVF, gamete donation, and gestational surrogacy are restricted in many countries. So are other medical procedures, such as stem-cell therapy, which is still considered experimental in the treatment of conditions such as Parkinson's disease or spinal-cord injuries. Patients suffering from these afflictions may head to India or China, which have become global hubs for stem-cell therapy.[33] Fourth, biomedical technology has rapidly diffused, making medical care more uniform and more available in a greater number of global locations. Whereas the thought of traveling to India or China for medical treatment might have seemed preposterous to a previous generation of Western patients, twenty-first-century biomedicalization has ensured higher standards of medical care and technical excellence in many countries,[34] including some of those in Asia, Latin America, and Eastern Europe, which are rapidly developing their medical tourism industries. Finally, globalization itself has led to medical travel. As discussed below, globalization has been accompanied by the movement of technology, people, finance, media, and ideas, making the thought of medical travel seem more reasonable to larger numbers of people. Medical travelers' access to the Internet—with thousands of medical tourism websites—is both a by-product of globalization and a facilitator of medical tourism as a growing global form.[35]

In this expanding global marketplace, medical travelers may be conceived of as savvy consumers, who make rational judgments based on the costs of procedures and related travel. Their travel is generally cast as being freely chosen, because the medical procedures they undertake are deemed elective.[36] Medical emergencies, by their very nature, must be handled at home, but elective procedures need not be. In the world of elective medicine, cosmetic surgery is the prototypical elective procedure, with vanity and narcissism deemed the motivating factors. However, such renderings of medical travel as selfishly elective are unfair, for they overlook the abject suffering that underlies much, if not most, medical travel. Heart disease, orthopedic problems, and cancer—conditions that are highly debilitating and often life-threatening—are, in fact, primary reasons for medical travel.[37] Embodied misery also accompanies organ transplantation for people with end-stage renal failure who are dependent on dialysis. Travel for bariatric surgery to overcome obesity, or corrective dental work to overcome painful and unsightly dental conditions, also brings its share of suffering. In addition, patients seeking experimental procedures, medications, or other treatments that are banned in home countries also travel overseas, sometimes to participate in the "offshoring" of clinical trials.[38]

Collectively, these various forms of medical travel have accelerated during the past decade. For example, in 2003, approximately 50,000 medical travelers left the United Kingdom, mostly to bypass long waiting lists in the NHS. In 2007 approximately 750,000 Americans—most of them belonging to the group of 46.6 million uninsured people—left the country for medical purposes. By 2010, the total number of medical travelers was estimated to be 6 million worldwide, with approximately 1 million heading to India, and another 1.2 million to Thailand. As of 2008 the total worldwide medical tourism market was estimated to be worth $60 billion; by 2020, the figure is expected to reach $100 billion.[39]

Interestingly, this new medical tourism is characterized as "reverse traffic."[40] That is, in an earlier day, "traditional" forms of international medical care involved the travel of wealthy elites from resource-poor countries to the medically "developed" countries of the West. However, in the contemporary era, the reverse is now true: Westerners are heading to third-world countries, where medical care has improved and can be purchased at bargain-basement prices. Take India, for example, the "poster child" for the new reverse traffic. Second only to Thailand in the number of medical travelers it attracts each year, Indian hospitals treated 450,000 foreign patients in 2007, when the country's medical tourism market was estimated to be worth $310 million. By 2012, that market had increased almost sevenfold to $2 billion, with an estimated annual growth rate of 30 percent. An Indian Medical Travel Association has been established to secure India's position as the world's leading global health care destination. Since 2006 the government has issued special M (for "medical") visas, as well as MX visas for accompanying spouses. Since 2009 the Indian Ministry of Tourism has worked to promote the accreditation of Indian hospitals through the Joint Commission International, an international accrediting organization, as well as India's National Accreditation Board for Hospitals. Able to boast of its accredited hospitals and English-speaking physicians (who have often trained in the United Kingdom or the United States), India delivers medicine at a fraction of what it would cost in the United States—for example, $10,000 versus $200,000 for heart valve replacement surgery, and $30,000 versus $100,000 for commercial gestational surrogacy. As a result, India has become a leading destination for medical travelers from many parts of the world.[41]

However, as we shall see in later chapters of this book, medical tourism in India has come at some cost to the local population. India is now estimated to spend nearly $50 billion on the private health care sector, including on medical tourism, but only $10 billion on public health care expenditures overall. Since neoliberal reforms began in the early 1990s, the Indian public health care system has sustained severe cuts, as have other forms of social-sector spending. As the health activist Amrita Sengupta has noted, "the dominance of the private sector not only denies access for poorer sectors of society but also skews the balance toward urban, tertiary-level health services with profitability overriding equity and rationality."[42] She reminds us that India's public health statistics are appalling. For example, only 17.3 percent of Indian women have had any contact with a health worker, and rates of maternal mortality remain extraordinarily high. In other words, neoliberal reforms in India have led to a two-tiered health care system: a failed public health sector for the poor, and a private sector with "world-class facilities built to cater to the elite—both Indian and foreign."[43]

In the world of IVF, India's self-promotion as a global medical tourism hub for foreign and Indian elites, including well-to-do Indians returning from the diaspora, has had some interesting and paradoxical side effects. For example, infertile Indian couples, especially in the middle class, may feel effectively barred from, or forced out, of the local IVF sector. As a result, hundreds if not thousands of infertile Indians fly to the nearby Emirates each year seeking assisted reproduction services. Furthermore, local Emiratis—who are often stereotyped as the kind of global elites who would travel to places like India to exploit the organs and wombs of the poor[44]—may, in fact, be loath to do so. As we will see, Emiratis, who are Sunni Muslims, are usually very concerned about following the religious mandates that disallow any form of third-party reproductive assistance. Thus, India is not a go-to site for most infertile Emiratis. In the Emirates, a very different story emerges about India and reproductive mobilities— one that challenges many assumptions about the poverty and misery in India and the comparative affluence and rapacious greed of Gulf Arabs. In the Emirates, for example, some of the world's wealthiest business people happen to be of Indian descent. In other words, India and "Arabia" are mutually imbricated in very direct, interesting, inextricable, and intimate ways in the Emirates—ways that often defy stereotypes about Gulf Arabs, South Asians, and their relative global positioning.

The medical anthropologist Beth Kangas, who was the first to conduct an ethnographic study of medical travel,[45] has taken great pains to challenge some of these circulating stereotypes about Gulf Arabs. She writes: "Stories of wealthy patients from Gulf countries who travel abroad for medical care often dwell on the extravagance—the large entourages and expansive accommodations. We miss the suffering that motivates the travel and the family members' concern for the patients. Similarly, medical travelers from developing countries are often discounted as the elite, as though we needed no additional details. Nonwealthy patients from the Gulf and developing countries are dehumanized when their travel is interpreted as an elite pattern."[46]

In her sensitive ethnographic portrayal of medical travelers from Yemen, Kangas shows that most Yemenis who travel for treatment are generally not from wealthy backgrounds. Furthermore, they pay dearly for their overseas medical care. In many cases, medical travelers' loved ones sell off precious family land and possessions in order to finance costly overseas medical interventions. Men in particular demonstrate their conjugal love and commitments to their wives by sending them abroad for treatment, even in hopeless cases of terminal illness. In general, Yemenis who venture abroad are forced to do so because of the poorly developed medical infrastructure in their home country,[47] which suggests the uneven pace of development within the Arab Gulf states.

Middle Eastern IVF Sojourns

The distribution of IVF services in the Middle East reflects this unevenness in medical infrastructure and support. Poor and increasingly war-torn countries such as Yemen, Syria, Sudan, and Iraq face major obstacles in the provision of successful IVF services, even though each of these countries has at least one IVF clinic. IVF absences in some Middle Eastern countries are counterbalanced by a profusion of clinics in most others. Overall, the Middle Eastern IVF industry is quite robust in terms of the sheer number of clinics.[48] For example, the three most populous nations in the region—Egypt, Iran, and Turkey—collectively now boast more than 250 IVF clinics. Furthermore, Iran and Shia-dominant Lebanon are becoming reprohubs for the Middle Eastern region, because they are the only two Muslim countries in the world where third-party donation of eggs, sperm, and embryos—as well as gestational surrogacy—are practiced. The reasons for this have to do with divergent Shia Muslim fatwas, emanating mainly from Iran, which have permitted donor technologies and surrogacy for Shia Muslim couples.[49] As a result, Tehran and Beirut have become Middle Eastern "hub cities" for reprotravelers from many parts of the region. Some of these reprotravelers are Shia Muslims, but many are Sunni Muslims, Druze, and Christians who are undertaking reprotravel primarily for egg donation, even though this practice is explicitly forbidden by most Middle Eastern religious authorities.

Within the Middle East, the actual regional scope of reprotravel remains unknown, largely because of the lack of development of a Latin American–style system of clinic registry. Registries are a fraught topic in the Middle East.[50] Due to the often fierce competition between IVF clinics, Middle Eastern IVF practitioners may be loath to disclose accurate clinical data on a voluntary basis. As a result, the political will and requisite authority to coordinate an IVF clinic registry and data collection system have been missing on both the national and regional levels. In other words, a most basic "social audit" of IVF clinics and their patients has never been performed in the Middle East as a whole.[51] This means that figures are missing for such important indicators as the number of IVF clinics, the number of IVF cycles performed annually, the annual number of IVF clinical pregnancies, the number of annual IVF births, and the number of patients traveling for IVF services each year.

Although these IVF statistics remain elusive, my own work on infertility and assisted reproduction in the Middle East suggests that Middle

Easterners have, in fact, been traveling for IVF ever since the first clinics opened in the region in 1986. In my earliest research on infertility in Egypt, which dates back to 1988, I tried to describe this Middle Eastern reproductive world in motion using language such as *quests, pilgrimages*, and *therapeutic transnationalism*. In my first book, *Quest for Conception: Gender, Infertility, and Egyptian Medical Traditions*,[52] I showed that traveling for conception—to saints' tombs, herbalists, healers, and holy men—had been going on in Egypt for centuries, with records dating back at least to the pharaonic period. Thus, reprotravel in the region was, in some senses, as old as conception itself.[53]

However, with the 1980 authorization of IVF by Egypt's leading Muslim cleric, a new specter of "test-tube baby making" arose on the Egyptian horizon. In 1986 the first IVF clinic opened in Cairo. In October 1988, when I headed to Alexandria, Egypt, to conduct my doctoral research, the newly opened infertility clinic of a public maternity hospital was promising state-subsidized IVF for the poor. I soon discovered that poor women were traveling from all over Egypt in the hopes of conceiving a test-tube baby. In 1991, one year after I left the country, the first Alexandrian IVF baby was born in that same public maternity hospital.

In 1996, when I returned to Egypt for a second period of field research, both Alexandria and Cairo were in the midst of an IVF boom. Ten clinics had opened in these cities, nine of them privately owned and operated. Interested in understanding local responses to this IVF globalization, I interviewed sixty-six Egyptian couples (most of whom were middle or upper class) at two private IVF clinics in Cairo. There I discovered patterns of reprotravel within the larger history of Egyptian labor migration, including the "brain drain" of educated Egyptians to white-collar jobs in the petroleum-rich Arab Gulf countries. Many of these dual-career couples were working overseas simply to earn the extra money needed to undertake IVF. Their trips back to Egypt during the summer months were motivated by their desire to make what they called "babies of the tubes." I came to think of their summer leaves as *IVF holidays*, since test-tube baby making was usually combined with much-anticipated visits back home to see their families. But I also noticed that Cairo's IVF clinics were flooded in the summer months with infertile couples from the Arab Gulf, who were also attempting to make a test-tube baby while on holiday in Egypt. Not knowing exactly what to call this, I wrote about the new *therapeutic transnationalism* in my book, *Local Babies, Global Science: Gender, Religion, and In Vitro Fertilization in Egypt*.[54]

I hoped to return to Egypt in 2003 to study the globalization of ICSI to the Middle East. I was interested in knowing whether infertile Arab men were traveling to Egypt to access this technology, which had first been introduced there in 1994.[55] However, research permission was refused by the *mukhabarat*, or secret police, who would not allow me to study anything related to "men," "masculinity," "infertility," or "Islam." These topics, I was told, were considered a "security risk." (The Egyptian *mukhabarat* were perhaps prescient. Eight years later, young men took to the streets in revolution. The number of infertile Egyptian men, of course, remains unknown.)

As I was unable to reenter Egypt, my colleagues convinced me to move my research to Lebanon, which had just reopened its Fulbright program after fifteen years of civil war, followed by ten years of Israeli occupation of southern Lebanon (1975–2000). I traveled to Lebanon with my family just before the outbreak of the US-led war in Iraq in March 2003. Fortunately, things were relatively calm in Lebanon, and I was able to conduct the first ethnographic study of male infertility and ICSI in two private IVF clinics in Beirut. As I would soon discover, these two clinics received numerous reprotravelers, mostly returning Lebanese migrants but also couples from neighboring Syria, Egypt, the Gulf States, and Palestinian men in the diaspora. Furthermore, several Lebanese men living in the United States and Canada were undertaking IVF and ICSI in Lebanon. I interviewed 220 men, fully one-quarter of whom had traveled across national and international borders to access ICSI. Most of these were Lebanese men living in the diaspora and combining their ICSI quests with family visits to Lebanon. Thus, I came to think of these men as "return reproductive tourists" on "ICSI holidays" back home.[56] However, notably, eighteen men in my study were from Syria and had secretly crossed the border into Lebanon to undergo IVF or ICSI with their wives. Rarely revealing the reason for their travel to anyone, they told curious relatives that they were "vacationing in Beirut." In describing these men in my book *The New Arab Man: Emergent Masculinities, Technologies, and Islam in the Middle East*,[57] I used the term "reproductive tourists" to describe these Syrian border crossers, but I noted that "reproductive exiles" might be the more appropriate descriptor, given that most of these Syrian men felt "forced out" of their home country by virtue of its impoverished and unreliable IVF services.

In some senses, it was my work with these Lebanese, Syrian, and to a lesser extent, Palestinian border crossers that led me to the Emirates. Many of the men in my study had lived and worked in either Abu Dhabi or Dubai, or in the less well-known emirate of Sharjah. Dubai, in particular, was evoked by Lebanese men as a kind of dream space, "the place where all young Arab guys want to go." When I asked why, I was told: "Because it is the best city in the Arab world!" As shown in the following chapter, Dubai may not be the "best" city in the Middle East—an evaluation that is entirely subjective and questioned by most scholars of the region.[58] However, Dubai may be the Middle East region's most "cosmopolitan" city, with a diverse population hailing from virtually every corner of the earth. Dubai is also the region's unparalleled shopping hub, with more than fifty major malls and more than thirty-five million travelers passing through Dubai International Airport (DBX) each year.[59]

Intrigued by such evocations of the Emirates, and encouraged by one of my Lebanese IVF colleagues (who was in the process of opening IVF clinics in Abu Dhabi and Dubai), I decided to undertake a study in the Emirates focusing on the intersection of reproductive travel and processes of globalization. I located my study in Conceive, the Emirates largest private IVF clinic, which is located strategically on the Sharjah-Dubai border. Over six months of fieldwork in 2007, I met and interviewed nearly 220 reprotravelers, representing 125 infertile couples, from 50 countries. Some were Arab reprotravelers coming from other parts of the Middle East, while others were "locals," or Emiratis, who had their own reasons for traveling across the Emirates or out of the country for IVF services. Many patients traveling to Conceive were South Asians, including many well-heeled professional Indian and Pakistani couples. In my study, Indians were the single largest group of reprotravelers, followed by Pakistanis, the latter of whom often bemoaned the relative dearth of IVF clinics in their home country, especially when compared to neighboring India.

Because relatively little is known about the men and women who engage in reprotravel to places like Conceive, this book attempts to shed light on their motivations and experiences, their dreams and difficulties. Who are they? Why did they travel? Why did they choose Dubai? Did they receive emotional and financial support? Were they satisfied with their experiences? What were the difficulties? And, ultimately, did the journey end with a "take home" baby?

A Reprolexicon

In order to answer these kinds of questions, this book relies on a conceptual vocabulary that I find useful in framing my ethnographic findings. I call it my *reprolexicon*, for it has helped me to think through what

I have discovered. Some of this reprolexicon is unabashedly derivative, inspired by the work of important globalization theorists in anthropology. However, other terms are original, designed to capture the dynamics, directionality, subjectivities, and affect associated with reprotravel. In subsequent chapters, I introduce several other key concepts, including *medical cosmopolitanism* (chapter 1), *IVF absences* (chapter 2), *reproductive outlaws* (chapter 3), and *reproductive damage* (chapter 4). Here, however, I would like to introduce five key tropes that animate this ethnography: *global reproductive assemblage, reproscapes, reproflows, reproductive constraints*, and *reprotravel stories*. I begin at the metalevel, describing the global configurations surrounding IVF and travel related to it. I end with the lived experiences of actual reprotravelers, for it is their stories that form the core of this ethnography.

GLOBAL REPRODUCTIVE ASSEMBLAGE

By this point it should be clear that reprotravel, and the larger world of IVF medicine in which it is embedded, constitutes a global form. If globalization can be defined as "the intensification of global interconnectedness, suggesting a world full of movement and mixture, contact and linkages, and persistent cultural interaction and exchange,"[60] then IVF and its associated movements constitute an example par excellence of globalization. IVF technologies have spread to most regions of the world, and with them have come increased mobilities (for example, of patients, physicians, embryos, gametes, and couriers), greater interconnectedness (for example between clinics, patient advocacy organizations, scholars, and websites), and global penetration of capital and labor (for example, by multinational drug companies, reproductive travel agencies, five-star hotels, and IVF clinic complexes).

According to Jonathan Xavier Inda and Renato Rosaldo, globalization consists of four characteristic elements: the speeding up of global flows; the intensification and regularization of links between different parts of the world; the making possible of action at a distance; and the entanglement of the global and the local, a process sometimes called "glocalization."[61] A great deal of anthropological work on globalization has been concerned with this final issue of local-global interaction. In response to one of the "grand statements" about globalization—namely, that the world is becoming increasingly culturally homogenized—anthropologists, working in a multitude of cultural settings, have taken great pains to demonstrate the pitfalls of this homogenization thesis.[62] In what now amounts to a vast corpus of work, anthropologists have demonstrated that cultural accommodations, creative hybridities, and outright resistances are likely to occur as humans encounter the global within their specific local cultural settings.

My work on the globalization of IVF and ICSI to Egypt—published in *Local Babies, Global Science*—was part of this earlier anthropological focus on locality.[63] In that book, I demonstrated how local factors served to shape the reception of new reproductive technologies in this cultural setting, especially given Egypt's own rich history of indigenous medicine dating back to the pharaonic period. Through my ethnographic research in Cairo's IVF clinics, I was able to show that in Egypt, many aspects of test-tube baby making—from the most mundane details of pharmaceutical purchases and injections to strongly held moral stances against third-party egg and sperm donation—are intimately shaped by local realities. Local theories of procreation, class hierarchies and accompanying stratifications in scientific literacy, gender relations and the varying embodiments of male and female infertility treatments, attitudes toward biomedicine and physician authority, and local theodicies and clerical decrees all matter greatly in the ways in which IVF medicine is practiced in Egypt. Indeed, the "local" is interwoven throughout the purportedly "global" science of IVF in the making of test-tube babies in Egypt.

Without completely abandoning this focus on locality, the attention of the anthropology of globalization seems to have shifted back in recent years to the global, with a primary analytical focus on the global movements of technology. To that end, Aihwa Ong and Stephen Collier, building upon Foucault's and Deleuze's analysis of "assemblage," have proposed the concept of the "global assemblage."[64] An "assemblage," according to Ong, is a "contingent ensemble of diverse practices and things that is divided along the axes of territoriality and deterritorialization."[65] Thus, a "global assemblage" can be thought of in the following way: "In relationship to 'the global,' the assemblage is not a 'locality' to which broader forces are counterposed. Nor is it the structural effect of such forces. An assemblage is the product of multiple determinations that are not reducible to a single logic. The temporality of an assemblage is emergent. It does not always involve new forms, but forms that are shifting, in formation, or at stake. As a composite concept, the term '*global* assemblage' suggests inherent tensions: global implies broadly encompassing, seamless, and mobile; assemblage implies heterogeneous, contingent, unstable, partial, and situated."[66] Among the range of phenomena that best reveal such assemblages, according to Collier and Ong, are "technoscience, circuits of licit and illicit exchange, systems of administration or governance, and regimes of ethics or values."[67]

The twenty-first-century movements of infertile couples to IVF clinics around the world could be conceived of, quite readily, as a *global reproductive assemblage*, involving the global diffusion of IVF and its underlying technoscience; international circuits of traveling people and, increasingly, their body parts (gametes, frozen embryos, and other biological substances); systems of administration involving both the medical and tourism industries; increasing regulatory governance, on the part of both nations and professional bodies; and growing ethical concerns about various forms of licit and illicit exchange, including unprecedented evasion of the law across national and international borders.

The concept of a global reproductive assemblage is also helpful in understanding how reprotravel as a global form is tied to larger political and economic structures, the underdevelopment of medical systems in some parts of the world, legacies of socialism and the postsocialist collapse of public health care systems in some countries, and ongoing postcolonial relations between certain nations (for example, the United Kingdom and India). In addition, imagining a global reproductive assemblage also sheds light on the growing overlap between two industries—the global IVF industry and the global tourism industry—with practices, profit motives, and ethical values that may or may not be convergent. Indeed, as a kind of metaconcept, the global reproductive assemblage brings together the many diverse elements operating on a global scale that make IVF and its associated mobilities a distinct form of global travel in the twenty-first century.

REPROSCAPES

Before the concept of global assemblages was introduced into academic discourse, the anthropologist Arjun Appadurai had already put forth his influential notion of "scapes."[68] In the mid-1990s, he outlined a "global cultural economy" and "imagined world" in which global movements operate through five pathways. According to Appadurai, globalization is characterized by the movement of people (ethnoscapes), technology (technoscapes), money (financescapes), images (mediascapes), and ideas (ideoscapes), which now follow increasingly complex trajectories, moving at different speeds across the globe. Appadurai reminded us that this transnational movement of people, goods, and ideas is both a deeply historical and inherently localizing process. In other words, globalization is not enacted in a uniform manner around the world, nor is it cultur- ally homogenizing in its effects. Furthermore, while acknowledging the importance of human agency—and especially the role of imagination in the social practices underlying globalization—Appadurai was also deeply concerned about the potential for disjuncture, even chaos, in the after- math of global movements and their deterritorializing effects.[69]

Appadurai's dynamic notion of scapes remains extremely provocative for thinking about reprotravel, for this form of global movement clearly involves two of Appadurai's five scapes—namely, ethnoscapes and techno- scapes. Ethnoscapes, according to Appadurai, involve "the landscape of persons who constitute the shifting world in which we live: tourists, im- migrants, refugees, exiles, guest workers, and other moving groups and individuals."[70] Technoscapes involve "the global configuration, also ever fluid, of technology and the fact that technology, both high and low, both mechanical and informational, now moves at high speeds across various kinds of previously impervious boundaries."[71]

The consideration of global reprotravel has the potential to extend Appadurai's theory of scapes. One scape of significant medical anthro- pological interest—namely, the *bioscape* of moving biological substances (such as blood and semen) and body parts (for example, gametes and organs)—might be added to Appadurai's list. Using Appadurai's language of scapes, global travel for IVF might also be thought of as a more com- plex *reproscape*—a kind of metascape combining numerous dimensions of globalization and global flows. That is, reprotravel occurs in a new world order characterized not only by circulating reproductive technologies (technoscapes) but also by circulating reproductive actors (ethnoscapes) and their gametes (bioscapes), leading to a large-scale global industry (financescapes), in which images (mediascapes) and ideas (ideoscapes) about making lovely babies while on vacation come into play.

This reproscape entails a discernible geography traversed by global flows of reproductive actors, technologies, body parts, money, and repro- ductive imaginaries (such as the birth of "miracle" babies).[72] In spatial terms, these global flows are also moving in particular directions, which may become quite regularized over time. For example, egg donors and recipients now head to Spain and Eastern Europe, while couples seeking surrogacy travel to India. As we shall see in this book, the Middle Eastern reproscape also entails a distinct geography traversed by global flows of reproductive actors, technologies, and their body parts. Within this re- gional reproscape, Middle Eastern couples needing donor gametes head to Iran and Lebanon, while the Emirates attract not only Middle Easterners but also many couples coming from places outside the region, including Asia, Africa, and Europe. (Perhaps because of the sheer distance, only infertile couples from Latin America and the Caribbean remain unrepresented within the reproscape that flows into the Emirates.)

In short, a reproscape is both spatial and dynamic, involving geography and movement. Whereas the global reproductive assemblage entails a coming together of diverse IVF elements, the notion of a reproscape is more dynamic, entailing the movements of reprotravel in a way that a global reproductive assemblage cannot. However, these movements are not unfettered. The adjective *stratified* might be added to the term *reproscape* to describe the inequalities, disjunctures, and obstacles that inhibit and even prevent flows of people, technology, and other forms across uneven global terrains.[73] To take but one example, elites from the Horn of Africa may come to the Emirates to undergo a single cycle of IVF. But the vast majority of infertile sub-Saharan African couples, from places like Somalia and Djibouti, will never take part in such global flows to the Arab Gulf. In other words, the *stratified reproscape* in which reproductive tourism takes place is an uneven terrain since some individuals, some communities, and some nations have achieved greater access to the fruits of reproductive globalization than others.

Furthermore, this reproscape is highly gendered, a feature of globalization requiring serious attention. Gender was not the focus of Appadurai's original work on global scapes. Yet the ethnoscape of moving peoples, the technoscape of moving technologies, the bioscape of moving body parts, and the ideoscape of moving procreative scenarios are rife with gender differences and disparities. For example, reproductive technologies such as IVF and ICSI are enacted on women's and men's bodies in highly differentiated ways. Furthermore, the global reproscape entails new forms of gendered reproductive labor (and disparities) among reproductive "assistants," most of whom are women and who undergo risky forms of hormonal stimulation, egg harvesting, pregnancy, and labor. Nonetheless, reproductive assistance also has the potential to create kin-like female alliances, including those between actual kin who donate their eggs or wombs to relatives and those between unrelated women who share their eggs with other women in infertility clinics or donate them for a fee.[74] Egg donation in particular invokes the notion of altruistic "gift exchange" between women, even though eggs are increasingly sold on the reproductive marketplace for up to $50,000, especially for "Ivy League" eggs of presumed superior intelligence and other ineffable qualities.[75] Indeed, the very term reproductive assistance is called into question when assistance comes at such a high cost. These variable measures of reproductive value are clear indicators of the stratified reproscape, in which some bodies are valued more than others.

REPROFLOWS

I propose the concept of *reproflows* to bring these bodies and body parts back into the discussion of IVF as a global form.[76] If a reproscape entails the geography and directionality of reproductive movements in space and time, then within each reproscape there are specific types of flows that are entirely unique to the world of IVF. The term reproflows alludes to embodied movements of many kinds—flows of reproductive actors, reproductive technologies, and reproductive substances as well as the mechanical and physiological movements of reproductive bodies themselves, which are required for the processes of assisted conception.

On one level, reproflows involve the movement of many kinds of human actors. These include the IVF scientists, physicians, embryologists and other kinds of IVF technicians who travel to and from sites of training, international conferences, and medical trade shows and to the countries and clinics where they provide their services. Among these reproductive actors are embryo couriers, who cross international borders carrying their precious cargos in carefully sealed cryopreservation tanks. Reproflows also involve the thousands upon thousands—perhaps millions—of men and women now flowing across national and international borders in their search for IVF technologies and related forms of reproductive assistance. Reproflows also include the reproductive assistants, including traveling gamete donors and surrogates, who may be flown across international borders in increasingly regularized circuits of reproductive exchange.

On another level, reproflows also engage nonhuman actors, which are crucial elements in the global reproscape.[77] Reproflows involve the movement of IVF technologies from the sites where they were developed (for example, England in the case of IVF and Belgium for ICSI) to many other countries around the world, flows that are made possible through processes of manufacture (in countries such as the United States and Italy) and global dispersion via medical trade shows and pharmaceutical representatives. Reproflows also involve many kinds of reproductive entities and substances, including the embryos passed from country to country through the work of embryo couriers; the frozen sperm samples, ready for use in donor insemination, which are posted through various international delivery services; and the reproductive hormones, or the costly medications used to stimulate women's ovaries into oocyte hyperproduction.

Finally, in the domain of reproductive physiology, reproflows speak to the quintessentially fluid nature of men's and women's bodies and to the biological movements of conception that take place every minute in IVF clinics and laboratories around the world.[78] For example, reproflows entail the flow of semen into plastic cups in IVF clinic bathrooms, as men are asked to masturbate themselves to ejaculation or to be masturbated by their wives. Reproflows include the flow of oocytes suctioned from women's ovaries and flushed from pipettes into waiting petri dishes in IVF laboratories, where they are handled and inspected by embryologists. Reproflows also involve the aspiration of semen from men's reproductive tracts, in the hopes of finding viable spermatozoa for the purposes of ICSI injection. And reproflows involve the flow of menstrual blood when conception is not achieved during a failed IVF cycle.

REPRODUCTIVE CONSTRAINTS

Reproflows speak to a world of moving technologies, bodies, gametes, embryos, and other reproductive substances—the very material and biological substrate on which the reproscape is founded. However, flows of bodies and body parts do not always occur in an unfettered fashion.[79] In the world of assisted reproduction, bodily flows are often blocked, hindered, or rendered inert. For example, reproductive hormones are injected without stimulating the maturation of eggs. Semen is ejaculated without yielding viable spermatozoa. Eggs are fertilized with sperm but do not become human embryos. Embryos are transferred into wombs but are not implanted in uterine walls. Pregnancy tests are positive but lead to negative outcomes, such as stillbirths and miscarriages. In short, biologically based *reproductive constraints* of many kinds continue to plague the embodied world of IVF—making IVF fail more often than not, thus seriously demoralizing those who have traveled to use it.

Biological obstacles are not the only deterrent to IVF successes. Indeed, there are numerous other arenas of constraint—structural, sociocultural, ideological, and practical obstacles and apprehensions—that may detract or deter IVF seekers from accessing assisted reproductive technologies within their home countries.[80] On a global level, the two most fundamental arenas of constraint are probably economic and legal. That is, IVF seekers may not be able to afford these services in their home countries, or they may be barred from accessing IVF because of various legal prohibitions. However, it is important to emphasize that economics and law are not the only arenas of constraint. Instead, a complex set of factors militates against access to IVF, thus setting in motion reprotravel across national and international borders. At least twelve arenas of constraint that serve as drivers of reprotravel have been identified in the literature:[81]

1. Specific IVF services may be exceptionally *costly*;
2. Specific IVF services may be *unavailable* because of a lack of clinical expertise or equipment;
3. Specific IVF services may be unavailable because of particular *shortages*, especially of donor gametes, which lead to long waiting lists;
4. Individual countries may proscribe specific IVF services based on *religious, moral, or ethical* concerns;
5. Individual countries may prohibit specific IVF services by *law*;
6. Certain *categories of individuals* may be excluded from receiving specific IVF services, especially at public expense, on the basis of age, marital status, citizenship, or sexual orientation;
7. Specific IVF services may be unavailable because of *safety* concerns or questions about risk;
8. Specific IVF services may be of *poor quality*;
9. Poor-quality IVF services may lead to *low success rates*;
10. Concerns over *medical confidentiality* and the desire for privacy may lead some IVF patients to travel abroad;
11. Linguistic and other *cultural barriers* in the delivery of IVF services may lead some IVF patients to seek services elsewhere; and
12. *Support* for patients (for example, from nurses, psychologists, health educators, support groups, or nearby family and friends) may be lacking.

These arenas of constraint can be grouped into four broad categories, namely, *resource considerations* (high costs; lack of expertise and equipment; resource shortages; and waiting lists, either for IVF itself or for donor gametes); *legal and religious prohibitions* (religious bans, national laws, and the denial of treatment to certain categories of persons); *quality and safety concerns* (unknown safety, poor-quality care, and low success rates); and *sociocultural issues* (confidentiality concerns, cultural and linguistic barriers, and lack of supportive services).[82]

In this book, these four broad categories are used as a general organizing framework for the chapters that follow, although not in the aforementioned order. Chapter 1 begins with the sociocultural domain, examining the various factors that are luring increasing numbers of infertile patients from their home countries to "medically cosmopolitan" Dubai. Chapter 2 focuses on various absences—of IVF clinics in some countries, of IVF cycles under rationed care in other countries, and of the money needed to pay for costly IVF services—which are forcing infertile couples to flee their home countries in search of IVF in the Emirates. Chapter 3 focuses on restrictions, particularly the legal and religious prohibitions that constrain access to specific IVF services within the Emirates, making the decisions regarding gamete donation, surrogacy, and multifetal pregnancy reduction (a form of abortion), quite difficult for some couples. Chapter 4 focuses on discomforts, or the kinds of physical risks and forms of outright medical harm that can occur in poor-quality IVF settings. When IVF patients experience or hear of "medical horror stories," they may travel abroad for more competent, successful, supportive, and culturally comforting care. For some, this may also entail the search for secrecy to avoid social stigma.

REPROTRAVEL STORIES

Each of these issues is perhaps best exemplified through stories of actual reprotravelers. During the course of my research I collected 125 *reprotravel stories*, some from men, others from women. However, most traveling couples spoke to me together in what I would like to characterize as a rather uncommon form of *marital ethnography*.[83] Throughout this book, I feature these reprotravelers' voices and their marital and reproductive stories as much as possible. I attempt to preserve the precise language and individual nuances and idioms with which people described their IVF sojourns to me. I also attempt to represent the global character of this study population, highlighting the voices of the nationally and religiously heterogeneous infertile couples who came to the Emirates from fifty different countries of origin. Because these reprotravel stories are often laden with medical language and descriptions of reproductive procedures and problems, I attempt to make the stories as meaningful and comprehensible as possible. However, I also provide a glossary of medical terms at the end of the volume to guide the reader.

Unlike Rahnia's reprotravel story, which I present in a verbatim transcription, all of the remaining reprotravel stories in this book are ethnographic hybrids, merging verbatim interview passages with story lines developed by me from the interview material. I cannot claim that these reprotravel stories—five of which follow each chapter—are totally representative of the larger sample of couples; of the Middle Eastern reproscape as a whole; or, on a more general level, of the dynamics surrounding reprotravel outside of the Middle East. However, the particular stories have been chosen precisely because they represent recurring themes that I discerned during hundreds of hours of listening, followed by careful rereading of thousands of pages of interview transcripts.

Ultimately, each ethnographer must find the best ways of bringing people to life in print. In this book, reprotravel stories are my attempt to portray both the sorrow and the hope that the infertile bring to their IVF sojourns. As an anthropologist, I place a premium on such stories. Stories are perhaps the best window into the world of infertility—a world that is replete with pain, fear, frustration, and longing for a desired child. Having focused on infertility as a global reproductive health issue for many years now, I continue to be moved by the local moral dilemmas and embodied suffering of infertile men and women such as Rahnia. Rahnia hoped that I would publish her story someday, so that others might learn from her trials and tribulations yet be inspired by her triumphant spirit. With this sense of moral obligation to Rahnia—and to the many other reprotravelers of my study—I do my best in the pages that follow to bring their stories to life.

HUBS

Medical Cosmopolitanism in the Emirates

A Clinic Called Conceive

In a converted showroom, across from a shopping mall, on the periphery of a busy traffic circle, in the emirate of Sharjah just over the border from Dubai, sits a clinic called Conceive. From the outside, the clinic is nondescript. Tinted showroom windows block the typically intense sun and increase patients' privacy. The clinic's sign provides the only hint of what occurs within, as the highlighted *o* in Conceive resembles an oocyte being penetrated by a single spermatozoon. The modest façade of this edifice (figure 1.1) belies the interior, for Conceive is a bustling, global IVF clinic, catering to infertile couples from five continents and nearly one-third of the world's nations. At Conceive, Muslim patients from Pakistan meet with Hindu physicians from India, are cared for by Catholic nurses from the Philippines, have their embryos handled by Greek Orthodox embryologists, and receive follow-up instructions from two African clinicians, both Muslims—one from Sudan and the other from Somalia. At the clinic entrance, infertile Arabs, Europeans, Africans, and South Asians are greeted by a smiling receptionist (figure 1.2), as well as by photographs of the rulers of the United Arab Emirates, which are prominently displayed in most businesses and hotels across the country. In this multiethnic, multireligious clinic, the clinical staff mingle across cultural divides, with friendships formed after many years of working together (figures 1.3, 1.4, and 1.5). The patient population is similarly diverse and multisectarian.

Although a glass wall is intended to separate the men and women in the waiting area, infertile couples from South Asia, Europe, North America, Australia, and Arab nations interact with each other across continental and gender divides, effectively ignoring the gender segregation instructions, which are printed in English. After all, English is the common language of the Emirates, where Arabic-speaking Emirati "locals," as they are often called, are outnumbered eight to one. As a result, all twenty-two clinic staff members at Conceive speak English, along with a variety of other languages, the most common of which are Arabic, Hindi, Tagalog, and Urdu. Conceive has developed a transcontinental reputation for delivering a wide spectrum of high-quality and effective IVF services within a multicultural clinical environment. These services are known by their acronyms and include intrauterine insemination (IUI), a kind of first step in the assisted reproductive journeys of many couples, in which the husband's sperm is injected directly into the wife's uterus in an attempt to overcome unexplained and less serious infertility problems; IVF to overcome female infertility; intracytoplasmic sperm injection (ICSI) to overcome male infertility; preimplantation genetic diagnosis (PGD) to test for genetic defects, check the overall quality of fertilized embryos, and sometimes select the sex of the embryo to be implanted; percutaneous epididymal sperm aspiration (PESA) and testicular sperm aspiration (TESA) to extract sperm from men's testicles in cases of severe male infertility or from men who have had vasectomies but who have decided that they want more children; cryopreservation or freezing of sperm, eggs, and embryos; and care of women with polycystic ovary syndrome (PCOS), which, as we will see, is a major cause of female infertility in the Arab Gulf and is increasing around the world as women become overweight and insulin resistant.

However, according to Emirati law, Conceive does not practice third-party reproductive assistance of any kind—not egg, sperm, or embryo donation, and not gestational surrogacy—nor does it practice multifetal pregnancy reduction, a form of selective abortion for high-order multiple pregnancies (those with triplets or more fetuses). These religiously inspired legal restrictions, while extremely prohibitive for some infertile couples, have not blunted patients' enthusiasm for undertaking assisted reproduction at Conceive. Infertile couples wanting to try IVF or ICSI using their own gametes (eggs and sperm) are traveling far and wide to reach Conceive, from places such as Afghanistan, Nigeria, Sri Lanka, and Canada.

Opened on July 4, 2004, which happened to coincide with America's Independence Day, Conceive is the brainchild of Dr. Pankaj Shrivastav, the clinic's physician director, who is widely revered as the "father of IVF in the UAE" (figure 1.6).[1] Born in India in the late 1950s, Dr. Pankaj (as he is known by both patients and colleagues) was destined for a career in medicine. The son of the director general of India's national health services, Dr. Pankaj was sent to India's most prestigious medical school, the Christian Medical College of Vellore, which was opened in the late 1800s by American missionaries and made famous a century later as the site of India's first open-heart surgery and kidney transplant. After completing his medical school training and American board certification in obstetrics and gynecology, Dr. Pankaj departed for London, where he undertook a three-year fellowship in infertility and IVF at the United Kingdom's largest private hospital. This was in the heady first decade following Louise Brown's IVF birth in England. IVF opportunities were opening up around the world, and clinics needed skilled physicians and embryologists. Thus, many British, North American, and other European-trained gynecologists began to serve as traveling "IVF troubadours,"[2] taking the art of assisted conception to other countries around the globe.

Dr. Pankaj is one such troubadour. After completing his fellowship, Dr. Pankaj was invited to follow his British mentor to Dubai, where the government hoped to open the UAE's first IVF unit as a kind of a "sister" program to its London counterpart. Until that point, all infertile Emiratis seeking IVF care were sent by the UAE government to London, an early form of reprotravel that was difficult for the UAE government to sustain financially over time. Thus, at the beginning of the 1990s, the Dubai Health Authority proposed to start its own IVF unit in the local government hospital, where Emiratis as well as expatriates could receive affordable infertility care. In May 1991, the Dubai Gynecology and Fertility Centre was opened at the government-run Rashid Hospital. Dr. Pankaj was asked to serve as the clinic's deputy director, a position that he held until 2004.

However, by the turn of the new millennium, the global landscape of reproductive medicine had begun to change. Across the Middle East, an "IVF boom" was occurring, with private IVF clinics opening in cities such as Beirut, Cairo, Casablanca, Damascus, Istanbul, Riyadh, Tehran, and Tunis. The Emirates were not immune to this technological globalization, nor to the concomitant privatization of most Middle Eastern medical services.[3] By 2005, the UAE was hosting seven IVF clinics, five of them private facilities located in the emirates of Abu Dhabi and Sharjah. By 2012, that number had increased to fourteen, twelve of them privately owned.

Dr. Pankaj was attracted by the promise and potential of running a private IVF clinic. With the encouragement of one of his patients—an infertile Emirati businessman, who volunteered to invest his own money and serve as the required local sponsor[4]—Dr. Pankaj decided to open a private clinic on the Dubai-Sharjah border.[5] He and his Emirati business partner rented an empty showroom and proceeded to create Conceive from scratch. "There was not a single wall," Dr. Pankaj explained to me. "We had to construct *everything*. So we started with half the current clinic. But then we found that we were running short of space, and at this point, we rented the second showroom next door and broke down the walls between them. By 2005, a year later, the entire clinic was completed."

Although neither the largest nor the smallest clinic in the UAE—the Middle East hosts IVF clinics ranging from huge, high-rise private hospital complexes in Amman and Abu Dhabi to tiny, cramped clinics tucked into the back alleys of Beirut and Cairo—Conceive can be fairly described as comparatively bright and spacious (figure 1.7). Perhaps because of the consistent sunlight, as well as the high ceilings of the former showroom, Conceive has a sunny feel, made even brighter by the numerous framed baby photos adorning the clinic's hallways (figure 1.8). The single-story structure consists of approximately a dozen connected rooms, including a combined reception and waiting area; rooms for patient history taking and ultrasound scanning connected by a long hallway; the office where Dr. Pankaj receives patients; a business office where patients pay their bills; an operating theater connected to an IVF laboratory; a recovery room with three beds for women still under anesthesia after returning from egg collection, which is connected to an anteroom with large, reclining lounge chairs for women who have undergone embryo transfer; a storage room that doubles as a staff kitchen; three unisex bathrooms that also serve as men's semen collection rooms; a small anteroom outside one of these bathrooms, where infertile men rest on gurneys following various genital operations; and a "VIP room" at the back of the clinic designated for Emirati "locals," who often desire secrecy when pursuing their IVF procedures. The VIP room, however, is more often used as a prayer room for Muslim patients and staff and as an extra office for clinical consultations. In 2007, it also served as the private interview room for my study.

In 2013, when I returned to the clinic for a follow-up research visit, it was clear that Conceive was going from strength to strength. Many of the

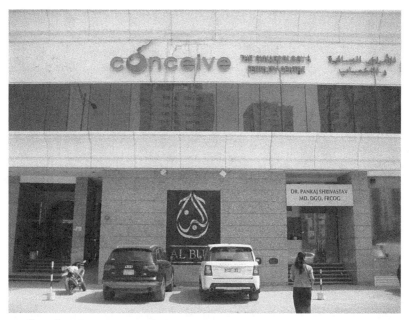

1.1 Conceive. PHOTOGRAPH BY JUSTINE HOOKS.

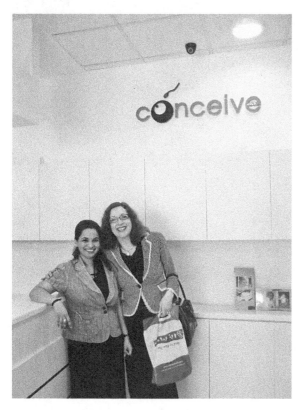

1.2 The author (right) at Conceive, with the receptionist. PHOTOGRAPH BY JUSTINE HOOKS.

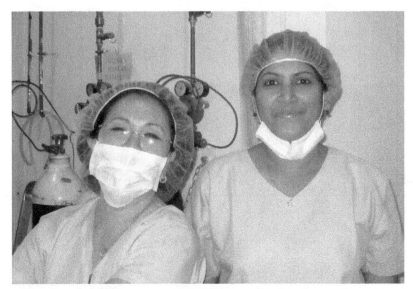

1.3 Two nurses, one from the Philippines and one from India, about to enter Conceive's operating theater. PHOTOGRAPH BY JUSTINE HOOKS.

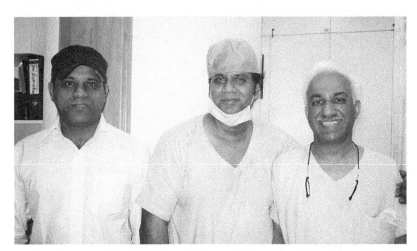

1.4 The three men of Conceive, from India and Pakistan, both Hindu and Muslim. PHOTOGRAPH BY JUSTINE HOOKS.

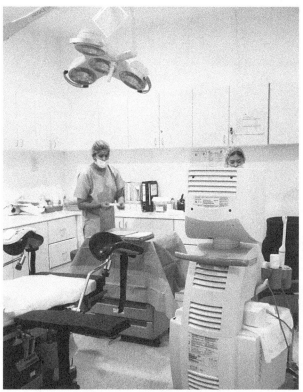

1.5 Nurses preparing Conceive's operating theater.
PHOTOGRAPH BY JUSTINE HOOKS.

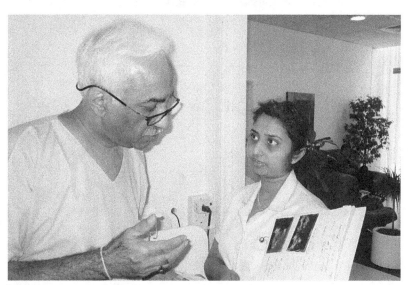

1.6 Dr. Pankaj Shrivastav consulting with a nurse in his Conceive office.
PHOTOGRAPH BY JUSTINE HOOKS.

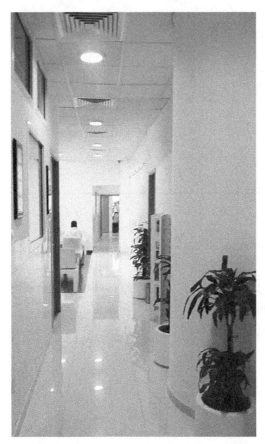

1.7 A hallway at Conceive.
PHOTOGRAPH BY JUSTINE
HOOKS.

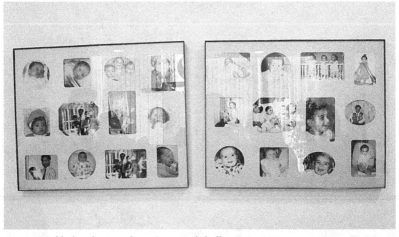

1.8 Framed baby photos adorn Conceive's hallways. PHOTOGRAPH BY JUSTINE HOOKS.

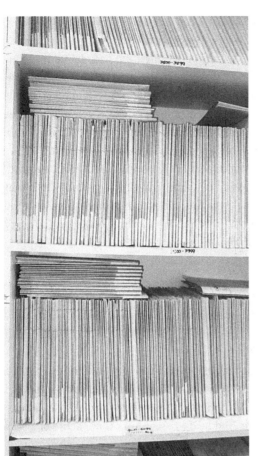

1.9 Conceive's thousands of medical files are carefully stored in cabinets. PHOTOGRAPH BY JUSTINE HOOKS.

1.10 Dr. Pankaj holding an Emirati IVF toddler, as Conceive's Sudanese IVF physician looks on. PHOTOGRAPH BY JUSTINE HOOKS.

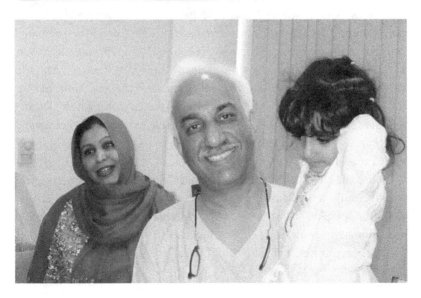

rooms, including the VIP room, had been further subdivided to add more office space for IVF consultations and storage cabinets for the burgeoning medical record files of the thousands of patients who had visited the clinic by that point (figure 1.9). Patients continued to come from many nations. On my first day back in the clinic, for example, I found a Sudanese couple and an Indian couple defying the gender segregation of the waiting area by sitting next to their spouses. I also saw a British couple waiting for an ultrasound scan and a happy Emirati couple returning to show off their IVF daughter to the clinic staff (figure 1.10). Wearing different national garb, speaking softly in different tongues, having traveled from vastly different geographical locations, these infertile patients had nonetheless found Conceive and were there on a bright Sunday morning—the beginning of the Emirates' work week—to make their test-tube babies.

Medical Cosmopolitanism

Conceive, I would argue, is a stunningly cosmopolitan IVF clinic. With more than twenty staff members hailing from the Middle East, Africa, South and Southeast Asia, and Western Europe, Conceive practices a kind of *global gynecology*, making infertile patients from abroad feel comfortable with the high quality of its IVF services and with its multicultural patient care, which can be delivered by co-nationals in Arabic, Hindi, Urdu, and several other languages. In the Middle East as a whole, the practice of global gynecology in a cosmopolitan clinic is unusual, perhaps even unique. Most clinics and hospitals in other countries are staffed by local Arab physicians, who treat mostly Arab IVF patients. For example, during my previous study in Beirut, I interviewed 220 IVF clinic patients (compared with 219 in the Emirates). But, in my Lebanon study, reprotravelers overwhelmingly hailed from two neighboring Arab countries—Syria and Palestine—or, to a much lesser extent, Egypt and the Arab Gulf. In contrast, Conceive provided a veritable object lesson in globalization. During the course of my research at Conceive, I was able to track the comings and goings of a diverse group of reprotravelers from 50 countries. Many of these travelers were Arab, but most were not.

To use the words of the anthropologist George Marcus, Conceive provided a "multi-sited sensibility" within a "strategically situated (single-site) ethnography."[6] That is, within this single clinic, both patients and practitioners were aware of coming together across vast cultural divides, thereby becoming part of something "global" in the enactment of a particular form of reproductive medicine. Their explicit attempts to overcome multiple differences—to be open to, and tolerant of, medical care delivered across geographic, ethnic, linguistic, religious, political, economic, gender, and cultural boundaries—provides a case study in medical cosmopolitanism. Conceive, I would therefore argue, is an example par excellence of twenty-first-century medical cosmopolitanism, a feature of health care delivery in the new millennium in a small, but growing, number of global hubs around the world.

What do I mean by *medical cosmopolitanism*? This term has two distinct but related meanings. First, it entails the concept of *cosmopolitan medicine*, a term that, as we shall see below, was originally used to signify the production of Western-based biomedicine and its rapid global spread.[7] The second meaning is related to the concept of *cultural cosmopolitanism*, or the coming together of people from many different nations at the point of medical consumption—namely, the actual delivery of clinical care. Medical cosmopolitanism signifies this double entendre—of the global production and consumption of Western, technoscientific medicine in places where the outlook of both practitioners and patient consumers is self-consciously cosmopolitan in nature.

Before I show how medical cosmopolitan is manifested at Conceive, it is useful to examine the original term, cosmopolitan medicine, which—although rarely invoked today—is still quite useful for thinking about the twenty-first-century phenomenon of medical cosmopolitanism. In addition, it is important to understand how recent theories of cultural cosmopolitanism relate to the delivery and consumption of medical care in the emerging cosmopolitan capitals of the world, of which Dubai, with its "health care city," is the Middle East's most salient example.

The physician-anthropologist Frederick Dunn coined the term cosmopolitan medicine in 1976, to refer to what was then being called "modern," "scientific," or "Western" medicine.[8] Dunn believed that those terms—often used in juxtaposition to "indigenous," "local," or "traditional" medicine—created an implicitly biased dualism. As he pointed out, "traditional" medical systems, such as Ayurvedic, Unani, or Chinese medicine, often included "scientific" elements. Similarly, Western medicine was as much "art" as science. Thus, claiming the mantle of science for one system but not the other was an error, according to Dunn.

In addition, Dunn favored the term cosmopolitan for its associated meaning of "cosmopolitanism." In "Traditional Asian Medicine and Cosmopolitan Medicine as Adaptive Systems," Dunn noted: "A dictionary definition of 'cosmopolitan' conveys the ideas of 'worldwide rather than limited or provincial in scope or bearing; involving persons in all or many parts of the world.'"[9] What interested Dunn most was the way that cosmopolitan medicine had achieved global ascendancy, even though the system was developed in the West and was then "transplanted" to other parts of the world. The rapid globalization of this system of medicine was clearly tied to capitalist expansion in the twentieth century.

Yet Dunn worried that a particular model of health care delivery—developed in the capitalist West, primarily for urban areas, with a strong focus on high-tech, curative medicine—was probably not "adaptive" in many other cultural settings. Although he noted that the cosmopolitan medical system was not globally homogeneous, manifesting significant local and regional variation, its transfer to other parts of the world might quickly lead to the subordination, even the demise, of local and regional forms. Dunn described cosmopolitan medicine as "global, largely urban," with an inherent appeal to scientifically educated "secondary elites." Furthermore, cosmopolitan medicine involved processes of professionalization and specialization, which could ultimately usurp the authority of local healers. Dunn cautioned that the cosmopolitan medical system might have a "profound impact" in non-Western settings, especially in poor, rural areas with little access to any system of medicine. He argued that cosmopolitan medicine often responded with biologically based solutions (such as vaccines and antibiotics) when the health care problems of the poor were, at their root, political and economic (and sometimes sociocultural or psychological) in nature.

Over time, and under the influence of the theories of Michel Foucault, the term cosmopolitan medicine gave way to the term "biomedicine"—a reflection of the centrality of Foucauldian "biopolitics" in Western thought, as well as the increasing importance of the "bio" (namely, the life sciences and biotechnologies such as IVF) in U.S. medicine, as noted by the medical sociologist Adele Clarke and her colleagues.[10] Today, the term biomedicine is used almost exclusively by scholars to signify Western, biotechnologically based medicine. However, I would argue that Dunn's earlier notion of cosmopolitan medicine signals the "global" in a way that the Foucauldian term biomedicine does not. What concerned Dunn—much more than Foucault—was the globalization and eventual hegemony of Western medicine around the world, concerns that were truly prescient. Four decades later, Western-invented, high-tech, urban-based curative medicine—Dunn's definition of cosmopolitan medicine—has, in fact, spread far and wide, including to the Middle East. To give just a few examples, Egypt, the site of my earliest research, now boasts twenty Western-style medical schools, almost as many schools of dentistry, and more than fifty IVF clinics, including five that are partially subsidized by the state. Saudi Arabia, a relative latecomer to the world of cosmopolitan medicine, now surpasses Egypt in the total number of medical colleges (twenty-one). Even tiny UAE (with a population of about nine million) now boasts four medical schools spread across the country, including one devoted exclusively to the training of female physicians (the Dubai Medical College for Girls).

As I would argue, the UAE—and particularly the emirate of Dubai—manifests the second distinct feature of medical cosmopolitanism. Namely, the country is the Middle East's most "cosmopolitan" nation, with Dubai the Middle East's only "global city."[11] Of all the cities in the Middle East, Dubai is the only one to have cultivated a reputation as a high-tech, global hub for medical treatment and consumption. Indeed, Dubai is now considered one of eight destinations for medical tourism within Asia (which includes the entire Arab Gulf).[12] Within the Middle East as a whole, Dubai is home to the region's only "medi-city." Called Dubai Healthcare City, this medi-city is registered as one of thirty-six tax-exempt "free zones" in the UAE, a list that also includes Dubai Silicon Oasis, Dubai Internet City, Dubai Academic City, Dubai Knowledge Village, International Media Production Zone, and, interestingly, International Humanitarian City. Dubai Healthcare City—which was initially developed with oversight by a Harvard University team called Partners Harvard Medical International—is said to include more than 100 medical facilities and more than 3,000 health care professionals. In addition, the Joint Commission International, the accrediting agency for the world's hospitals, has opened a regional office in Dubai to oversee the hospitals in Dubai Healthcare City. Despite some setbacks associated with the economic downturn of 2008–9 (for example, the Mayo Clinic closed its Dubai Healthcare City branch in 2010), the medi-city has nonetheless become a destination point for medical travelers from around the world and hopes to increasingly "compete for foreign patients."[13] It has also served to staunch the flow of wealthy Gulf Arabs patients out of the region, who, in prior years, would have traveled abroad for medical treatment.

Dubai Healthcare City is part of a much larger attempt by the Dubai government to create the Middle East's first global "techno-hub,"[14] attracting the biotechnology industry and other high-tech industries to this part of the world. For example, one free zone is called Dubai Biotech Research Park and is designed to bring the biotech industry to the UAE. Beginning in 2012, Dubai began hosting an annual Biotechnology World Congress, with the stated mission of "promoting the translational nature of modern biotechnological research, with emphasis on both the basic science in industry and academia as well as its practical and clinical applications . . . the principal goal of this symposium will be to present the world with the breakthroughs in Biotechnology and bring together both young and experienced scientists from all regions of the world to open up avenues for their meaningful collaboration at [the] regional and global level."[15] Dubai's attempt to bring biotechnology to the Arab world, including in the aftermath of the Arab revolutions, is quite significant. As Rana Dajani noted in an opinion piece in *Nature*, "science is not a high priority for countries that have just rid themselves of dictators, but in the wake of the uprisings and protests it is natural for researchers in those nations and colleagues abroad to see opportunities to improve the generally abysmal state of science in Arab countries."[16] Hence, the biotechnology conferences must be seen in this light—as an Emirati attempt to establish technoscientific leadership on a "regional and global level" in the aftermath of economic crisis and revolution.

Cultural Cosmopolitanism in the Emirates

Dubai's attempt to signal its medical cosmopolitanism at the turn of the twenty-first century is part and parcel of larger state-sponsored efforts in the Emirates to showcase a particular brand of cultural cosmopolitanism.[17] Cultural cosmopolitanism has been characterized as a style of living in transnational spaces and social fields—a willingness to engage in the world with cultural "others."[18] Described by some as a kind of "globalization from *within*," as opposed to globalization taking place "out there,"[19] cultural cosmopolitanism has been called a way of "being" in the twenty-first century, particularly in global cities such as Dubai.

However, Dubai's cosmopolitanism, or the bringing together of diverse constituencies from around the world, has a much longer history. Formerly part of the Trucial States—a loose confederation with the neighboring emirates of Abu Dhabi, Ajman, Fujairah, Ras al-Khaimah, Sharjah, and Umm al-Quwain—Dubai was known as a cosmopolitan trading hub and a place of Arab, Persian, and Indian hybridity.[20] During its colonial period as a British protectorate—which began in 1892 and ended in 1971—the coastal town of Dubai was the most thriving, trade-friendly, free port of the lower Arab Gulf.[21] As a result of this early openness, large populations of South Asians and Iranians settled in Dubai, many of them middle-class and wealthy merchants.

With the founding of the Emirati nation-state on December 2, 1971, the influx of foreigners into the country was heightened by a period of hyperdevelopment—particularly in Dubai, but also in Abu Dhabi, the largest and most petroleum-rich emirate, and the nation's new capital. Since then, the UAE has become known as one of the largest migrant-receiving countries in the world,[22] in which Indians and Pakistanis in particular have found work as day laborers in the booming construction industry.[23] Today, the nation of seven confederated emirates is decidedly multinational and multicultural. Of the more than 9.44 million people living in the country in 2014, according to official reports,[24] only about 13 percent are Emirati (and this may be an overestimate, based on the underreporting of other nationalities). The largest single group is South Asians, who, at approximately 58 percent of the total population, are nearly equally divided between Indians and Pakistanis (the former slightly outnumber the latter). Other Asians and Arabs from many nations—primarily Lebanon, Syria, Palestine, Egypt, and Sudan—make up about 17 percent of the country's population. The remaining 8.5 percent are primarily Western expatriates (or "expats"), as well as a growing number of migrants from various parts of Africa.[25] The only continent not well represented in the Emirates today is South America.

Dubai is the Emirates' largest city, with a population of nearly 2 million and more than 70 nationalities represented.[26] According to most commentators, Dubai is now the Middle East's only cosmopolitan metropolis— although, as the anthropologist Ahmed Kanna has put it more skeptically, Dubai has become a "fashionable global city," a "neoliberal enclave," and a "zone of exception" for certain "privileged foreigners," including a "multinational capitalist class" of globalized middle- and upper-middle-class expatriate workers.[27] No longer dependent on the petroleum industry, Dubai's economy has significantly diversified, with main revenues coming from three interrelated sources: the global financial services industry, a luxury real estate sector (including many high-rise apartments and luxury homes on the man-made Palm Island), and the international tourist industry.

The tourist industry bears special mention here. Not only is tourism the main engine of Dubai's economy—thereby distinguishing Dubai from the other emirates—but it is also what undergirds the "lure of Dubai" for medical travelers, who can gain easy access to hotel accommodations and can generally receive month-long visitors' visas, extendable for up to three months, before they are required to leave the country. Given the well-developed tourist infrastructure and the relatively lax criteria for getting a visa, it is not surprising that Dubai was the eighth most visited city in the world in 2012 (thereby displacing Rome), and at the top of the top-ten "destination cities" in the Middle East and Africa, according to a *Forbes* survey.[28] As a tourist destination, Dubai is famous for its iconic architecture—including the sail-boat-shaped Burj al-Arab, which is the world's only seven-star hotel, and the sparkling, stalagmite-shaped Burj Khalifa, which is now the world's tallest building (figures 1.11 and 1.12). However, what attracts most tourists to Dubai is the shopping. With more than seventy malls—including the Dubai Mall, the world's largest, and the Mall of the Emirates, with its mind-boggling indoor ski slope—Dubai has been called the "shopping capital of the Middle East."[29] It is a veritable mecca of consumption, with shoppers coming from Western and Eastern Europe; South, Central, and Southeast Asia; East, West, and South Africa; and most of the Arab world, including all of the countries in the Gulf Cooperation Council[30] (figures 1.13 and 1.14). As part of its Destination Dubai Initiative, Dubai also hosts annual shopping festivals and an international outdoor shopping bazaar called the Global Village, which is advertised as a space "where the world comes together" to buy and sell goods from many nations (figures 1.15 and 1.16). Dubai also hosts many other internationally themed conferences and touristic events, such as sports competitions, art and literature exhibitions, and both Western and Islamic fashion shows.

Given Dubai's "brand" as a hub for global tourism and shopping, it is not surprising that in 2012 it was rated the twenty-second most expensive city in the world and the most expensive city in the Middle East.[31] Nonetheless, Dubai has also been rated as one of the best places to live in the Middle East. For example, the American consulting firm Mercer gave Dubai top billing for the region in 2011.[32] The well-known Middle East journalist Thomas Friedman has famously extolled Dubai in various media reports as "an enclave of Arab progress," "orientalism in reverse"[33] and "the sort of decent, modernizing model we should be trying to nurture in the Arab-Muslim world."[34] Indeed, according to Friedman, "Dubai is where we should want the Arab world to go."[35]

However, this unabashed enthusiasm for Dubai is questioned by a host of recent scholars who have pointed to the "dark side" of Dubai, particu-

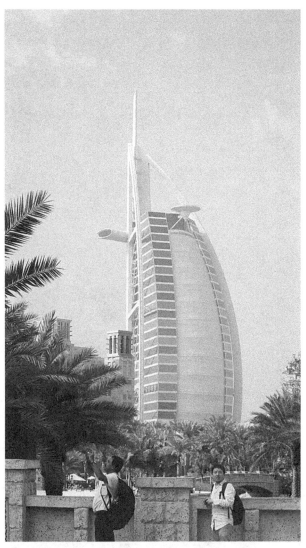

1.11 Dubai's Burj al-Arab, the world's only seven-star hotel.
PHOTOGRAPH BY JUSTINE HOOKS.

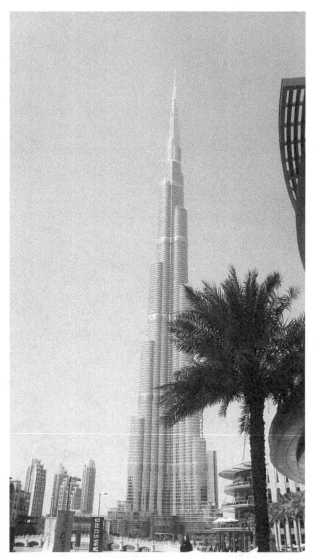

1.12 Dubai's Burj Khalifa, the world's tallest building.
PHOTOGRAPH BY JUSTINE HOOKS.

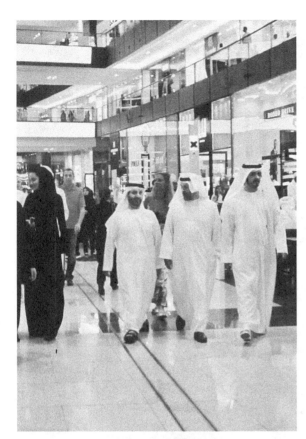

1.13 Gulf Arabs shopping at Dubai Mall, the world's largest. PHOTOGRAPH BY JUSTINE HOOKS.

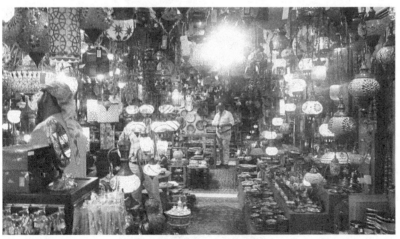

1.14 A Middle Eastern artisanal shop in the Emirates.
PHOTOGRAPH BY JUSTINE HOOKS.

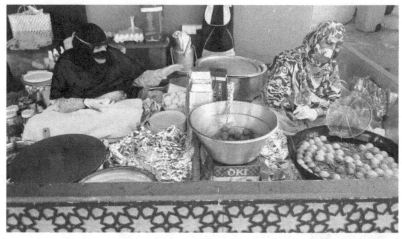

1.15 Emirati women preparing traditional foods for visitors to Dubai's Global Village, an international shopping bazaar with pavilions from many nations.
PHOTOGRAPH BY JUSTINE HOOKS.

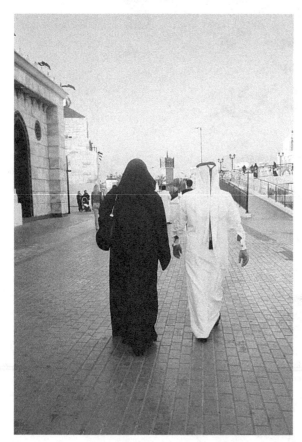

1.16 An Emirati couple at Dubai's Global Village.
PHOTOGRAPH BY JUSTINE HOOKS.

larly following the spectacular economic crash of the emirate in 2008–9 and its partial "rescue" by the petroleum-rich "big brother," Abu Dhabi. In his comprehensive book, *Dubai: The Vulnerability of Success*, the political scientist Christopher Davidson has chronicled a host of recent problems in the emirate, despite its considerable achievements and successes.[36] First, Davidson challenges the notion that Dubai is cosmopolitan in the same way that other international cities are (for example, London, Hong Kong, New York, and Singapore). Cosmopolitanism in these other cities developed organically, but in the Emirates it has been created by state policies of importing workers.[37] As Davidson points out, Emiratis and foreigners rarely intermingle socially. He calls Dubai a place of "fragmented ethnic enclaves," with a very unbalanced sex ratio caused by a mostly male workforce (76 percent). Second, the UAE's "ruling bargain" provides generous welfare benefits for Emirati citizens at the expense of their political freedoms. In return for the rulers' largesse, Emiratis are expected to be politically quiescent and are harshly punished if they "insult" the rulers through political activism. In other words, the Emirates' "unwritten social contract," which is similar to that found throughout the Gulf monarchies, is political acquiescence in exchange for wealth distribution.[38] Third, only local Emiratis (of Arab Bedouin or Persian *ajami* origin) are automatically entitled to citizenship. It is rare for foreign residents—including members of the large South Asian population—to become naturalized, even in the case of those who were born in the country after their families had resided there for generations. Without citizenship, most foreigners do not own property, renting their accommodations from Emirati nationals, who serve as wealthy landlords. Furthermore, all businesses opened by noncitizens in the Emirates must have a *kafil* (local sponsor), who, as a "sleeping partner," generally does not work in the business, but draws off at least 51 percent of the profits.[39] As a wealthy "rentier elite," Emiratis now face the "vulnerability" of their extractive system, which comes in the form of "rentier pathologies," according to Davidson, or what he calls "the Dubai Paradox." In other words, young Emiratis, especially young men, are generally undereducated in the low-quality government school system, are economically unproductive, and are voluntarily unemployed—a kind of "slacker" generation prone to lassitude and chronic overconsumption.[40] Some of this consumption, furthermore, is religiously illicit. Davidson points out that Dubai has become "Sin City"—the home of alcohol in the midst of a "dry" region and a site for gambling, international criminal and terrorist organizations, human trafficking, homosexuality, and sex tourism.

Intrigued by these post-2009 depictions of Dubai as a den of iniquity, the anthropologist Pardis Mahdavi set out to study human trafficking and prostitution in the Emirates. In her recent book, *Gridlock: Labor, Migration, and Human Trafficking in Dubai*, she challenges the assumption that Dubai is the regional hub of human trafficking.[41] Focusing her ethnographic study on sex workers, she shows that many women make economically motivated decisions to undertake sex work, often absconding from the traditional female "care industries" (that is, domestic work, nursing, and child care) after they arrive in Dubai and work for some time there. The problem for many of these foreign women is that they find it difficult to leave, eventually becoming "stuck" in a marginalized profession. Mahdavi also shows that sex workers are rated and compensated according to rigid ethnoracial and national hierarchies, which are found in Emirati society as a whole. For example, lighter-skinned Arab and Persian women, who can "talk dirty" in Arabic and Farsi, are often deemed more desirable than darker-skinned South Asian women, who, like the thousands of male day laborers from India and Pakistan, constitute an oppressed migrant population in the country.[42]

Such ethnic stratification—and particularly the position of South Asians in Dubai—is discussed in a sophisticated manner by Kanna. In his recent book, *Dubai: The City as Corporation*, he describes Dubai as an "ethnocracy"—a society governed by an exclusive, ruling tribal "ethnie," whose members have a common descent and who view all groups of foreigners as subordinate.[43] In this ethnocracy, Emiratis worry about their "cultural integrity," seeing it as threatened. Thus, Emiratis are reluctant to open up to outsiders, worrying that "cosmopolitanism has gone too far" in Dubai, where 95 percent of the workforce is made up of foreigners.

Kanna points out that Dubai has the largest South Asian population in the Middle East—what he calls "Indian Ocean Dubai." Thus, among South Asians, Dubai is viewed as either "the most South Asian major Middle Eastern city," or "the westernmost Indian city," depending upon one's vantage point. Furthermore, one's experience as a South Asian living in Dubai depends largely on one's class position. Although the majority of the South Asian workers are low-paid migrant laborers living in sometimes abominable conditions in remote desert labor camps,[44] Dubai is also home to many middle-class professional South Asians. These were Kanna's main informants, and they shared a "neoliberal identification" with Dubai as a cosmopolitan hub and a "freemarket space of economic opportunity."[45] Kanna notes that much of the literature on the Arab Gulf ignores these middle-class foreigners and their central role in societies such as the Emirates.[46] This theme is also taken up by the anthropologist Neha Vora, whose recent book, *Impossible Citizens: Dubai's Indian Diaspora*,[47] is important in understanding the interethnic dynamics of Conceive, to be described later in chapter 4.

Suffice it to say here that at Conceive, South Asian professional couples were at the core of my study. But so were other transnationally sophisticated, highly educated, dual-career couples from many nations—some of whom were making a life in the Emirates as "prospering professionals,"[48] while others had simply traveled to the Emirates for IVF care in a comfortable, cosmopolitan milieu. In general, these infertile couples were connected by their shared outlook on life—a certain "cosmopolitan disposition,"[49] or "a conscious openness to the world and to cultural differences."[50] Thus, I came to think of most of these couples as cosmopolitans—"boundaryless global citizens"[51]—who were attracted to Dubai because of its reputation as a cosmopolitan hub. Like the young Arab men in my earlier study in Lebanon, many of these infertile couples told me, with apparent sincerity, that Dubai was "the best place in the Middle East." Others were even more emphatic, saying that it was "the only place" they would ever consider visiting or living in an otherwise war-torn region. Consider this response from Hans, a thirty-six-year-old Dutch man, when I asked him simply, "Do you think that Dubai is a good place to come for treatment?":

European people, if they know [sic] about it, they would flock to this place! Treatment is very cheap here for Europeans, compared to Europe, where it's bloody expensive! The only minor problem is that they feel threatened by the Middle East, afraid even to fly to the Middle East. Three years ago, on my trip to Holland, I was on Emirates Air on my way to Dusseldorf (I speak German as well). This German guy, when we reached Turkey [from the Emirates], he dialed his wife: "I'm out of the war zone now. I'm safe now." I couldn't understand what he was saying! When visitors from Holland come here [to Dubai], they say, "I can't believe this country is like this!" It's far from their perceptions. For them, the whole Middle East is a backwater, a war zone. In fact, a big part of the Middle East *is* back at the turn of the century. Saudi Arabia, for example, it's like 100 years back in time. But this country *is* exceptional.

Hans was not alone in highlighting the "exceptionalism" of Dubai and in regarding the Emirates more generally as a "safe haven" in the midst of a culturally conservative, violent war zone. Most of my interlocutors felt comfortable in Dubai because of the "global" (as opposed to the exclusively "Arab") nature of the place. They extolled the virtues of Dubai's international workforce and potential for cross-cultural friendships. They complimented the rulers of Dubai for their cultural tolerance and economic foresight. They compared Dubai favorably with other cities they knew in Europe, America, and Asia. And they explained that Dubai was an excellent place to seek medical treatment, including for IVF, because of its multiculturalism. I came to think of this discourse emanating from my study population as the *lure of Dubai*. It provided a powerful incentive for my informants to seek IVF in the Emirates. Interestingly, the most powerful pro-Dubai endorsements were generally expressed by men, even though wives often concurred with their husbands' sentiments. For example, Akil, a young entrepreneur from India, extolled the virtues of Dubai to me in this way:

Akil: It's the most modern city—up there with any other city in the US. Dubai definitely would compare favorably, not necessarily in the same medical terms, but in the attitudes and minds of the people. It's essential to building a young economy. It's a young government, very young. The federation is hardly thirty years old. But lots of credit goes to the ruling family.

Marcia: So the ruler of Dubai has done a good job?

Akil: Dubai has gone berserk! As Thomas Friedman has said, "Dubai is Singapore on steroids."

Marcia: Really?

Akil: Absolutely! Singapore *and* Shanghai. This place *is* on steroids. [Formerly] two-lane roads now have six lanes. Two other highways will be transformed from two lanes to eighteen lanes in less than two years. Buildings are coming up over here, including this building [Conceive]. In less than five years—this building is five years old. What's really changed the entire situation is 9/11, September 11. With the US and Europe freezing assets for Arabs, they had to park their assets in an Arab country. Lebanon has civil war. Iran and Iraq are unstable. Saudi Arabia is a bit too conservative. The only place left is the Emirates.

Marcia: What about Egypt [as of 2007, the time of our interview]?

Akil: Hosni Mubarak is a dictator. Not that the ruling family here isn't. But the fact is, Dubai is the only place for companies like Microsoft, SYSCO, IBM, GE. Huge American companies and IT [information technology] companies. Their investment base was *in* Dubai. . . . It's the last holdout for *very* large American companies, American schools, American universities, a very prominent American hospital, and a large and prominent American community.

Cosmopolitans in the Clinic

Akil's level of enthusiasm for Dubai was shared by many reprotravelers, who had come to Conceive from far and wide. Having worked exclusively in Arab-serving clinics in Arab countries, I had never before grasped the meaning of "infertility around the globe," even though I had used this phrase as the title of a volume I had coedited.[52] At Conceive I truly witnessed the global scope of infertility as a reproductive health problem. I met infertile couples from many nations, some of whom were living in the Emirates and some of whom were visiting from their home countries. In addition, I met a significant number of infertile Emirati couples, who are referred to as "nationals" in Arabic (*muwatinun*), or as "locals" in English. Often, these Emirati couples were traveling across the Emirates in the hope of receiving IVF services away from the peering eyes of friends and family in their home communities.

During six months (January–June 2007) of intensive field research at Conceive, I conducted in-depth, unstructured, ethnographic interviews with 219 IVF-seeking patients from 50 different countries of origin. As shown in table 1.1 and map 1.1, couples in the study hailed from an equal number of Middle Eastern (fifteen) and European nations (fifteen), followed by an almost equal number of Asian (nine) and African (eight) countries. The United States, Canada, and Australia were also represented, with Latin America being the only part of the world entirely absent from this otherwise global study population. It became clear to me during my study—which involved follow-up trips to Conceive in 2009, 2010, and 2013 and follow-up interviews with clinic staff members in 2012 and 2013— that Conceive is situated in the center of a global reproscape comprising four major territorial reproflows: a Middle Eastern reproflow heading east into the Arab Gulf; a European reproflow beginning in England and heading east across western Europe; an East African reproflow heading northwest from the Horn of Africa; and a South Asian reproflow heading southwest from India and Pakistan (maps 1.2 and 1.3).

The Indian Ocean reproflow was the most prominent in this study, and was clearly influenced by the fact that Dr. Pankaj himself hailed from India. Infertile South Asian couples comprised the main patient population

Table 1.1. **The Global Reproscape of Conceive** Fifty Nations of Origin among the Study Population

Middle East	Europe	Asia	Africa	Other
Afghanistan	Belarus	China	Djibouti	Australia
Bahrain	Bulgaria	India* (59)	Eritrea	Canada
Egypt	England* (15)	Korea	Ethiopia	USA* (6)
Iran	Finland	Malaysia	Nigeria	
Iraq	France	Pakistan* (17)	Somalia	
Israel	Georgia	Philippines* (7)	South Africa	
Jordan	Germany	Singapore	Sudan* (11)	
Kuwait	Hungary	Sri Lanka	Tanzania	
Lebanon* (17)	Ireland	Uzbekistan		
Morocco* (5)	Italy			
Oman	Netherlands* (5)			
Palestine* (10)	Poland			
Syria* (8)	Romania			
Turkey	Russia			
UAE* (14)	Sweden* (6)			

Indicates a country with five or more study participants; the number of individual participants is included in parentheses.

at Conceive and were the single largest cohort of participants in my study. To be precise, I interviewed seventy-eight South Asians, representing forty-three couples. (Although all of these couples were married, I sometimes interviewed husbands or wives alone, rather than as couples.) The majority were Indian, followed by Pakistanis. One couple hailed from Sri Lanka and another couple identified themselves as Kashmiri, although they were citizens of India. Interestingly, this was a religiously mixed population. Twenty-seven of the thirty-three Indian couples in my study were Hindu, six were Muslim (including the Kashmiri couple), and three were Christian. All of the Pakistani couples were Muslim, as was the only Sri Lankan couple (who explained to me that their ancestors hailed from Malaysia). Most had taken up residence in one of the seven emirates, some having relocated there for the explicit purpose of conception—a phenomenon that I have come to think of as *reproductive resettlement*. Many of the UAE-based South Asian couples had traveled across the emirates seeking treatment at Conceive. Furthermore, many couples had come directly to Conceive from India and Pakistan, while a few had arrived from diasporic communities in the United Kingdom, the United States, and China. These South Asian couples often stayed in the UAE on tourist visas during the weeks and even months of treatment at Conceive, returning home after

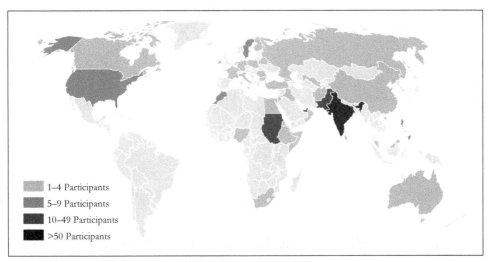

Map 1.1 The fifty nations of origin of reprotravelers to Conceive. MAP MADE BY NICK ALLEN.

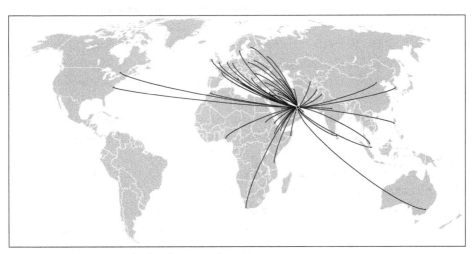

Map 1.2 Reprotravelers' pathways to the UAE. MAP MADE BY NICK ALLEN.

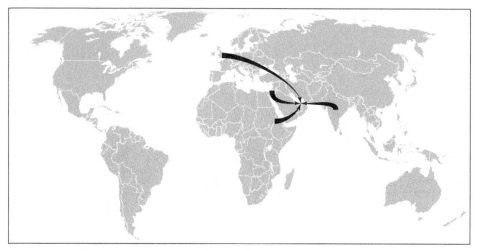

Map 1.3 Four major reproflows to the UAE from Europe, the Middle East, East Africa, and South Asia. MAP MADE BY NICK ALLEN.

an IVF cycle had been completed and a pregnancy confirmed or its failure accepted.

In addition to South Asian reprotravelers, there were many infertile Arab patients in my study, especially from the Levantine countries of Lebanon, Palestine, and Syria. Europeans in the study came primarily from England, the Netherlands, and Sweden. The majority of African patients at Conceive hailed from Sudan, but several infertile couples in my study had traveled from as far as Nigeria or Tanzania in the hopes of conceiving in Dubai.

The only criterion for inclusion in my study was a history of reprotravel across borders. All of the couples in my study had traveled—the spouses journeying together or alone—in search of assisted conception. Such reprotravel generally took four major forms. The first form was *incoming reprotravel* across international borders. Like Rahnia, many of the reprotravelers in my study had flown into Dubai International Airport from other countries to try IVF or ICSI at Conceive. A second major form was *outgoing reprotravel* from the UAE. Many of the foreign expatriates living in the Emirates had attempted to access IVF or ICSI outside the country, only to return to the Emirates—and Conceive specifically—when their outbound attempts at conception had failed. Much of this outbound travel occurred during annual leaves, and usually involved visits back home with family.[53] A third major form was *bidirectional reprotravel*. Many of the couples in my study had sought assisted reproductive services both in and out of the Emirates, sometimes traveling back and forth many times. The reasons for these bidirectional flows are multifarious and will be explored in later chapters. Suffice it to say here that frequent bidirectional reprotravel may result in very fragmented care, including the life-threatening complications experienced by Rahnia in the opening story of this book. A fourth and final form was *inter-Emirates reprotravel*. This type of reprotravel, usually by car or bus, was necessitated by the fact that only three of the seven emirates—Abu Dhabi, Dubai, and Sharjah—offer IVF services. The four other emirates—Ajman, Fujairah, Ras al-Khaimah, and Umm al-Quwain—do not.

Obtaining detailed reprotravel stories from the 125 patient couples involved in-depth interviews, each one lasting about one to three hours. (By the end of my study, I had collected nearly 1,700 pages of interview transcripts.) Ninety-four interviews were undertaken with infertile couples together, since marriage—as shown by a valid marriage license— is strictly required for IVF by the UAE Ministry of Health. However, I also interviewed thirty-one men and women alone, either because they had traveled by themselves that day, or because they were waiting for their spouses to complete various medical procedures in the clinic. In some of these solo interviews, men and women used their time with me as an opportunity for catharsis. I heard painful histories of war, refugeeism, male infertility, and complicated reprotravel stories, especially from the Middle Eastern–born men in my study. In a few cases, men and women shared their secrets of sexual dysfunction, infidelity, or polygamy for the first time. Indeed, seven marriages in the study—all of them among couples from the Middle East or Africa—were under extreme duress.

However, it is very important to stress that the vast majority of couples in this study claimed to have successful marriages, despite their vexing problems of infertility. The average length of marriage was 6.2 years, but the range was quite wide. One-quarter of the couples in the study (thirty-two) had been married less than three years and were often seeking IVF due to fears that they would "age out" of their fertility. The majority of couples (forty-one, or one-third of the couples) had been married between four and six years. However, longer marriages were quite common: 22 percent (twenty-seven couples) had been married between seven and nine years; 12 percent (fifteen couples) between ten and twelve years; 4 percent (five couples) between thirteen and fifteen years; and 2 percent (three couples) for more than fifteen years, with eighteen years being the longest marriage in the study.[54] In most cases, husbands were older than their wives, although in sixteen marriages (13 percent), wives were older than their husbands. The average age of husbands in the study was 35.6 years, with nearly half of all men (sixty-nine) in their thirties. About one-third of men (thirty-six) were in their forties, and the rest were either still in their twenties (eight) or in their fifties (four). Women's ages varied less, given the inherent limits of the human female reproductive life cycle. The average age of the women in the study was 32.7, with the vast majority of women (eighty) being in their thirties. One-quarter of the women (thirty) in the study were still in their twenties, with the youngest age being twenty-three (she had been married for five years to an azoospermic husband). A dozen women in the study were in their forties, with two women aged forty-five. In the case of these older women, traveling for IVF was usually a race against time, with their husbands aiding and abetting the journey.

At Conceive, men's commitment to both their marriages and their cross-border treatment quests was quite clear, as will be shown in many of the reprotravel stories presented throughout the book. I often sat with husbands in clinic waiting areas or with them at their wives' bedsides. As women slept, many men talked about their infertile wives with great fondness and affection. This was especially impressive in the case of a few men in arranged marriages, who explained to me that they had never set eyes on their wives until their wedding days. However, the vast majority of marriages in this study were between men and women who had chosen each other and married for love. Among the Westerners in the study, most couples explained that they had "been together" for some time before marriage, often relying on oral contraceptives and condoms to prevent pregnancy. Some of these couples had met in Dubai, or had moved or traveled there following marriages in their home countries. Interestingly, twenty-one couples in the study had "mixed" marriages, meaning that husbands and wives hailed from different countries. These included marriages between European women and Arab men, European men and South or Southeast Asian women, and Arab men and women from different countries, many of whom had met each other while working overseas. Among the couples in the study, the vast majority (114) were in their first marriages; only eleven men and one woman had been married previously. Among those in first marriages, the prevailing sentiments expressed by both spouses in the interviews were feelings of love, commitment, and support, despite the hardships of infertility. These marital commitments were at the heart of much of what I witnessed at Conceive,

Table 1.2. **Global Cosmopolitans** Top Ten Professions of Men and Women in the Study, in Rank Order

Men	Women
1. Business owners and managers	1. Teachers
2. Information technology professionals	2. Administrative assistants
3. Engineers and architects	3. Designers (fashion, art, or interior)
4. Financial analysts and bankers	4. Physicians
5. Petroleum industry managers	5. Allied health professionals
6. Shipping and logistics professionals	6. Financial analysts and bankers
7. Construction and real estate agents	7. Travel and hotel industry specialists
8. Pilots and airline industry managers	8. Beauty industry professionals
9. Media and telecommunications specialists	9. Media and publishing specialists
10. Salesmen	10. Airline and shipping industry specialists

including the complex choreography of work, travel, and treatment, all of which were tightly intertwined.

How would I characterize the couples in my study? As suggested earlier, I came to think of them as "global cosmopolitans"[55] or "global mobiles"— mostly middle- to upper-middle-class, highly educated professionals who were committed to their careers, were comfortable with international travel, had friends and coworkers from many countries, and in some cases had established themselves in the Emirates' multinational expatriate workforce as high-tech nomadic workers. These global cosmopolitans were not truly elite in their lifestyles and attitudes, nor were they part of the global migrant, working-class labor force that includes domestics and construction workers.[56] Instead, with only a few exceptions, the men and women in my study were socially situated in between these extremes: they were internationally well-traveled, middle-class professionals, who were attempting to balance their meaningful careers with their desires to become parents.

In general, work was very important to both the men and the women in the study. As shown in table 1.2, men and women occupied a wide variety of professions, most of which had required a college education or a professional degree. Among men, business, finance, IT, engineering, and construction management were prominent career paths, as were various professional positions within the airline and petroleum industries, given the study's location in the Arab Gulf. Among women, health and education were the prominent career trajectories, with many teachers, physicians, and nurses in the study. In addition, given the study's location in a hub of global travel, tourism, and shopping, many women in the study worked for airlines, hotels, and the beauty or fashion industry, as well as in international shipping. A few of the women in the study held high-powered positions in multinational corporations or in the financial sector.

Only seventeen of the women in the study had never worked, and most of them were either from South Asia or the Middle East. Yet it is important to note that many of the Indian, Pakistani, Emirati, Sudanese, and other Arab women in the study had impressive career trajectories. Among them were Sudanese physicians and professors, Emirati meteorologists and certified financial analysts, Pakistani artists and designers, and Indian IT engineers and small business owners. Furthermore, some of these women had met their husbands while pursuing higher education abroad, including in the United States and United Kingdom. Happy to meet an American anthropologist, some couples reminisced fondly about their American college days or about their various trips for business and leisure to the United States.

One of the many remarkable career women I met at Conceive was Aziza, a thirty-year-old ethnic Turkmen woman from Afghanistan, whose family had fled as refugees to the United States when she was only six years old. Educated in California and living independently since her late teens, Aziza defied every stereotype of the subservient Afghan woman. Four years before I met her at Conceive, Aziza had married Saaleh, an Afghan refugee from Germany. He accepted and encouraged Aziza's desire for independence and a fulfilling career. Considering each other "best friends, actually," the couple moved to Kabul to start a telecommunications business and to invest in a new Afghan airline. Working together out of a home-based office, Aziza and Saaleh were "making good money," with which they were supporting many of the less fortunate members of their large families. But in Kabul, Aziza also saw the opportunity to help Afghan women more generally, including adolescent girls from impoverished families who were faced with early marriage and widows who needed income to support their children. Aziza applied to German funding agencies and received generous grants to start two women's microenterprise NGOs. One allowed Afghan widows to tailor hospital and school uniforms in the relative safety of their own homes, while the other taught young Afghan women computer skills. In general, Aziza said that she wanted to help Afghan society—especially Afghan women—to circumvent the

Taliban, whom she called "people with no brains." Aziza was proud of her considerable accomplishments in Afghanistan, commenting that "the way I'm working in Afghanistan, being a woman, no one will believe me!"

As an Afghan woman, however, Aziza was still expected to have children, and Saaleh's family had begun to pressure her relentlessly. "His family is chasing me for a baby, you know, because I am considered 'very old' by Afghan standards," she explained. Saaleh's mother had recently spent two months with them in Kabul, which Aziza described as "a terrible time." Saaleh defended Aziza from his mother, saying that any infertility problem was probably due to his reckless youth in Germany as a "party animal with multiple girlfriends." Yet Aziza complained: "They think nothing can be wrong with a man—the typical Islamic mentality. His mother—oof! I'm sick of her! Every day, it was, 'I want five Turkish boys from you!'" The daily barrage unsettled Aziza, and she began to inquire about doctors in the two small European-run hospitals operating in Kabul. After failing to find any infertility specialists there—let alone IVF clinics—Aziza soon became a reprotraveler to the Emirates. For the three months before I met her, she had flown from Kabul to Dubai every ten days and then stayed two to three days in the Dubai apartment that she had owned since before her marriage. She used these short visits for ultrasound scanning and infertility treatments at Conceive.

Aziza was notable in that she continued to run her businesses, despite these frequent sojourns in Dubai. Unfortunately, not all career women were as fortunate as Aziza. One of the most striking findings of my study was the relatively high percentage of women who had given up their careers, at least temporarily, in their international quests for conception. Nearly one-third of women in the study had left their jobs to manage the complex choreography of infertility treatment and reprotravel. Not a single husband in the study was unemployed. But the relatively high unemployment rate among women—44 percent overall, including both those who had never worked and those who had quit work for treatment—was one of the great burdens resting on the shoulders of childless women in this study. Although the disruption in men's work schedules was frequently lamented during interviews—especially among a group of men whom I call the "traveling husbands"—it was the "traveling wives" in this study who had sacrificed their careers in order to become mothers. "Quit work for IVF" is what I typically coded in my notes. Yet these women were generally much more eloquent about the career disruptions engendered by infertility treatment and travel, explaining that undergoing IVF, especially with the accompanying travel, was "like a job" or a "major project" that took them away from their professional employment.

Shilpa, a thirty-eight-year-old Indian physician, described the "break" she had taken from work in a busy medical clinic in order to pursue IVF: "I've taken a break from work because of my treatment. Where I work, it is very busy, and mentally, it is too much stress trying to work and going through this treatment. The whole time, going through this and that, and also thinking about work, it becomes too stressful. Mentally, I have to be here [at Conceive]. So I quit my job for now, but I *will* get back to my work someday."

Laura, a thirty-nine-year-old Canadian flight attendant, described her race against time, first to marry and then to conceive. Fortunate to find both a husband and to learn that she was now five weeks pregnant with twins, she explained why she had chosen to quit work in order to pursue IVF within the first six months of her marriage:

> I used to work as the manager of the first-class cabin, but this had to go. I am not actively working at the moment. I was trying to pursue treatment while doing contract work, but there was too much coming and going. I wanted to see what the future held in terms of children. If it held, then we would give it a chance. I always wanted children. The week after I met my [British] husband, Tony, I told him, "I want children, so if you're not interested, then don't waste my time!" He just laughed. He said, "I've never met someone so honest." But you see, I'm not getting younger, so I might as well be honest. I'm too old to waste time. And now that I'm pregnant, I know that it is a lot of hard work to have twins, which is why I didn't go right to work again [after IVF] and get my job back. I've done a lot of things that I've wanted to do, and I think this may be true for other women who are going through these things [infertility and IVF] later in life. I've traveled, I've enjoyed my life. I started flying as cabin crew when I was eighteen. Although the last four years with [a particular airline] was a grand job, I was willing to give it up. I've seen a lot of places, more than most people. So I don't feel that I've missed anything. I've done more than most people. I don't come from a well-off family, so this was my way to enjoy life, to get paid and travel. I would still love to do something as in "a job," but it needs to be something different, which I still enjoy doing. I need to be there for my children. Fortunately, Tony has a good job. While money is not flowing in, we're not at the poverty level.

Women such as Laura were sometimes forced to travel alone because their husbands were unable to escape demanding jobs. For many of the men in the study, taking time off from work was a major problem, especially given the constraints of their busy professional lives. Men often made noble attempts to combine reprotravel with the demands of their professions. However, reprotravel was seen as jeopardizing men's as well as women's work, because it required time off—either as vacation and sick days or as unpaid leave. Permissions had to be sought, thereby revealing infertility problems to employers. With the global economic downturn beginning at the time of my study, many men felt that their jobs were less secure than before, making the prospect of taking time off seem especially threatening. Even though most of the infertile couples in my study wanted to stay together, literally and figuratively, during the entire IVF treatment process, reprotravel often pulled them apart, with wives often forging ahead on their own and their traveling husbands trailing behind them.

Professional women such as Shilpa and Laura typically found their ways to Conceive through circuitous routes. At the time of my study in 2007, Conceive was three years old but had yet to develop a fully operational website. Throughout my study, Internet-savvy men and women told me that Conceive's website was still "under construction" and needed to be completed, which they believed would serve to attract even more patients from around the world. Shortly after I left, Conceive did develop an interactive website (www.conceiveuae.net), complete with a baby photo gallery, an "Ask the Doc" space for e-mailed questions, information about the most common types of infertility and their treatment, and region-specific infertility issues addressed by Dr. Pankaj through short feature videos on the website. However, at the time of my study, this joyful "making you a family" website had yet to be launched at Conceive. Thus, many couples in the study described spending hours searching the web, scrolling through various IVF locations before ultimately arriving at Conceive.

The importance of Internet research among this population of tech-savvy global cosmopolitans cannot be underestimated. Being an "Internet researcher" was a major theme of interviews with both men and women, who prided themselves on having found Conceive, sometimes "by accident" or through following specific Internet research links, which led them to Dr. Pankaj and his record as the UAE's first IVF physician and an innovator in the development of PESA to overcome male infertility. Nearly half of the couples who had made their way to Conceive had done so by using the Internet—specifically by following various links, listening to other satisfied patients in Internet chat rooms, reading academic literature to learn about Dr. Pankaj's scientific credentials, and generally surveying the global landscape of IVF to make calculated decisions about where to travel. For example, a South African women named Nellie described how she had come across a website (www.expatwoman.com) which was designed just for women living in the Emirates, particularly Dubai. Infertility and its treatment was a main topic in the chat room and on the website's bulletin board. "The things people said about Dr. Pankaj," Nellie remarked, "made me realize that he is, for some people, a god."

Like Nellie, other computer-owning, tech-savvy women and their husbands agreed that the Internet had allowed them to become somewhat scientifically literate about the causes and treatment of infertility. A man named Nelson explained: "Although I'm Australian, I've gone to a lot of websites in the US to see what they're saying. I've done a lot of research, all on the web. The web has been a *great* resource. I don't know how people managed *before* the web. Anything—if you put it in Google, hundreds if not thousands of references will appear." But, as Nelson and others suggested, the web could also be misleading, confusing, even "scary," presenting horror stories and worst-case scenarios. Thus, the Internet alone was often not enough to bring patients across great distances to Conceive.

Rather, as became clear to me during my study, Conceive largely operated through a global network of word-of-mouth referrals, with Conceive situated in the center of a vast regional reproscape. Because of its location on the border of the Middle East's most global city, Conceive received patients from many parts of the world, and when satisfied, they told their friends and physicians back home about their experiences at the clinic. Over time, global chains of referral developed, with local gynecologists in places like Dar es Salaam, Karachi, London, Montreal, and Mumbai telling their infertile patients to consider traveling to Conceive if they hoped to achieve IVF success at comparatively affordable prices. Furthermore, Dr. Pankaj was widely acclaimed within local gynecology circles as the founding figure of IVF in the country. Thus, many UAE-based gynecologists who did not specialize in infertility referred their infertile patients directly to him.

Because of these kinds of local and global physician referrals, the power of the Internet, and the "grapevine" of recommendations from friends, family, and employers in many countries, Conceive was full of reprotravelers, many of whom had learned about the clinic through multiple sources. For example, an Indian man named Vinay pronounced it "unbelievable" that twelve of his friends had referred him to Conceive, suggesting that they, too, were infertile. One of the few lower-class women in my study, a Filipina factory worker named Anabel, described how her sympathetic Indian boss had called Conceive directly to make an appointment for her. Similarly, a Pakistani woman named Parveen described how a Latina physician working in an Iranian hospital in Dubai wrote a letter of referral for her to take to Dr. Pankaj at Conceive. Parveen explained:

> I didn't take it seriously, I don't know why. Then I was going through my files and I saw this letter and said, "Oh my God!" I had just seen my friend, an old college friend, at the airport. It had been five years since we'd met, and after finding out that I didn't have children yet, he said, "I'll tell you about a clinic. Me and my wife went there." And then I met another doctor back in Pakistan who referred me here. So everyone was saying, "Dr. Pankaj, Dr. Pankaj," and it pushed me, because I wasn't doing anything, just sitting at home.

Similarly, a forty-five-year-old Sudanese woman, Samira, visited her gynecologist in Khartoum, who made a "full investigation" and gave her a report to take to a gynecologist in Abu Dhabi, where she was living and working as a security manager. As Samira explained: "So I went in March and met him [the doctor in Abu Dhabi], and he advised me to come here [to Conceive]. He said, 'You have to gain your time, with your age, your egg problems. Gain your time. Go to Dr. Pankaj straight away. He is a very good guy. Even women half your age are going to him. Open your file with this Pankaj, and everything will be okay.'"

Cosmopolitan Lifestyles and Consequences

Samira, Laura, and Shilpa—ages forty-five, thirty-nine, and thirty-eight, respectively—were among the many highly educated professional women in my study who had delayed having children in pursuit of their careers. Fertility postponement among career women is a growing global trend—described by some as women's concession to an unforgiving labor market in which women must attempt to balance their work with motherhood.[57] The results of fertility postponement have been documented for many Western and some East Asian countries. These include significant increases in age at first marriage; significant increases in age at first birth (to nearly thirty in most Western European countries); smaller family sizes; below-replacement fertility levels in many nations; increasing levels of age-related infertility among women; and women's risk of permanent biological childlessness.[58] In fact, studies show that highly educated, professional women face a true "fertility penalty."[59] For example, in corporate America, nearly one-half (49 percent) of high-earning women over age forty are childless, even though 86 percent of them indicate that they want (or would have wanted) children.[60] Similarly, in the United Kingdom, which currently has the highest European age at first birth, 28 percent of women with college degrees were childless at the end of their childbearing years.[61] Overall, only about half of women who postpone childbearing until their thirties will conceive in the following six years, an indication of women's "difficult choices about what to prioritize at different times in their lives—children, education or career."[62]

Silvija, a thirty-two-year-old Bulgarian woman in my study, who had experienced meteoric career success in hotel services management, was stunned to discover that her inability to become pregnant after more than a decade of marriage was due to premature menopause. As her husband Grigor sat quietly by her side, she lamented:

> For the last ten years, every time we spoke to our families, they would say, "We're waiting for a baby. We're waiting for a baby." And every time, I would tell them that I wanted to do my career. So it's mostly *my* fault. *I* wanted to do a career, and now he's suffering because of me. It's not easy for him. He wanted a baby ten years ago, but I said, "Wait one more year, one more year." I have a very stressful job, with lots of pressure, so I wanted to wait. But in the end, it was too late.

Professional women such as Silvija often do not realize that oocyte (egg) quality significantly diminishes over time, a process that begins in the late twenties and rapidly accelerates after age thirty-five. By age forty, a woman has less than a 5 percent chance of becoming pregnant naturally, and chromosomal abnormalities will lead to miscarriage in one-third of all pregnancies.[63] The outcome is age-related infertility, or what is known in the medical literature as "advanced maternal age" (AMA).[64] IVF clinics around the world are now filled with such older career women who have delayed their childbearing and who are suffering from AMA-related infertility.[65] This was certainly true at Conceive. As noted above, eighty of the women in my study were in their thirties and twelve were in their forties. The women's average age was almost thirty-three, with the oldest two women (including Samira) aged forty-five. Fifteen of these women had been told that the major factor underlying their infertility was AMA, which women themselves often perceived as the "ticking of the biological clock." The clinical statistics among this group of fifteen women were grim. Altogether, they had undertaken twenty-seven IVF or ICSI cycles, experienced ten miscarriages, and had one life-threatening ectopic (tubal) pregnancy. Only two women were pregnant at the time of the study—one because she had used donor eggs at an IVF clinic in Cyprus on her ninth IVF attempt.

"Aging out" of one's fertility was thus a major concern expressed by many women in their thirties and forties. A thirty-five-year-old Filipina woman named Luz, married to a German husband, put it this way: "Maybe this is an interesting fact for your study. It is the biological clock which is really . . . which will push you to alternative countries—traveling around the globe, even, to find the right kind of treatment. In your twenties, you might not think of doing this. But more and more the push of age will lead you to look to some exotic kinds of things, like going abroad."

Another woman, Meera, had grown up in the Indian community in Dubai, had gone to college in the United States, and then met her Irish husband, Sean. They had moved together to Australia to pursue their professional careers but recently returned to Dubai so that Meera could take over the family shipping business. Married for six years, Meera was now forty, and she realized that she could postpone her childbearing no longer. Meera and Sean had this to say about fertility postponement, which they viewed as a widespread problem in their group of professional friends:

Meera: There's a lot of demand for IVF in Australia, because people are having children later, and later, and later.

Sean: I think everywhere—I can't really say, but it seems to be more prominent, that couples are waiting and then having problems, like endometriosis, and guys with sperm problems. Maybe from "the lifestyle," or the agriculture and the chemicals in the food and air.

Meera: And age. Women's age.

Sean: I don't think that people of our parents' age had these problems. They sneezed the wrong way, and they're pregnant! We know someone who said, "I used to throw my underpants on the bed and my wife was pregnant!"

Meera: But I think in our circle of friends, half a dozen people, females, have these sort of problems, all kinds of issues going on. I have a friend, Louise, who has ovulation problems, and she's only thirty-two.

As suggested by Sean, "lifestyle" was also deemed a potential causal factor in infertility. Many men and women at Conceive were skeptical about their own lifestyles, which they linked to their infertility problems.[66] My infertile interlocutors confessed to me, with clear feelings of guilt and shame, that they were leading unhealthy lives. Both men and women told me: "I don't have the healthiest life." "I'm a workaholic, and I'm overweight and I get no exercise." "I have a lot of work stress and I travel too much. I also love to eat and I get home late after going out for dinner." "My vices are smoking and drinking. I've tried to stop smoking, but now I am a social smoker only." "I'm a nervous wreck. I have work stress, travel pressure, and I can't sleep."

To wit, men and women engaging in high-octane, money-generating, travel-filled, restaurant-dining, late-night lives felt that the fast pace of the "high life" was taking its toll on their reproductive bodies. They enjoyed, but also lamented, this cosmopolitan way of being, believing that it had diminished their fertility over time. Throughout my interviews, I heard about the pressures of work—working too much, for too many hours, and to the point of workaholism and exhaustion. I listened to stories about frenetic travel schedules—lives spent "in transit," working from hotels and airports, sitting in traffic jams (notorious during Dubai's rush hours), breathing in polluted air, often in high heat. I heard about the overconsumption of food—nights spent out dining at different restaurants, enjoying global cuisines, but also consuming too much food, some of it unhealthy. I also listened to guilty admissions about vices—particularly smoking and drinking among men, sometimes to excess, even to the point of alcoholism. In general, in this cosmopolitan population, life was out of balance. Too much work, too much travel, too much eating and drinking, and too much stress led to too little sleep, too little attention to diet, too little exercise, and too little bodily self-care. Although I never asked sensitive questions about actual or perceived weight problems, many men and women volunteered to me that they were overweight, sometimes significantly so, and some of them had developed diabetes and/or hypertension.[67]

For example, Chitra, a twenty-seven-year-old Indian teacher at a private school, who had already lived in two other countries (Nigeria and the United Kingdom) before marrying into the affluent Sindhi Indian community of Dubai, had this to say about lifestyle and infertility:

Infertility is *very* common in my community. It's not like they talk about the specific problems, but more like, "How come you're not planning?" They are talking about this [infertility]. It's definitely common, and also a lifestyle problem perhaps. Dubai is a very hectic society, especially in the community I live in. I'm in the Sindhi community. We're all from India, but it depends where you're from. I'm from the Sindhi community and the lifestyle is very flamboyant! It's very common for some people to go out, to eat out, five times a week! Also, the lifestyle, it's an effort to exercise. You don't go walking outside because there are no sidewalks. People are not walking. So you have to go to the gym. There's no naturally occurring exercise—that is, among those who are quite affluent. We just sit on our asses all day and do nothing! No wonder we're getting sick! Not just Sindhis, everyone!

Similarly, Fakhira, a thirty-one-year-old Pakistani interior designer, who had just flown into Dubai from Karachi, had this to say about work, stress, and infertility:

Fakhira: I'm an interior designer and I just stopped working two months ago. I need to relax and take time out, because I've been working and traveling a lot, and he [her husband] travels a lot, too. I've been to China, Thailand, Italy, Malaysia, Canada, America, sometimes for work and sometimes for holidays. He travels a lot to the Middle East, Asia, the States, the UK for his job in the IT sector, in satellite communications. So we have a hectic lifestyle. I didn't even think about having a baby the first three to four years [of marriage].
Marcia: Were you using contraception?
Fakhira: No contraception. No nothing! But no pregnancy either. So when we found out it was him [male infertility], he felt like—initially, when he found out, he was miserable. He felt it *a lot*, and he was crying. But we're more like friends, and I never brought it up, that this is "because of him." It's just a medical problem, and now I found out that *I* have a problem [PCOS]. So it's not his fault, actually, and there's no medical cure, and no cause. It's a strange thing—his sperm count is variable. Sometimes the sperm tests are much better than other times. I think this is because he's so busy at work. There's a lot of work stress. He *is stressed*. When he's relaxed, he's in a good mood and up to doing something [an ICSI cycle]. But he is mostly overworked and a little overweight, also.

Fakhira's case speaks to the two main infertility problems I encountered at Conceive: male infertility and PCOS. Both of these problems have a genetic basis, and both are linked to lifestyle factors.[68] To begin with male infertility, it is now recognized that microdeletions of the long arm of the *Y* chromosome are the most frequent genetic cause of infertility in men.[69] In men with such *Y* microdeletions, the spermatozoa will always be infertile because these genetic alterations are incurable and persist throughout a man's lifetime. Such deletions are manifest in a variety of sperm defects, including oligozoospermia (low sperm count), asthenozoospermia (poor sperm motility, or movement), oligoasthenozoospermia (low count and poor motility), teratozoospermia (abnormal sperm morphology, or shape), and azoospermia (absence of sperm in the ejaculate).

However, lifestyle factors can also diminish sperm profiles in men who are not genetically infertile. A major risk factor is smoking (and other forms of tobacco consumption such as traditional Middle Eastern waterpipe smoking). Recent studies have shown the negative, spermatotoxic effects of cigarette smoking on sperm count, motility, and morphology, resulting in impaired sperm function. Furthermore, sperm count and morphology may decrease over time, with each additional year of smoking.[70] Secondhand smoking may also affect a woman's reproductive health by impairing fertilization, decreasing embryo quality and implantation rates, and resulting in early miscarriage.[71] In the context of IVF, the odds that fertilized embryos will become implanted in a woman's womb may be affected by the ambient tobacco smoke in her environment.

Unfortunately, male smoking is widespread in the Middle East (38 percent of men smoke) and in the world more generally (36 percent of men overall; 35 percent in developed countries, 50 percent in developing countries).[72] Of the world's billion smokers, 81 percent are men,[73] which suggests that male smoking is a truly widespread lifestyle issue, not only in cosmopolitan settings such as Dubai but also in most other parts of the world. At Conceive, I did not collect specific information on smoking, but some men and a few women in my study told me that they were smokers. In some cases, they had tried or hoped to quit, and the need to quit was a message that was reinforced vigorously in the clinic. Indeed, I observed Dr. Pankaj on several occasions giving firm lectures, even commands, to male patients to stop smoking, especially if they hoped to improve their sperm quality or the chances of embryo implantation. Men were often at a loss about what to do, especially those who admitted to being "addicted" to cigarettes. Take, for example, this interaction, which I witnessed between Dr. Pankaj and Mike, the husband of a long-term infertile British woman, who had undergone many grueling IVF cycles in the United Kingdom without any success:

Dr. Pankaj: Once her embryos are inside, I don't want any nicotine around her.

Mike: I only smoke outside.

Dr. Pankaj [turning to the wife]: I can smell the nicotine now! I'm not putting those embryos back in till he assures me he's not smoking. I'm wasting your embryos otherwise. There is a significantly lower rate of IVF success in women whose husbands smoke. Okay?

Mike: Okay.

Dr. Pankaj: Nicotine can affect your embryos. So you've got two days to stop. On the 31st is your embryo transfer. [Turning to the wife] I'm not going to put your embryos back if he's still smoking then.

Mike: Have you ever smoked?

Dr. Pankaj: Of course, I have!

Mike: Then you know how difficult it is to stop.

Dr. Pankaj: There will be drama in your household, but you have two days. Enjoy it!

Although I was a bit taken aback by this bedside ultimatum, Dr. Pankaj was proud of his smoking-cessation lecture. "Did you hear me telling him not to smoke?" he asked. I answered, "Yes, and I'm totally antitobacco. But would you really not do the embryo transfer?" Dr. Pankaj replied, "Of course, I'll do it. But now his wife will put pressure on him to quit!"[74]

Whether women undergoing the stresses of IVF can make their husbands stop smoking is very uncertain. It is especially doubtful given that women themselves are often under incredible pressure to lose weight prior to IVF, especially those women diagnosed with PCOS. PCOS is a condition related to weight gain, and it was a widespread problem among women in my study. This genetically based metabolic disorder is linked to insulin resistance and diabetes.[75] Like diabetes, PCOS is considered to be a "lifestyle disease with a genetic predisposition."[76] In other words, a woman may have a genetic predisposition to PCOS, but a "lifestyle" factor—namely, overeating, sedentarism, and subsequent weight gain—may be necessary to trigger the onset of the condition.[77]

On a clinical level, women with PCOS are generally (although not necessarily) overweight, and sometimes obese.[78] Because of hormonal disruptions leading to excess androgen (testosterone), women with PCOS often have unwanted facial or body hair (hirsutism), and thinning or loss of hair from the scalp, resembling male balding. Oily skin with a mild form of disseminated acne is also a telltale sign of PCOS. Most important in the infertility diagnosis, women with PCOS have so-called "polycystic ova-ries." Instead of producing one dominant follicle around a mature egg as part of the normal menstrual cycle, polycystic ovaries contain many small cysts, which are egg-containing follicles that have not developed properly due to a number of hormonal irregularities. These multiple cysts can be seen in an ultrasound scan and are a key finding in the differential diag-nosis of PCOS.

Worldwide, 6 to 8 percent of women are estimated to have PCOS.[79] However, the rates of PCOS in some parts of the world, including the Arab Gulf and South Asia, have been shown to be much higher. The UAE sits squarely in what could be called the world's *diabetes-obesity-PCOS belt*. Di-abetes rates throughout the Arab Gulf are among the highest in the world, with an overall prevalence of 19 percent in the Emirates and 23.9 percent in Kuwait, which now has the highest rate of diabetes in the region.[80] With respect to diabetes in the Emirates, a national survey called the Emirates National Committee on Adult Diabetes (ENCAD) study was conducted jointly by the World Health Organization and the UAE Ministry of Health between 1998 and 2000.[81] The study involved the random screening of 6,609 women of all ages—2,363 Emirati nationals and 4,246 foreign resi-dents. The researchers determined that 40 percent of the women were overweight, 33 percent were obese, 20.6 percent had impaired glucose tolerance, and 22.3 had diabetes. Among women in the study of reproduc-tive age (ages 20–44), the rates of impaired glucose tolerance (27 percent) and diabetes (35 percent) were even higher. In short, the study proved what many physicians already suspected—that lifestyle changes leading to weight gain and diabetes were taking their toll on Emirati society.

But what about PCOS? A study conducted at Conceive between Sep-tember 2005 and July 2009 confirmed the relationship of PCOS to the earlier ENCAD findings.[82] The Conceive study involved 501 female part-ners of infertile husbands, who were randomly selected and screened for PCOS. PCOS was highly prevalent in the Conceive clinical population, oc-curring in 23.5 percent of European or American women, 39.4 percent of Gulf Arab women, and 42.5 percent of South Asian women in the study. Across all three groups, menstrual irregularities, excess androgen levels, and polycystic ovaries were detected. Insulin resistance was also a key find-ing among the South Asian (96.5 percent) and Gulf Arab (80.9 percent) women diagnosed with PCOS, although it was less common among the European or American women in the study (18.8 percent).

Women in the Conceive study were also overweight, based on body mass index (BMI). Normal BMIs range from 18.5 to 24.9 for women; 25 is considered overweight, and 30 is obese. Average BMIs in the Conceive study were 24.7 for European or American women, 27.5 for South Asian women, and 28.8 for Gulf Arab women. Women whose weight was followed annually showed an average gain of 5.63 kilograms (12.41 pounds) with each passing year.[83]

In short, the Emirates is now a global hub for a triad of linked problems, including *overweight/obesity, insulin resistance/diabetes*, and *PCOS/infertility*. Attempting to reverse this trend, Dubai began a campaign on July 19, 2013, to encourage weight loss among city residents, more than half of whom were overweight, but less than a quarter of whom admitted to having a weight problem.[84] For every kilogram (2.2 pounds) lost, Dubai promised to give residents one gram of gold (the equivalent of $45 in 2013 prices), and the "biggest losers" had the opportunity to win more than $5,000 in a lottery. The reward increased to two grams of gold for every kilogram that a family lost during the summer of 2014—a campaign that focused on Dubai's increasingly obese youth.[85] Health care commentators responding to this public health campaign were skeptical. One noted that "Dubai residents are already so rich (the UAE has a GDP per capita of over $45,000 per year) that getting a couple hundred bucks for giving up the convenience of McDonald's may not be an attractive enough incentive."[86]

As a physician working on the front lines of the obesity, diabetes, and PCOS epidemic in the Emirates, Dr. Pankaj is deeply troubled by what he observes on a daily basis in his own clinic. He considers PCOS to be an "epidemic"—one of the emerging "lifestyle diseases" of the Emirates. As he explained to me, "70 percent of our female patients have PCOS, either as a primary or associated cause of their infertility. It is a genetic problem of insulin resistance *plus* lifestyle changes. It's *much* higher here in the UAE than in India or the UK. Yet many women do not know that they suffer from this problem."

Women's lack of a PCOS diagnosis before coming to Conceive was a huge issue in my study. For example, Aarti was a thirty-year-old Indian teacher who had been married for nine years without conception. Frustrated, she came to Conceive on the recommendation of a friend: "Dr. Pankaj was the one who diagnosed it [PCOS]. He told me to do a lot of things. He was the one who checked me out really well. I've been with him now nearly two, two-and-a-half years. I'm really grateful, because initially, someone [an Indian physician] told me, 'You're PCO[S], but it's not so important.' Dr. Pankaj said, 'Who said it's not important?' The first doctor had said I'm not 'highly PCO[S].' But Dr. Pankaj said, 'PCO[S] is a case. You're a PCO[S] case. It has nothing to do with 'highly' or not.'"

Aarti was one of the fifty-two women in my study who had been diagnosed with PCOS. PCOS and male infertility were the two most common infertility factors in my study: 42 percent of women suffered from the first problem, and 42 percent of men suffered from the second. Furthermore, twenty-two of the couples in my study (18 percent) suffered from both PCOS and male infertility, making their cases doubly difficult to manage and overcome. PCOS treatment often involves extended regimens of medication to regulate insulin levels as well as weight reduction—the latter deemed difficult by most women. For example, Josephine, a thirty-five-year-old Christian Indian woman, who had recently moved to the Emirates with her husband, had been diagnosed with PCOS by a female physician in Dubai. She explained:

In fact, Dr. Pankaj was pretty happy with the previous doctor's prescriptions. She had started to treat my irregular periods, and she was on the right track, Dr. Pankaj told us. I really didn't know how common PCOS is. But in this part of the world, it's pretty common. Maybe it's the water, the lifestyle. We can't figure it out. Two out of three women seem to have PCOS. At social get-togethers, you hear people talking about that. Dr. Pankaj said it has to do with weight gain. He told me that I needed to reduce by seventeen kilos [37.5 pounds]. I was seventy-six kilos [167.5 pounds], and I was supposed to be fifty-nine [130 pounds]. So he asked us to join a gym. He said there were two things that needed to be done. First, the insulin, which was in his hands. The other was with us, to reduce the weight. I would love to join a gym, but my work schedule is bad. I get home late, and I'm pretty exhausted and tired. We used to go for walks together, but our work is pretty stressful. We came here to get financial stability, then we'll move back home. That's the main reason for being here. But the lifestyle—there is so much pressure.

As Josephine suggests in her final remark, the relationship between infertility and lifestyle is beginning to be understood by a growing number of cosmopolitan couples. At this point, let us listen to the stories of some of these cosmopolitans who have chosen Dubai as a venue for treatment. Their reprotravel to Conceive reflects their global mobility, their cosmopolitan lifestyles, and their attraction to Dubai as a multicultural metropolis and a medically cosmopolitan reprohub.

HUBS: Reprotravel Stories

• A Traveling Husband

Fuad was a brooding but loquacious Lebanese man, who told me, somewhat apologetically, that "I talk a lot."[87] A member of one of many internationally "mixed" couples at Conceive,[88] Fuad was seated at the bedside of his Russian wife, Tatiana, who was stunningly beautiful even in a hospital cap and gown. When I asked the less attractive Fuad how he had met his wife, he told me a story that was familiar to me from my prior work in Lebanon. Like 55,000 other young Lebanese men of the "war generation" (those who came of age during the 1975–90 civil war), Fuad had been sent to college in the former Soviet Union through a scholarship provided by a left-leaning Lebanese political party. As a student in Moscow, he learned to speak fluent Russian. Later he married Tatiana, who was a divorceé and the mother of a nine-year-old daughter, Aleksandra. In an attempt to make a comfortable life for his bicultural family, Fuad settled Tatiana and Aleksandra in Dubai, which he perceived to be the best possible option in the Middle Eastern region. But living in Dubai was expensive, forcing Fuad to take a more lucrative telecommunications position in Riyadh, Saudi Arabia. Not wanting his beloved Tatiana to move again—and especially not to a more conservative country—Fuad moved alone to Saudi Arabia, beginning his career as a "frequent flyer" across the Gulf.

Like many other Lebanese men, Fuad had also set in motion the family's immigration to Canada. His stepdaughter Aleksandra, eighteen years old, had recently started college in Toronto, and Fuad hoped that she would make her future life there. Fuad had cut his ties to Lebanon, especially after the 2006 summer war with Israel. Nonetheless, as the only son, he was expected to support his aging parents, making him effectively responsible for four households—his parents' home in Beirut, his wife's apartment in Dubai, his stepdaughter's dormitory in Toronto, and his own townhouse in a "foreigners' compound" in Riyadh. In addition, he and Tatiana were contributing a small amount to her parents' upkeep in Grozny, Russia. Fuad admitted that he no longer enjoyed traveling to Grozny through Moscow, where "they hassle me. I look like a Chechen. They hate Chechens."

Through a lengthy and wide-ranging interview, I came to think of Fuad as a "global cosmopolitan"—one of the new generation of educated, middle-class

Arab businessmen, whose lives are decidedly transnational, exceptionally mobile, markedly multicultural and multilingual, and at times extremely stressful. Fuad was eager to narrate to me his tale of stress and woe, in which he punctuated the pathos with moments of ribald humor.

On the side of pathos, Fuad and Tatiana had struggled with long-term reproductive troubles. After nine years of "togetherness"—seven of them as a married couple—Fuad and Tatiana had still produced no child of their own. Fuad blamed this barrenness on his dislocation in Saudi Arabia, as well as both spouses' infertility problems, which he described to me from Tatiana's bedside. As he explained:

> We were not thinking about it—pregnancy—or when it will come. But then we had an "incident" in 2000—an ectopic pregnancy, "outside the uterus" [that is, with the fetus developing in the fallopian tube]. We were there in Lebanon, meeting my parents for the first time, and then we were supposed to go to Germany, through Berlin, to stay with my uncle. But she had severe pain, and it was an ectopic emergency, so we stayed in Beirut, where they treated her. Before that time, her [fallopian] tubes were fine. But now we discovered that one of her tubes is blocked, and we have to do IVF.
>
> On the initial test, the first test, my count was also low, like 18 million, with 90 percent abnormal sperm.[89] This is because of my "lifestyle." I'm smoking and consuming spirits. I'm a social drinker, but I have a lot of opportunity to drink! So I was tested again this year, and I started going over things, treating myself with vitamins. I decreased my intake of spirits. But I couldn't stop smoking. I still smoke one pack a day. But with these changes, my count was raised from 18 million to 45 million to 55 million. On the day of insemination, it was 113 million, but still 85 percent abnormal.
>
> You know what? I'm not the first one with these [infertility] problems. I'm understanding that it's a common problem in the Middle East. It's the lifestyle, the stress, the money issues, and the lifestyle again. Most guys now have high blood pressure. Like me, I have high blood pressure, and for two years, I've been on medication. People in the [United] States and in Canada, they walk, they play sports daily. They go to work, change their clothes at work, and go to the gym while working. Like it's a must—daily exercise. But here, it's a crazy society because of the weather [high heat] and traffic jams. People don't have time to exercise. People don't follow hobbies, and when they do, they don't really work on them. But it's worse in Saudi Arabia. I'm living in Riyadh, and it's the worst place. It's landlocked, and there's no beach. I have economic reasons for being there, but it's not nice at all. For couples, espe-

cially expatriates, they can survive if they're both working. Otherwise, you'll be dying from doing nothing at home! You will gain weight as a woman, and so you have to work. You go inside a compound [for expatriates], and it's not a healthy environment. I live in a compound, and I'm the only Arab there! You drink the local stuff, the local spirits, which are not good for your health. So now I'm stopping all of this. In fact, I want to stop my job in Saudi Arabia, even though I can't afford to right now. I would prefer to have a Canadian passport but to stay here [in Dubai]. There are a million and a half Lebanese in Quebec alone! But it is better to be there if you're young, right after graduation. Not at this age. It's too late for me now, to start all over again from zero. If I were twenty-two or twenty-four, I would go there. It's a good place for the freshly graduated. I could stay six or seven years there, and then move to the Gulf. But we did the opposite!

As I soon came to realize, Fuad and Tatiana were living "betwixt and between" three continents and five countries—the Emirates, Saudi Arabia, Lebanon, Russia, and Canada. Thus, deciding where to pursue assisted reproduction was a difficult calculation: "We did a *lot* of research, and not only on the Internet. We did Internet research about the process, all the IVF procedures and this ICSI. We did our own research on the doctors who do this. She has a beauty parlor in Dubai. She's a beautician, and so a lot of people come in there, and they told us why they had chosen to come here. It was word of mouth that got us to Conceive." But "getting to" Conceive was not so easy. Consequently, Fuad was quite grumpy on the day of our conversation:

We did an insemination two weeks ago, and it was not a success. This is why I am pissed today. We were supposed to do IVF on February 25, but first she needs an operation to block the tube. It is filled with water, and it needs to be blocked so that [the fluid] will not leak into the uterus.[90] But then we have to wait for one more month before we can do IVF. So they should have checked the tube *before* insemination, because it was a wasted process—and a waste of money and time. I don't find flights easily from Saudi Arabia. I just arrived last night, and I'm leaving again in three hours.

Fuad was a "man on a mission"—to fly across the Gulf in time to deposit his semen in the IVF laboratory and to support Tatiana through her various assisted reproductive procedures. Fuad's difficult commute between Riyadh and Dubai made the thought of trying assisted reproduction elsewhere seem highly impractical. Although IVF cycles in both Russia and Canada are partially subsidized by the state, Fuad and Tatiana did not have full citizenship rights in either country.

Furthermore, they had already experienced long waiting times and the lack of individualized medical attention in previous visits to public clinics in those countries. Coupled with the long flights, travel costs, and lost work days, they decided that reprotravel to either Moscow or Toronto was simply not worth it.

When I asked Fuad whether he considered himself to be a "reproductive tourist," he had this to say:

> At the end of the day, you don't want to say, "This is it. We give up." We need to feel that we're doing something [to have a baby]. But it's not a straightforward procedure. You can't mix "tourism" in the title for this. I'm finding that it's difficult to travel like this. It's not about the money. It's about finding the right time. Today I should be working, but instead I'm coming here. And this has happened time and time again. I don't know how some people can afford it, because medicine and travel are expensive. I *can* understand if you go to Slovakia, for example. I heard about hot tubs, mineral waters, like a "spa." Two- to three-day trips there. But this, we're talking about two weeks of daily injections, for example, and staying without sex. Doing this test, the semen test. So imagine if you are flying! It is madness, and it's depressing. People usually fly to have fun, not this. It's *not* tourism. Even for those who stay in a hotel. Do you think they are having a nice time? At night, he should not touch her, because he has to come in the morning and shake his thing [masturbate into a plastic cup]!

I asked Fuad what he hoped to achieve at Conceive. "I hope to have two—twins," he said. "But one is enough. If we have to repeat a procedure like this again, then we don't have time for two. But if two come at the same time, this will be a blessing." When I asked Fuad if he preferred boys or girls, he exclaimed, "Boys!" When I asked him why, he explained: "Because we have a girl already. I've raised her as my stepdaughter since she was nine years old. But this is a family issue—who will take the family name? In my [natal] family, there are three girls, and I'm the only boy. All over my family—my aunts, cousins, and uncles—each one of them has only one boy and a lot of girls."

I then asked Fuad if he would ever consider egg or sperm donation, practices that can increase the success rates of IVF and ICSI but that have been banned by the Sunni Islamic religious authorities, including in the UAE, which eventually passed a law against them. He explained:

> I'm Muslim, Sunni, but this is only on my ID card. I'm not practicing. I'm not a religious guy at all, since I drink. But I heard about it a lot—that you can have different eggs from different women. But, you see, I'm against it. It's not about

religion, it's about DNA! And we have a kid already. We prefer to get our daughter married, and then she will have her own children. It's better than having another person serve as a donor for us. I'll tell you who would do that—those who need the "sensation" of kids. But we have that already because of our daughter. For me, it's not a moral issue. It's not a sentimental issue. I need the DNA! My family's name! And it's the same with adoption. When thinking about alternatives and different steps to having children, the last one is adoption. I won't go through with that. I'm not Angelina Jolie! We need *our* DNA. It's a good match!

As we looked down at Tatiana, who was resting quietly, I felt compelled to mention to Fuad that she was certainly a beautiful woman. "Yes," he confirmed. "But even more from the inside than the outside." Tatiana, who spoke little English, was soon to be moved into the operating theater for a diagnostic procedure to visualize the inner recesses of her barren womb. Whether she and Fuad went on to conceive the child of their dreams is unknown, for I only encountered them one more time in the clinic—and they were not yet pregnant.

• **A Frozen Embryo Checkup**

Fuad was one of many traveling husbands in my study. Generally, the men I met at Conceive were on the go—often for work but also because they hoped to make a baby with their beloved wives and were willing to travel to do so. Whereas Fuad had returned to Dubai to reunite with Tatiana, other men whose wives lived outside of the Emirates had come to Conceive alone as male reprotravelers. I met many of these solo traveling husbands in the clinic—men who had come from far and wide to deposit their semen into plastic cups, to settle their IVF accounts, and to undertake clinical consultations with Dr. Pankaj, particularly regarding male infertility.

One day I saw a European man sitting by himself in the ultrasound scanning area, and I asked him if he would be willing to participate in my study. He said he was happy to do so, after having a brief meeting with Dr. Pankaj. As it turned out, Marku was Romanian and was "passing through" Dubai to check on the status of his four frozen embryos. We spent several hours together, with Marku telling me at the end of his interview that he had "needed that"—that I was "like a psychologist" to whom he had just unburdened himself.

In the course of our conversation, I learned that Marku and Doina, his wife of ten years, had been together since their teens as university students in Romania. Now in their late thirties, Marku said that he could not possibly imagine life without Doina, even though they were living apart—Doina in Romania and Marku in Qatar, where, as a petrochemical engineer, he worked twenty-eight days on and then several weeks off an oil rig in the middle of the Persian Gulf. Marku considered this lifestyle to be "an adventure" and in general professed his love of travel, hotels, and new experiences. The only problem was that the Qatar job offered "no family status." When I asked Marku what that meant, he explained, "I have no flat, no home, where they pay utilities or offer facilities for a family." This was in marked contrast to an earlier job he had had in Abu Dhabi, where Doina had been able to join him because the company had offered housing and other benefits for trailing spouses.

However, the Abu Dhabi years had been difficult ones for Doina. She had become pregnant "by surprise" but experienced an ectopic emergency, with the fetus stuck in the fallopian tube. According to Marku, the doctors in Abu Dhabi had been "so afraid of not doing the right thing" that they had probably over-reacted, undertaking a major surgery to remove the affected fallopian tube. In retrospect, Marku realized that an ectopic pregnancy could be removed through medication, which would have spared Doina's fallopian tube for future conception.[91] "This was the start of our trial," Marku explained:

We started following up on the Internet—*everything* we could find. We sent letters by e-mail to some doctors in Romania and asked them to answer us. Some answered us, telling us what to expect, what chances we have. So, looking around here, we found this doctor [Dr. Pankaj]. At first, we found some doctors in Abu Dhabi. We went to two hospitals there, a few hospitals, but we were not so happy about the information we got from them. They did not convince me. But we finally found this doctor [Dr. Pankaj]. One of my wife's colleagues told her about the clinic and gave her the phone number. We put this doctor's name on the Internet. We were searching the Internet with his name. And we found that he is involved in some conferences and activities. He has published scientifically. We saw that he is quite professional. So we came here, directly here, because we were a little disappointed with our experiences in Abu Dhabi.

To be honest, I cannot distinguish them [the clinic staff at Conceive] in the beginning. They looked completely the same in the beginning, and so I had a hard time in the beginning remembering them. And my English is very poor, so when they're speaking, I didn't understand that it's English! And then I had almost the same shock when I heard people in the clinic at that time speaking Scottish, and it was quite hard for me to understand. But you get used to it. Because actually, coming here—even before the first trial, we got used to this clinic a long time ago. Here, we meet everybody, white, black, from all areas. It's one big Babylon here! I don't know where else you can find this—maybe in the US?

Within this Conceive "Babylon," Marku and Doina were among the first cohort of patients to undertake IVF following the clinic's opening in 2004. Although their two IVF attempts were unsuccessful, four extra embryos were fertilized and put in a cryopreservation tank at Conceive for long-term storage and future use. However, at this point, Doina was discouraged and homesick, so Marku encouraged her to move back to Romania to receive support from both of their families. This also freed Marku to take the higher-paying position in Qatar. But it also marked the beginning of Marku's reprotravel. Back and forth between the airports in Doha and Bucharest, Marku traveled many times to be with Doina through painful medical procedures in Romania, including the removal of her second damaged fallopian tube.

Marku soon realized that Romania itself was becoming an Eastern European hub for IVF with donor eggs. Although Marku and Doina had never contemplated using donor eggs, they noted that many newly opened IVF clinics in Romania were advertising this form of reproductive assistance. They decided to try IVF in Romania with the country's foremost IVF physician—one who, according to Marku, had helped a sixty-seven-year-old woman to conceive and had ended up in the *Guinness Book of World Records*. Already feeling reproductively elderly at age thirty-seven, Doina sought out this doctor, who practiced out of a government IVF clinic in the gynecology ward of a large, overcrowded state hospital, where patient care was minimal. After two failed IVF attempts there, Marku and Doina decided never to return. After a total of four failed IVF attempts—two in the Emirates, two in Romania—Marku described Doina's demoralization in this way:

> She feels that she has no time at all. She's already thirty-seven. She's in a kind of bad psychological state now. We can manage, but always in the back of her mind she thinks, "I'm losing my time." She believes that she's too old, the eldest woman, and she's not happy at all. The sooner you do this IVF, the better, because the counter is running against you! So she's not working at all right now. She was offered a job [as a teacher], but she is staying at home. She refused a job because she is following her treatment. She told me, "I can accept a job, but I have to go to treatment. I have to stay home. I have to stay and rest. At work, they would just refuse if I had to take more than a day off." So her psychological shape is a little bit bad. She's gotten a little bit fed up. She's not eating so much. She's kind of depressed. How many pills she has taken? How many injections has she gotten? One in the morning, one in the

afternoon, every single day. So I feel so guilty. I'm not there all the time to support her, and she always needs some support from me. I feel guilty, because I'm not there all the time. But we have to survive economically somehow.

According to Marku, the only bright light in Doina's reproductive quest has been the Internet. Doina has found considerable solace in a Romanian chat room, where infertile women pose and answer questions for each other and generally give and receive support. Marku expressed pride in Doina's role as a chat room authority figure:

Some of the women, they are doing IVF for the first time, and they are so scared. They are asking, "How do I start this?" My wife is like a veteran of that! She's like a consultant now! She's at home, and she's online all the time, answering these questions for others in the forum. It's good for her, too, to be helping other women. The last time, I was so impressed. We failed our last [IVF] cycle only one month ago. In Romania, they do these IVF cycles in groups, so the women get to know each other. In that group, my wife failed, and one other woman failed, and one other woman *did* get pregnant on her first trial. This woman, the one who got pregnant, was so scared to do IVF. She was trembling; she couldn't manage herself. So my wife, she forgot all of her pain, and went to that woman to comfort her. And afterward, when the woman got pregnant, my wife posted her congratulations. I was so *proud* of my wife. She passed through her pain and just supported that woman. She didn't feel any jealousy or anything. I'm so proud of her.

Marku explained that he would happily adopt a child, as would Doina. They "opened a file" with an adoption agency in Romania. However, changes in the country's once liberal adoption law have made it virtually impossible for foreigners to adopt a Romanian child, and almost as difficult for infertile Romanian couples to do so. Marku explained that poor Romanian mothers are now discouraged from putting their children up for adoption and instead receive child-support benefits from the state. Furthermore, children in foster care can be released for adoption only once all known biological relatives have been contacted and given up their guardianship rights. Marku explained that these new protections are in place to prevent the international trafficking of children and to end Romania's bleak history of "prison-like" orphanages. Yet for pro-adoption infertile couples like Marku and Doina, adoption reform has been a mixed blessing, making this avenue to parenthood much less feasible than before.

The question for Marku, then, is what to do? As a man of "adventure" and action, he could not sit still and let the possibility of parenthood pass them by.

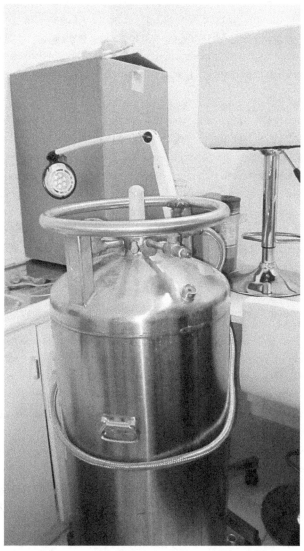

1.17 A liquid nitrogen dewar tank to cryopreserve embryos in the back room of Conceive. PHOTOGRAPH BY JUSTINE HOOKS.

Thus, on a bright winter day in January, Marku "made shore" from the Qatari oil rig, hopped into his car, drove down the Arabian coastal highway from Doha to Dubai, and turned up unannounced at Conceive, where I happened to meet him. His goal, he told me, was to "check up" on his four frozen embryos—which, according to Dr. Pankaj, were still safely stored in a large liquid nitrogen dewar tank in a back room of Conceive (figure 1.17). Knowing that his and Doina's embryos were safe and sound, Marku felt both determined and relieved:

> The next trial, if we do it, it will be here with Dr. Pankaj. Because it's just a small treatment. We already have our embryos, and it was a big struggle to get them! Doina has gotten very concerned that she can't produce any more eggs, that her eggs are "going down." She believes it's because of her age, and she's so stressed. So I came here to find out about our frozen embryos. Three are in good shape—type A.[92] Two out of the three have eight cells, and the third has six cells. The fourth has only four cells. I will explain this to her, and she will decide. Only by herself can she make this decision. We can do it now or later. The embryos can stay in the freezer. They can wait for us. The last solution is here—waiting for us in the freezer.

• **Race against Time**

Doina's stress over her reproductive aging speaks to the race against time that faced many of the older professional women I met at Conceive. Min was one such woman. Hailing from Singapore and married for four years to an Australian architect named Peter, Min looked youthful and radiant. Thus, when she told me that she was already forty, I was quite surprised. Min explained, quietly and matter-of-factly, that "time isn't on my side."

I learned from Min that she had met Peter in Singapore, where he had spent eight years of his professional career before they had married. But Peter had also lived for one year in Dubai, and he was eager to return there to take on an exciting airport architectural project. Min also believed that a change of scenery might be therapeutic. She had been trying to get pregnant since her first day of marriage to Peter, and she secretly believed that the stress of her busy job in corporate communications was affecting her ability to conceive. Although Min had visited a gynecologist in Singapore, he had been nondirective. "I basically had to pester him to hurry it along," Min complained, "and he finally recommended some ovulation tablets."

Moving to Dubai, then, provided a fresh start on Min's path to fertility. No longer working, and taking pleasure in decorating their Dubai apartment, Min felt a "peace of mind" that she had not experienced in years. Furthermore, Min soon discovered that Dubai was home to several major hospital complexes, including Dubai Healthcare City. She soon made an appointment with a female Indian gynecologist, who prescribed a syncretic blend of ovulation induction medication and herbal supplements. Within a month of the doctor's appointment, Min became pregnant. Overjoyed, she planned their Christmas trip home to Singapore and Australia, where she and Peter planned to break the happy news to their families.

All was well until the return flight to Dubai. Stopping in Singapore on their way back from Australia, Min began to feel unwell: "I was fine until I traveled. I was twelve weeks pregnant, and I had some sort of infection, bacterial vaginosis, a swelling of sorts. So I saw a gynecologist in Singapore. She took care of me before I left, and she cleared me for travel. But two to three weeks later, when I was back in Dubai, I went to the hospital with PROM—premature rupture of the membranes—and I miscarried at fourteen weeks."[93]

Min went onto describe how the miscarriage was significantly affected by Dubai's restrictive abortion law:[94] "Under Dubai law, we couldn't do anything. We came up against the anti-abortion law. We both knew the case was hopeless, and we would have opted for an abortion. But we were forced to wait for the fetal heartbeat to stop—seven days of waiting in the hospital until it happened."

After this unfortunate event, Min did not become pregnant again. Reluctant to view herself as infertile, Min nonetheless decided to visit a fertility specialist. "I guess I was at the point to move on with it," she explained. "I'm forty, and I feel pressure to move forward with this." In what she called her "race against time," Min's first meeting with Dr. Pankaj proved fortuitous. Following a thorough medical history of both partners, an analysis of Peter's semen, blood tests, a physical examination, and an ultrasound scan of Min's ovaries, Dr. Pankaj delivered some surprising news:

Min: One of the first things [Dr. Pankaj] said, just by looking at me and my oily skin and acne, is that I probably have PCOS.
Peter: It's quite frustrating, really . . . he scanned her ovaries to confirm what he saw ten minutes earlier. The relative obviousness of the whole thing is a bit frustrating.
Min: My gynecologist in [the Dubai hospital], she *did* scan me and did some tests, but she couldn't detect anything.
Peter: That's why you need a fertility specialist! That is the way to reconcile it. PCOS doesn't flash up in lights. You need a specialist to detect it.

Min: My gynecologist, she *was* telling me that I was not ovulating every month. And I did go for blood tests. I was worried at the time that I was having pre-menopausal kinds of symptoms! I always had oily skin and a little bit of acne.

Peter: It got better in the last year or so. But now we know that this was all obviously PCOS-related.

With Dr. Pankaj attempting to mitigate the ovulatory problems associated with Min's PCOS, Min and Peter were weighing the pros and cons of undertaking IVF. In their view, they had three countries to consider—the UAE, Australia, and Singapore. They discussed the advantages and disadvantages of each:

Peter: Obviously, staying at Conceive is the more practical option, because there's the element of support from me. Min's family is in Singapore, so there is support there, too.

Min: [Dr. Pankaj] said that here [at Conceive], there is a 40 percent success rate. That's pretty high. In Singapore, it's 26 percent—in the twenties . . . but in Singapore, one of my colleagues was in her early thirties, and she did IVF and it was successful.

Peter: Because Singapore, in that part of the world, is relatively developed. It's very much like Dubai is to the Middle East.

Min: Plus, the government is putting in lots of funding for health care research. Lately, the news from Singapore shows a lot of high-profile cases. For example, they worked on separating conjoined twins a couple of years ago. They successfully split them. Before that, a few years back, they did successful research on the same thing I had—ruptured membranes. They were trying to develop an artificial membrane for such cases.

There's a lot of attention to these cases. So the facilities in Singapore have been attracting people from the surrounding countries—from Indonesia, Malaysia, Philippines, Thailand, and also Brunei, which is very rich.

Marcia: What about Australia?

Peter: In Australia—any time I've been in the hospital or worried about my health—they have a pretty good standard. But they have waiting lists. For IVF proper, I really have no idea, to be honest. But I suspect they have a waiting list for IVF as well.

Min: But there is also private medicine in Australia. The extra benefit is shorter wait times, but you pay more for that.

Min and Peter were unclear whether they qualified for state-sponsored IVF in either Singapore or Australia because they were no longer living there as residents and taxpayers. The logistics of return reprotravel to their home countries also seemed daunting. Peter considered this to be the main reason for trying IVF in the Emirates. As he explained:

> **Peter:** My primary concern, obviously, you know, if we were to do IVF back in Singapore, my primary concern is that I wouldn't be there all the time. I wouldn't be able to support her, unless I quit my job. The sort of work I do, construction, you have to be reasonably quick around here! And, typically, the only vacation breaks we get are two trips of two to two-and-a-half weeks each year.
>
> **Min:** Just being separated during IVF would be hard. I know I will be more comfortable with him around if there are decisions to be made.
>
> **Peter:** Having to make a *family* decision, so to speak, is obviously important. Although it would be great to have, in Min's case, the rest of her family around, these aren't the kinds of issues you can sort out with them. There's another element, too. IVF hasn't been the focus of our vacations back home. I'm not certain how compressible the whole process is. And if you have to do IVF the whole time you're there, from a stability point of view, this could be very stressful. It seems better if you can do IVF where you live, versus doing it on a vacation.

At this point in the conversation, it seemed appropriate for me to ask Min and Peter if they would consider IVF-related travel to be "reproductive tourism":

> **Peter:** I just find the term "reproductive tourism" to be encapsulating Dubai or the UAE in many ways. Although maybe it's been helpful in putting it up as a headline, so to speak, with a degree of sensitivity, it is all quite sort of gimmicky. A new gimmick, the same way you hear of every new development in Dubai. I just saw the leaflet on the table [my study ad]. I'm happy to go get it, because it gave me a little bit of a laugh. The heading said, "Reproductive Tourism." [He left to get the ad from the waiting room.]
>
> **Min:** It's just that, when you hear the subject "tourism," it is transient and a term having something to do more for leisure. I think for women who do travel to go for IVF, or reproductive assistance, it's something personal, a personal decision, a personal problem. Tourism just doesn't come into it.
>
> **Peter [having returned]:** A lot of this is happening by default, people choosing to go to the UAE for treatment. Of course, reproductive tourism may be accurate and everything, but I don't quite see putting it up as a headline for the UAE.
>
> **Min:** Having a child is so important to families here. Look at the cultures of the Middle East. I'm not sure that traveling far and wide to have a child

is "tourism." . . . Reproductive tourism sounds like something selfish. But people are coming to places like this because they have no choice.

• Inter-Asian ICSI

Min and Peter were among the many older professional couples I encountered at Conceive. But younger couples—some of them facing serious infertility problems—were traveling to the clinic as well. Gandhali and Paavan were one such couple. I met them in the clinic's ultrasound scanning area, where they volunteered for my study, explaining that they had traveled from China to overcome their infertility problem. Both twenty-eight years old and married for seven years, Gandhali and Paavan were a young, college-educated, highly successful Indian couple, who had married for love—Gandhali moving from Mumbai after marriage to join Paavan and his family in Dubai's affluent Sindhi merchant community. After marriage, Gandhali, who had a bachelor's degree in communication studies, opened a Dubai-based advertising agency. Paavan, meanwhile, had started a successful import-export business with China, and, four years after marriage, the couple decided to relocate to Guangzhou, the capital of Guangdong Province, to expand the business. In this respect, Gandhali and Paavan were representative of many of the young, dual-career Indian couples in my study. Highly educated, professionally ambitious, with entrepreneurial aspirations, these middle- to upper-middle-class Indian couples were global mobiles, traveling frequently to take advantage of family ties, business connections, and entrepreneurial opportunities in the growing global hub cities across South, East, and Southeast Asia.

Gandhali and Paavan had homes in three Asian cities: their main residence in a foreigners' high-rise apartment complex in Guangzhou, an unoccupied house that they owned in Mumbai, and their apartment in Dubai, where they had lived at the beginning of their marriage and where they stayed when returning to Dubai for business, family visits, and now infertility treatments. Their infertility had come as a great surprise. Assuming that they were young and fertile, and more interested in building businesses than a family, Gandhali and Paavan had used condoms for the first four years of marriage. But when they stopped using contraception, Gandhali did not become pregnant. Puzzled, the couple considered seeking a diagnosis at the American hospital in Guangzhou, a city of eleven million people. Although Gandhali believed that she might find a fertility specialist in that hospital, Paavan was highly skeptical about the general quality of medicine in China. In a vibrant couple's interview—filled with animated dialogue—they explained their treatment decision making in this way:

Gandhali: We don't trust medicine there [in China].

Paavan: We've never heard bad things about it, but there is the language barrier.

Gandhali: I got a cold, and my maid got a syringe! I don't want to take any medicine for a cold!

Paavan: And a lot of Chinese still rely on herbal medicines. Even urban, educated people still prefer traditional to Western medicine. Their mentality is completely different.

Gandhali: So we decided that we needed to come here or go to India.

Paavan: The thing with India is, we've never lived in India, or rather I've never lived there, and I'm not very comfortable there. We have a house in Bombay, but we would have to get it cleaned and settled in before we could use it. I can't take fifteen to twenty days out in India. There's not good access to the Internet as frequently, and I haven't really lived there.

Gandhali: Just as important, here we have family. The clinic here does the same thing as in India, but there is much cheaper! It's 10 percent of the cost.

Paavan: The quality of Indian clinics is very good, but it's not 10 percent.

Gandhali: Here, it's 25,000 dirhams [$6,807] to do IVF. Over there, it's maximum 100,000 rupees [$2,275].

Paavan: So that's maybe 8,000 dirhams [$2,178], one-third of the cost.

Gandhali: Plus, a few people we know got some treatment from Dr. Pankaj. One couple in our building here has twins from Dr. Pankaj. So that kind of motivated us to have trust.

Marcia: They told you that their twins were from IVF?

Paavan: We don't know the full story. Indian couples with fertility problems don't really discuss much. It's more like, "My mother found out from someone." It's through the grapevine.

Based on these perceptions of IVF in the three countries, Gandhali and Paavan decided to travel from China to Conceive in May 2005. At Conceive, Paavan undertook his first semen analysis, and learned that his sperm count was less than one million, when a count of fifteen million is diagnostic of male infertility. Only twenty-six at the time, Paavan was devastated:

Paavan: They said our only option is ICSI. I was affected pretty badly by the news. . . . Really, it just hits you. Your confidence level goes down. I was very bad for maybe four to five months after that, feeling depressed. And in India, there's lots of alternative medicine there. My parents are kind of into that. So for maybe six to seven months, I was doing, I don't know exactly what I was taking, some tablets, some weird concoctions that came from India! But I went for a semen test again, and it was the same thing. My first test was in 2005, and ever since, it's been the same. I've got sperm, but the numbers are really low, the motility is pretty low, and the sperm quality overall is D+.

Marcia: But you know that ICSI was designed for these kinds of problems?

Paavan: Yes, ICSI, we've read a lot about it as well on the Internet, and the doctors explained what happens with ICSI. But what really affected me is that if I was ten years older—ten years ago ICSI wasn't there. So there would have been no option for me. But then again, I've been thinking a lot recently. I'm not really a believer in God per se. But nature doesn't intend for me to be a father. So I don't know how right this is, morally speaking, to do ICSI. I feel like I'm doing this because of a lot of pressure from my family, my friends, and my wife. I would have preferred, left to my own decision, to adopt or maybe use a sperm donor. I've been told the possibility that if we have a boy with ICSI, the same problem will be carried into him as well. Actually, my right testicle is 50 percent of the normal size, and the doctor told me that this could happen to my son. And since ICSI is fairly new, I heard that there could be abnormalities in the child. ICSI is relatively new, so very little is known about that. So you know what concerns me is the whole question, philosophically, it's bothering me a little bit, that "nature doesn't want me to have" [a child].

Paavan was not the only man in my study who was worried about siring an "abnormal child" through ICSI. As Dr. Pankaj often warned patients with severe male-factor infertility problems, ICSI could, in fact, perpetuate genetically based male infertility problems into the next generation of male offspring. In some cases, Dr. Pankaj recommended to couples that they transfer only female embryos if they wanted to avoid such outcomes.[95] Paavan found the ethical implications of passing on male infertility to any future son deeply troubling. Yet Gandhali's desire to become a mother outweighed her concerns:

Gandhali: I don't actually believe this. I've heard nothing really about the health of children from ICSI. Frankly, all my friends are getting pregnant, one by one, except me. I just want to get pregnant! I want *his* child, so I don't want to use a sperm donor, even if it's available over here.

Paavan: I don't think it is, although we've never looked into it seriously.

Gandhali: We'll do the ICSI, no matter what! Believe me, as soon as you get married, the pressure is on—immediately! My mom . . .

Paavan: Her parents, my parents.

Gandhali: The uncles, the aunts.

Paavan: And nowadays, any relative we meet, any relative we meet after a long time, the first question is: "When are you going to get good news?"

Anywhere we go, in China, in Dubai, in India. My friends who married in the last three to four years are very much after me, too. They're starting to get pregnant.

Gandhali: Now I wish I would have done ICSI several years ago. We would have had a baby by now! The thing is, my friends are having kids before me, even if they got married after me. It's the "social eye" that looks at you!

Paavan: Every couple that becomes pregnant, there's that much more pressure on us. What especially bothered me is that my grandfather had never said anything. But in the last five to six months, even he's asked!

Gandhali: In India where he lives, women are completely pressured.

Paavan: But even more so in the UAE, I think. It's worse here among our local friends [Emiratis]. It's the first question they've asked us from the time of our marriage. This is how it starts: "Are you married?" "Do you have kids?" "No! Why?" That's the way it is with locals, or any Arab for that matter. There is *so much stigma* attached to this. Even with my best friends, I *never* talk to them about this.

Gandhali: You can't talk to anyone.

Paavan: I'm *very* close to my sister, and I never told her, and she just found out.

Marcia: How?

Paavan: Through my mother.

Gandhali [turning to Marcia]: No, *I* told his sister that. *I* told her.

Paavan [surprised]: You did? Why?

Gandhali: Maybe I was depressed. I just told her. I don't know.

Marcia: How did she respond?

Paavan: Actually, she was very pissed at me. She lives in the US, and she was feeling cut off from the family. She wanted me to tell her this directly.

Gandhali: But he didn't want me to tell anybody except "the moms."

Marcia: Why just the moms?

Gandhali: We are attached to our moms more than our fathers.

Paavan: I *should* tell my mother. She will want to know what's wrong. And she suggested coming here. It's the same with your mother.

Gandhali: Since the first year, it's been, "Why haven't you had babies? Tests should be done!" Every day, the whole year. When we found out, I told her, and she was upset for a day or two. But then she began pushing us to start treatment, and we kept delaying it.

Paavan: Initially, it was alternative medicines we tried. That was the initial thing. But afterwards, we decided to give it a break. We took a vacation.

Gandhali: And we settled in China.

Although relocating to China was like taking the lid off an infertility pressure cooker for Gandhali and Paavan, the move was also culturally jarring. The young couple felt "cut off from the cultural mainstream" in a country where *Newsweek*, *Time*, CNN, BBC, and Wikipedia were still blocked by the government. Unable to speak fluent Chinese, Gandhali and Paavan also found their ability to enjoy life in China quite limited. Gandhali admitted that she spent most of her time at Starbucks, which was conveniently located next to their apartment complex. "It's just coffee, massages, and eating," Gandhali complained. Most important from a fertility perspective, "overindulging" in various "vices" in China had caused her to gain weight—five to six kilograms—which had triggered a new diagnosis of PCOS:

Gandhali: Dr. Pankaj told me to reduce my weight the first time I came for treatment. . . . In China, I used to drink a lot. We all used to drink. And after that, my insulin was up pretty high. When I came back to start treatment, he put me on Metformin and told me to come back after I lost five to six kilograms.[96] There's a lot of eating and drinking there. I've stopped drinking completely, because it's not okay at all. Sindhis aren't supposed to drink. Our parents didn't know that I drink. And just the week before, I told his mother, when she asked me where we went, I told her, "We went out to a pub." "A pub! So what? You all drink alcohol? You drink whiskey or what?" You see, you can't drink or smoke in front of Sindhi parents. There are very few who are open-minded about that.

Paavan: And they're vegetarians, our families. Even though Sindhis are not strict vegetarians, they hardly ever eat meat. But you *can't* be a vegetarian in China! To be a vegetarian, I couldn't eat! They say in Cantonese: "Anything with a back facing the sun can be eaten."

Gandhali: And he started smoking, because of depression.

Paavan: That has to do with China.

Gandhali: After every little bit, he runs out to smoke.

Paavan: That started with China, really. *A lot* of men smoke there. A lot! When you're conducting business, you almost feel to get closer and to make a deal you *must* smoke and drink. In the office, it's mostly smoking. But in lots of cases, you go to a function and the boss comes with cigarettes packaged as a gift and it's rude to say no. I used to smoke in college, but I was able to stop pretty quickly. So I can cut down any time.

Gandhali: Knowing the treatment, you shouldn't be smoking! I can't take smoking. I hate the smell.

Given that smoking can negatively affect ICSI outcomes, Gandhali was probably right to admonish Paavan about his smoking. I, too, told the couple that smoking is generally bad for male reproductive health. I asked Gandhali and Paavan if they planned to return to "smoky China" at the completion of their ICSI cycle:

Gandhali: As soon as I get pregnant.
Paavan: I'm going back next week.
Gandhali: Thanks for telling me! I didn't know that.
Paavan: I have to go back. I have work waiting for me there.

Despite the couple's bickering, it was clear that Gandhali and Paavan loved each other very much, and viewed their childlessness as a shared struggle. Because they were such a loquacious and forthcoming young couple, I decided to ask them at the end of the interview: "How's your marriage holding up?" Gandhali answered for both of them: "Now, since the treatment started, he's been more depressed. He's been a little aloof because of the treatment. And because of the [hormonal] medicine, I'm getting a little finicky, picking some fights without reason. In the first few days, I was crying all day. But every time we travel for treatment, we're getting closer. We're young, and it's like we're growing up together."

• Cosmopolitan Activism

In my many years of interviewing infertile couples across the Middle East, anonymity and confidentiality have generally been key concerns. Most of my infertile interlocutors have wanted reassurances that I am not a journalist and that their real names will never be used in any future publication. Thus, it seems exceptional to end this chapter "on the record" with Nathalie Brousseau and Amer Attar—a quintessentially cosmopolitan, Dubai-based couple, who allowed their names, story, and photos to be published.

Nathalie can only be described as the Emirates' most influential IVF twin activist. Over the years, she has used her own difficult experiences—including infertility, multiple ICSI cycles, the premature births of three children (including a set of twins), long stays in neonatal intensive care units (NICUS), and all of the decision making surrounding which country, IVF clinic, doctor, treatment, birth strategy, and care for preemies to trust—to help other couples facing these problems in the Emirates. With Amer's blessing and support, Nathalie first launched a website to provide a full range of informational services for both infertile couples and new parents in the UAE. In 2012, she also organized Dubai's first annual Twins Plus Festival, bringing together the country twins and triplets of many different nationalities (figure 1.18). Many of the children's parents are former patients of Dr. Pankaj, who is treated as an honored guest at the festival.

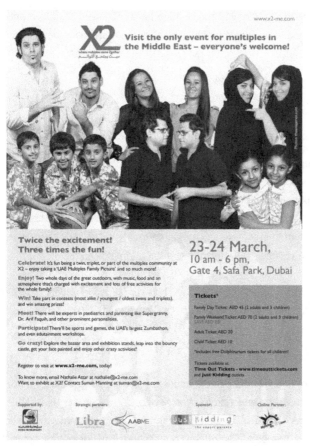

1.18 A flyer announcing Dubai's second annual IVF twin festival. COURTESY OF NATHALIE BROUSSEAU.

When I met Nathalie and Amer in 2007, they had been married for seven years, but their infertility journey was just beginning. They told me the story of their unlikely meeting and how becoming pregnant was not their first priority, as they attempted to forge a multinational, multicultural life for themselves. Amer hailed from Syria, but had left the country at age eighteen with the help of his uncles living in the United States. Working his way through college, Amer eventually landed a position in Silicon Valley, where he worked for sixteen years on the business side of the IT industry. On a trip to Germany, Amer met Nathalie, who was working there even though she was a French citizen. After carrying on a long-distance relationship for one-and-a-half years, Amer and Nathalie decided to marry—first in a civil ceremony in California for visa purposes, then in religious weddings with their families in a church in France and a mosque in Syria. Nathalie joked with me that she had had "many marriages to the same man!"

Hoping to fit into her wedding dress with each celebration, Nathalie did not want to get pregnant right away. Furthermore, their future in the United States was uncertain. Although Amer had gained citizenship there, he had heard glowing reports from many of his Syrian friends about the excellent IT opportunities to be found in Dubai. Nathalie had never traveled to the Middle East but was willing to move, and she secured an excellent position in Dubai with an international moving and storage company. As young, educated professionals living in a growing global hub, Nathalie and Amer worked long hours, but they also loved the multicultural atmosphere and nightlife of Dubai:

> **Amer:** It's the most modern Arab country. I have personally traveled all over the Middle East, and I will never be able to live anywhere else other than here. It's a boomtown, which means that living here is a mighty traffic mess, and the cost of living has increased dramatically over the past four years.
> **Nathalie:** But, personally, I still love it. The life is still easy.
> **Amer:** The social life here is very, very different from the US or even Europe. It's much better, actually. Different means better. We have friends from a lot of different countries
> **Nathalie:** You do have the chance to make friends here. I think people are more open to friendships, because all the people are in the same boat. So we've had good luck meeting nice people.

At the time of their move to Dubai, Nathalie and Amer had been married for three years, so they decided to start "trying for a baby" almost as soon as they reached the Emirates. During this early phase, Nathalie missed her period for twenty-five days and was quite hopeful that she might be pregnant. Because several home pregnancy tests had come back negative, she went to a female gynecologist's office for a more sensitive pregnancy blood test. Nathalie described the physician's interpersonal skills as horrendous: "She didn't call, and she didn't call. So I was a little forceful over the phone. So then she sent me a message—an SOS in big boldface letters: 'YOU ARE NOT PREGNANT!' If I had not known this from the home pregnancy tests, it would have been very demoralizing. It was very tactless."

Amer, meanwhile, underwent his first semen analysis. The test clearly indicated a low sperm count, but the doctor was nonchalant, chalking it up to "stress." Not knowing what to do, the couple decided to seek second opinions. Nathalie was advised to visit the female gynecologist serving the French expatriate community in Dubai. Amer found a urologist in a major Dubai hospital. Amer's sperm count was even lower on the second semen analysis—having dropped from fourteen million to five million. This time, the urologist was directive, telling Amer that he needed to "look at other options," including ICSI.

With their very mixed experiences in the Dubai health care system, Nathalie and Amer's first reaction was to travel outside the country for ICSI—ideally to France, where Nathalie could be close to her parents. However, they soon discovered that trying to coordinate an ICSI cycle in France was not at all straightforward. They described it to me in this way:

> **Nathalie:** Obviously, you need to have a place to stay. So I looked at the two cities closest to my parents, and found four clinics there. I started communicating with them by e-mails, but the response was not great, because French people don't go by e-mail. They prefer to have phone calls, or people just walk in. If I have to have my parents go there for me, it's okay.
>
> **Amer:** But what made me worry a little bit was the stress—you know the stress that Nathalie is going through is not an easy stress. Financially, also, is another aspect, because this is not a cheap process. What we're looking at, with the travel, also the time off from her work and my work.
>
> **Marcia:** Isn't IVF free in France?
>
> **Nathalie:** In France, it is covered by the government—four to seven times, do you believe that!? But I don't live there. I'm not part of the social security system, because I'm not a resident. Unless I want to move back to France, I would have to pay for it on my own.
>
> **Amer [joking]:** Maybe that would be the next option. You go over there, I stay here. And then I suppose I can send you my sperm by FedEx! E-mail them to you!
>
> **Nathalie [smiling]:** Actually, for me to be away for two to three months didn't make a whole lot of sense. We were thinking of doing the scans and tests and injections here, and just flying to France for the procedure. But after a series of scans, I knew this was ridiculous.
>
> **Amer:** It wouldn't work, in all likelihood.
>
> **Nathalie:** And you have to build a relationship with your doctor—not just on the day of the procedure.
>
> **Amer:** This doctor [Dr. Pankaj], on the first day we met him, we felt comfortable with him, and so we scrapped going to Europe.
>
> **Nathalie:** It's probably *not* good to fly the first three months if you're just pregnant. And I cannot stay at my parents' home for three months and stay sane! I love them, but I need my space.

Amer: I love it there!

Nathalie: Because you love their food, and they're not your parents!

Amer: The food, the wine, the cheese!

Nathalie: Honestly, it would be really hard to travel, although we seriously contemplated it. Between the traveling, the time off, staying out there for a long time, and the coordination of it all, it just seemed too difficult.

Although Nathalie and Amer quickly ruled out reprotravel to France, they were fortunate to discover a "fantastic French website" for people seeking IVF services in that country. The website contained a complete registry of IVF clinics, a discussion of IVF and ICSI success rates, and a great deal of information about the basic processes underlying these procedures. As tech-savvy professionals, Nathalie and Amer were attracted to the Internet as the best place to learn about ICSI. Thus, the dearth of information on ICSI in the Emirates was quite frustrating. Even Conceive's website was "under construction," which surprised Nathalie:

It's too bad they don't have a good website. They have so many success stories! They should share the stories about why people are coming here. They need basic information, some simple information, such as, "If you're bleeding, this is what you should do. If you're going through this or that should happen, you should contact us." Right now, to even get the doctor on the phone is not easy! Every time you call, it's busy or the message says to call back. So they need a good website. To have such a professional place like this, it's a shame people don't know about it. Definitely, it would look more professional to have a website.

Despite these complaints, Nathalie and Amer felt relieved to be starting ICSI at Conceive. They felt especially comfortable with the clinical staff, who delivered sensitive, multicultural care. Nathalie described the Conceive staff in effusive terms. "They are so nice, so personable, absolutely adorable, each one of them, completely amazing, so human, which makes a huge difference when you're going through it."

Although Nathalie often found Dr. Pankaj to be brutally honest to the point of brusqueness, she and Amer had the utmost confidence in his clinical acumen. In their case, he had performed multiple semen and hormonal analysis tests on Amer, which consistently showed a low sperm count, poor sperm motility, and a high percentage of abnormally shaped spermatozoa. Although these kinds of severe male infertility problems are common across the Arab world, Amer seemed to blame himself for his sperm defects, telling me apologetically that "I don't have the healthiest life." Nathalie immediately interjected, attempting to diffuse the blame and to take some of the responsibility off Amer's shoulders. I, too, intervened.

> **Nathalie:** But you have pretty much stopped smoking. I did, too. You smoke five to six cigarettes a day, never heavy.
> **Amer:** Well, some nights I go over ten to fifteen. I *do* smoke on the weekends. I'm a "social smoker," but now only small cigars.
> **Nathalie:** He didn't use to do sports, but he started two months ago, heavily, with a personal trainer, two to three times a week.
> **Amer:** But, still, we know that the sperm count is low, the movement, the mobility, is also very low, and the sperm shape is not good. It's abnormal. But last time, they still found quite a lot of good ones, even though a lot were abnormal. And only 20 percent of my sperm have mobility.
> **Nathalie:** This could be stress. You *are* a stressed person. You stress easily, and it goes into your body. You live with your stress!
> **Amer:** Is that true?
> **Nathalie:** Absolutely!
> **Amer [joking]:** If my wife said it, it must be true! I *do* have my days.
> **Nathalie:** You're the worrier. You sleep very lightly, because you think about things a lot.
> **Marcia:** Actually, there's a lot of male infertility in the Middle East, so you're definitely not alone.
> **Nathalie:** It's because of the weather!
> **Amer:** And the male domination. I think that most Arab men can't actually handle this. The perception is "He's not a man!" It has to do with a lot with his honor.
> **Nathalie:** I think it's everywhere. If you want a child, you just have to put your ego on the side and start looking at options.

Accepting the fact that they were facing a serious male infertility problem, Amer and Nathalie decided to undergo ICSI at Conceive. On their first attempt, Nathalie produced thirteen healthy eggs, with Amer joking that she was "going for some kind of record"! Ten eggs were fertilized, but only three embryos were of high enough quality to put back in Nathalie's uterus. Sadly, Nathalie did not become pregnant.

Demoralized but not completely daunted, Nathalie and Amer rebounded quickly, asking both of their families and all of their friends to "pray for us." Nathalie's Catholic priest and her "extremely religious" parents were supportive, even though they all realized that the Vatican opposed the practice of IVF (and hence ICSI) as "unnatural." However, Nathalie said that she disagreed with this position and wished that she could tell the Pope. "Personally, I believe I'm not playing God," she stated. "It's not like I'm doing an offense. It's not easy for two people trying to have children. There is just a health problem that we're trying to fix." Amer described himself as a Sunni Muslim "in spirit," although he rarely prayed or went to the mosque. As a result, he had never looked into any Islamic fatwas on assisted reproduction. However, he assumed that IVF and ICSI must be condoned by Islam, since they are practiced in the Emirates. Although the nation-state as a whole was officially Muslim, Nathalie and Amer appreciated the fact that people like them—from different faith traditions—could live and worship freely in Dubai:

> **Amer:** I mean, how many gods and different religions must be present here? There are Druze, Shia Muslims, Catholics, even Mormons, all here in Dubai.
>
> **Nathalie:** Different religions, different skin colors, different ways of living, different cultures. Just the names: Paul, John, Kate, Rohan, Pankaj. They can be together, and it's lovely!
>
> **Amer [joking]:** Thank God that Muslim people go to the mosque on Friday, and church is on Saturday here. So our kids can go to the mosque on Friday and church on Saturday!
>
> **Nathalie:** I think it's going to be interesting for them to grow up with both religions living together, side by side. They can see that they don't have to fight with each other.
>
> **Amer:** And then they can go and teach that to the rest of the world.
>
> **Nathalie:** I think it's going to be challenging to raise our kids anyway, no matter the religion. Even if the parents are both French, both Catholic, they could still have issues about how strictly to raise the child. In our marriage, we're a little bit more careful, more aware of the chance of misunderstanding. It's probably brought us closer. People from the same culture are able to take it for granted that it's going to be smooth, and it often isn't.
>
> **Amer:** I wouldn't actually say that it's brought us closer. We're just pretty good at living through tough things together—making problems "ours" together. We're probably closer because of that.

This approach to life—the sharing of problems as a committed, multicultural couple—was probably what led Nathalie and Amer to keep on trying ICSI. Within four months of their initial failure, they were back at Conceive, "starting over" again with a second cycle. They hoped for twins—with Amer joking, "Can we do two and get one for free? Do two IVFs, and get one free, like frequent flyers!"

On the day of the egg collection, I sat with Amer at Nathalie's bedside. Dr. Pankaj stopped by to report that eight eggs had been retrieved from Nathalie's

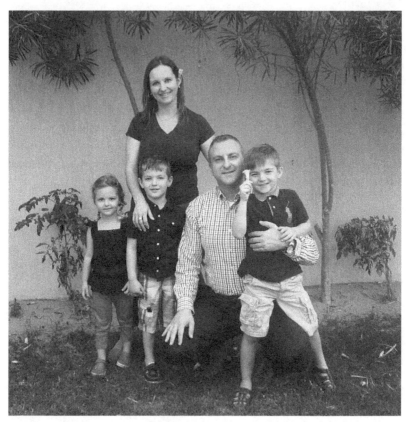

1.19 The Attar family: IVF activist Nathalie Brousseau; her husband, Amer Attar; and their three IVF children, Alexandre and twins Adam and Aliya. PHOTOGRAPH BY JUSTINE HOOKS.

ovaries, and Amer's sperm count was twenty-five million, the highest on record in Amer's file. Dr. Pankaj joked with Nathalie, "I don't know what you fed him!" But then turning more serious, he added, "But there are a high number of abnormal sperm, 95 percent, and only 20 percent are alive. So we'll be doing ICSI anyway." He ended by telling Nathalie, "Today, just stay at home. Stay in bed. But tomorrow you can be completely normal, not resting. Except that you must refrain from intercourse. I'll see you back on Sunday morning for your embryo transfer."

I did not see Nathalie and Amer on the morning of their embryo transfer, but we did exchange e-mail addresses and promised to stay in touch. Exactly two months later, I received an e-mail message from an ecstatic Nathalie, telling me that she was twelve weeks pregnant. Although there had been some initial concerns about the small size of the fetus, her latest ultrasound scan had been very encouraging. Dr. Pankaj had thus referred her to an obstetrician for follow-up prenatal care and eventual delivery.[97] Their baby boy, Alexandre, was born via natural childbirth on October 14, 2007, six weeks premature, with his first days spent in a Dubai hospital NICU.

Three-and-a-half years later, in March 2011, Nathalie e-mailed me again to say that another successful ICSI cycle at Conceive had resulted in the birth of twins, a son, Adam, and a daughter, Aliya, who, after a long stay in the NICU, were now healthy toddlers, having just turned eighteen months old. "Our family is (hopefully) complete and we feel so blessed to have our dream come true," Nathalie wrote. She also described her new website, "entirely dedicated to making parenthood in the UAE a little simpler for people like us."

On a return trip to the Emirates in March 2013, my fourteen-year-old daughter, Justine, and I visited Nathalie, Amer, and their three frolicking ICSI children, as they played in the garden of their Dubai townhome (figure 1.19). Alexandre, the oldest, was in school, and while Nathalie worked on organizing the upcoming Emirati twin festival, her three-year-old twins were being looked after by a French au pair and Amer's mother, who had come from war-torn Syria to live with her son's family. Amer told me that he was also supporting his sister's family in Beirut— including her husband and six teenage children—because they had been forced to flee from Damascus. As the eldest son and the family "worrier," Amer realized how lucky he was to be living in Dubai rather than Syria. Indeed, in Dubai, Amer and Nathalie had been able to forge a wonderful, cosmopolitan life for their three precious, multilingual, multicultural, interfaith ICSI children. Moreover, with Amer's support, Nathalie had become something of a local IVF hero, helping others to achieve their "Dubai dreams" through her informational website and her dissemination of resources for parents of IVF multiples. Such local IVF activism is exemplary of the new twenty-first-century global movement to make IVF more widely known and accessible to non-Western couples. In the next chapter, we will see why such IVF activism truly matters—especially for women and especially for those coming from places of IVF absence.

ABSENCES

Resource Shortages and Waiting Lists

The Announcement

On Sunday, July 7, 2013, Great Britain rejoiced as Andy Murray won the men's tennis championship at Wimbledon, reclaiming the trophy for the United Kingdom after seventy-seven years. But in another part of the country, a different kind of victory was unfolding. On Monday, July 8, the European Society for Human Reproduction and Embryology (ESHRE)— then holding its massive annual meeting in London for thousands of in vitro fertilization (IVF) practitioners from around the globe—issued a press release titled "IVF for 200 Euro per Cycle: First Real-Life Proof of Principle That IVF Is Feasible and Effective for Developing Countries."[1] Very shortly afterward, British news outlets, including the BBC and Radio 4, were using headlines such as "IVF as cheap as LE170, doctors claim."[2] On July 10, Dr. Geeta Nargund, an IVF practitioner at St. George's Hospital in London, explained on BBC television why bringing down the cost of IVF to 200 euros ($253) per cycle was so important: less than 10 percent of the world's infertile population had access to IVF; the cost of an average IVF cycle was $12,000 in the United States, $7,500 in the United Kingdom, and $3,500 in India; the new IVF procedure had a 30 percent success rate, equivalent to conventional IVF; and twelve healthy IVF babies had already been born.[3]

The announcement of low-cost IVF (LCIVF) in London that day attracted far less attention than Murray's victory at Wimbledon. But I would argue that the LCIVF announcement was much more momentous. Throughout its thirty-five-year history, IVF has been far too expensive for most infertile couples in both "developed" and "developing" countries. For example, less than 1 percent of infertile couples are able to use IVF in China, India, Pakistan, Indonesia, and Egypt.[4] Less than 10 percent have access to it in Russia, Argentina, and Italy.[5] Furthermore, because of the high price tag, few governments have been able or willing to subsidize the cost of IVF in their national health insurance schemes, meaning that IVF exists primarily in the private medical sector. Problems of accessibility, cost, and rationing create "an almost insurmountable obstacle to adequate reproductive health care."[6] In short, although about 95 percent of the world's people express the desire to have children at some point in their lives, only half of those who are infertile are able to seek medical care, and less than a quarter actually obtain it.[7]

The move to create LCIVF harkens back to the 1948 United Nations Declaration of Human Rights, which states in Article 16.1: "Men and women of full age, without any limitation due to race, nationality or religion, have the right to marry and found a family."[8] LCIVF thus represents an attempt by activists in the new millennium to bring reproductive justice to the world's infertile, most of whom are located in resource-poor countries where the world's highest rates of infertility cause untold suffering among both men and women.[9] The LCIVF movement has been more than a decade in the making and has involved many prominent IVF practitioners.[10] However, the driving force behind the London announcement was Dr. Willem Ombelet of the Genk Institute for Fertility Technology, in Genk, Belgium. Ombelet has been a tireless advocate for infertile couples around the globe.[11] As the coordinator of ESHRE's Special Task Force on Developing Countries and Infertility, he has been a leader in the recent efforts to prioritize infertility as a global reproductive health problem and to innovate solutions through LCIVF.[12] It was Ombelet's nonprofit organization, The Walking Egg, that invented the LCIVF method first announced in London. Ombelet explained to reporters: "We succeeded with an almost Alka-Selzer like technique. Our first results suggest it is at least as good as normal IVF and now we have 12 healthy babies born."[13]

LCIVF essentially bypasses the need for a costly IVF laboratory by simplifying embryo culture methods and eliminating high-end equipment. The "tWE lab IVF culture system" developed by scientists at The Walking Egg is "designed for simple assembly and to fit within a container for transport."[14] The savings in lab costs are thus passed along to patients.[15] However, LCIVF cannot mitigate the high costs of intracytoplasmic sperm injection (ICSI)—the variant of IVF designed to overcome male infertility. With ICSI, single spermatozoa are injected directly into oocytes through delicate micromanipulation techniques under a high-powered microscope.[16] ICSI requires use of expensive laboratory equipment and trained personnel, as well as physicians who are sometimes required to extract spermatozoa directly from the testicles. Because ICSI may never become "low cost" for the world's infertile men—who contribute to more than half of all cases of childlessness[17]—the announcement of LCIVF must be viewed as a kind of half measure. Furthermore, other IVF scientists have cautioned that the LCIVF method must be "replicated in different laboratories and under field conditions," must be assessed for long-term safety issues and hidden costs, and must involve training of experienced embryologists in low-resource settings, who might otherwise fail to embrace LCIVF for fear "that some of their skills may become largely redundant."[18]

Nonetheless, LCIVF holds out great promise for the world's infertile women, who number in the hundreds of millions, who bear the major social burden of infertility in their societies, and who are the reason why IVF was developed in the first place—namely, to overcome the problem of women's blocked fallopian tubes. Indeed, the global metrics of infertility, which are simply staggering, suggest why infertile women matter, and why LCIVF is a potentially monumental development in overcoming gendered suffering around the globe, especially in Africa.

Global Metrics

The global metrics of infertility shine a glaring light on the nature of the gendered inequalities and reproductive injustices that the LCIVF movement is attempting to overcome. Six demographic realities speak to the need for LCIVF. First, although infertility is rarely acknowledged by global health agencies as an important reproductive health problem, millions of people around the globe suffer from the condition.[19] The total worldwide population of infertile people is very difficult to estimate, but three studies carried out since 2000 put the figures in the many millions, with estimates ranging widely from 48.5 million to 186 million.[20] The most recent global survey, carried out with support of the World Health Organization (WHO), suggests that the absolute number of infertile couples around the world has increased only slightly between 1990 and 2010, probably because global fertility rates have dropped significantly—that is, fewer people are trying to have children, and population growth has slowed as a result.[21] However, unlike fertility rates, infertility rates have not dropped over the past two decades. Infertility affects 8–12 percent of reproductive-age couples in most populations, with 9 percent currently cited as the probable global average.[22] However, in some regions of the world, the percentages may be much higher, reaching nearly 30 percent in some cases.[23] Infertility prevalence rates are especially high in South Asia, sub-Saharan Africa, the Middle East and North Africa, Central and Eastern Europe, and Central Asia, in that order.[24]

Second, women in the global South disproportionately suffer the consequences of both "primary" and "secondary" infertility. Primary infertility is the inability to conceive in the absence of a prior history of pregnancy (the so-called "base form" of infertility). Secondary infertility is the inability to conceive following a pregnancy (whether that pregnancy ended in abortion, miscarriage, stillbirth, or the birth of a child). Secondary infertility is the most common form of female infertility around the globe, and it is usually due to sterilizing reproductive tract infections, which damage or destroy a woman's fallopian tubes. Secondary infertility is most common in regions of the world with high rates of unsafe abortion and poor maternity care, which lead to post-abortive and postpartum infections. The good news is that the problem of secondary infertility seems to have diminished substantially over the past two decades.[25] However, parts of sub-Saharan Africa, Latin America, South and Central Asia, and Central and Eastern Europe remain global "hot spots" of secondary infertility, with rates exceeding 16 percent, or one in every six women.[26] In fourteen of twenty-three sub-Saharan African countries participating in a regional study, the percentage of women with secondary infertility was greater than 25 percent.[27] In Zimbabwe alone, the percentage of women ages 25–49 with secondary infertility was estimated at 62 percent, or nearly two-thirds of all women.[28]

Third, Africa is the continent that is most afflicted with infertility. Repeated cross-national surveys have demonstrated the existence of very high rates of infertility in parts of West, Central, and Southern Africa, with comparatively lower rates in North and East Africa.[29] Demographers of sub-Saharan African have described what they call an "infertility belt" across central Africa, with very high rates of both primary and secondary infertility in Angola, Cameroon, the Central African Republic, Equatorial

Guinea, Gabon, Liberia, Mozambique, and Sierra Leone.[30] High rates of African infertility are largely due to sterilizing infections; more than 85 percent of infertile women in sub-Saharan Africa have a diagnosis attributable to an infection, compared with 33 percent of women worldwide.[31] It is estimated that approximately 70 percent of sterilizing pelvic infections are due to sexually transmitted infections (STIs), while the rest are due to pregnancy-related sepsis—that is, postpartum, post-abortive, and iatrogenic or medically induced infections.[32] Furthermore, STIs—primarily gonorrhea and chlamydia—can also lead to male infertility, due to resulting obstructions of the seminal vessels needed for sperm transport. Almost half of men in sub-Saharan Africa have a medical history of STIs, a rate that is two to four times higher than in the rest of the world.[33] Although rates of both primary and secondary infertility seem to have diminished in sub-Saharan Africa during the past two decades, the high rates of infertility overall represent a regional tragedy—especially given that most cases are preventable with early detection and antibiotic treatment of the infections that cause them.

Fourth, in Africa, high rates of infertility coexist with high rates of fertility—a demographic paradox known as "barrenness amid plenty."[34] Sub-Saharan Africa has the world's highest total fertility rates, even in the midst of high rates of infertility and life-threatening HIV infection. Because children are greatly desired in high-fertility societies, women and men are less likely to use barrier forms of contraception, thus exposing themselves to the risk of sterilizing infections as well as HIV and AIDS.[35] Sadly, studies have shown that infertile women in sub-Saharan Africa are at significantly increased risk of HIV infection, and women who are already infected by HIV have diminished fertility, for reasons that are not well understood.[36] Furthermore, many anthropological studies have shown the daily suffering of infertile women in African communities where large families are the social norm.[37] One review noted: "Women who are unable to bear children are rejected by their husbands and ostracized by society, often living as outcasts and perceived as inferior and useless."[38] Whereas HIV leads to physical death for many reproductive-age women in Africa, infertility leads to a kind of social death, which is why access to both kinds of ARTs—antiretroviral therapies and assisted reproductive technologies—is so vital.

Fifth, lack of infertility prevention and treatment services in Africa and in other parts of the global South are justified as a form of population control. Infertility is often invoked as the "solution to overpopulation" or, more benevolently, as a "low-priority" issue in the context of scarce health care resources, poor medical infrastructure, and the heavy burden of other life-threatening problems such as HIV and AIDS, malaria, and maternal mortality.[39] Although these concerns raise major questions about prioritizing infertility as a reproductive health issue, they may also reflect a tacit eugenic view that infertile people in developing countries are unworthy of treatment; thus, overcoming infertility problems for most of the global South, including through provision of IVF services, contradicts Western interests in population control.

Finally, those parts of the world with the highest rates of infertility are least likely to offer IVF. A cruel demography is at play here, whereby those with the greatest "unmet need" for IVF (to use the language of public health) are often those with the least access to this technology.[40] To reiterate an important point, IVF was designed to overcome blocked fallopian tubes—the major form of female infertility in many developing countries. Yet these are the very nations that are least likely to be served by IVF clinics. Not surprisingly, this is especially true in sub-Saharan Africa and Central Asia, two vast regions of the world that, as we will see, seem to have been bypassed in the new millennium's race to IVF.

IVF Absences

Little is known about either infertility or IVF in Central Asia, whereas much has been written about sub-Saharan Africa as an infertility-plagued continent devoid of IVF services. Sub-Saharan Africa has a huge unmet need for IVF, yet it represents a veritable IVF lacuna—a mostly blank space in the global topography of rapidly spreading IVF services. This grim reality is why the LCIVF movement has focused almost exclusively on Africa, holding its inaugural meeting in Tanzania and launching its first clinical field trials in countries such as Ghana, South Africa, Uganda, and Zambia.[41] As of this writing, few African nations offer any conventional IVF services, let alone those at low cost. IVF services, when present in urban areas, are neither accessible nor affordable for most infertile African couples. And the region as a whole now lags significantly behind the rest of the world in terms of IVF globalization.

The anthropologist James Ferguson has coined the term "global shadows" to focus attention on the places and spaces where the fruits of globalization are largely absent.[42] With some degree of despair, Ferguson notes that the literature on globalization is "oddly out of place in Africa,"[43] where globalization is highly selective, discontinuous, and characterized by widespread disconnections and exclusions.[44] Ferguson condemns the "relentless negativity" with which Africa continues to be described.[45] Yet he concludes that much evidence supports these kinds of characterizations— namely, the "lacks and absences, failings and problems, plagues and catastrophes."[46] For example, in the realm of health, he notes: "Modern social and medical services, where they exist at all, are more likely to be provided by transnational NGOs than by states—and this at a time that the AIDS epidemic is creating unprecedented need for such services."[47]

In terms of IVF, neither NGOs, African states, nor the private sector have stepped forward to meet the need. Thus, for most infertile African couples, marginal economies, political violence, and the underdevelopment of medical infrastructures render IVF an impossible luxury in their home countries. The notion of "stratified reproduction"—introduced by Shelee Colen,[48] and then endorsed by the medical anthropologists Faye Ginsburg and Rayna Rapp two decades ago[49]—still comes closest to evoking the global inequalities that make it possible for some couples to achieve their reproductive desires, including through IVF, while others may be disadvantaged, devalued, or even harmed, physically or socially, in their attempts to conceive. In other words, recourse to IVF takes place on an uneven playing field, with some individuals, communities, and nations benefitting much more than others from the fruits of technological globalization.[50]

The inherent unevenness of IVF globalization, particularly in Africa, has been carefully documented by a group called the International Federation of Fertility Societies (IFFS). Since 1998 IFFS has undertaken an international surveillance project every three years in an attempt to assess the number of clinics (if any) in each country, the services offered, and the nature of each country's ART legal and regulatory environment.[51] The IFFS surveillance project has provided invaluable information on the inexorable global growth of the IVF sector in some places and not others.

As of 2002, IVF and ICSI services were available in about one-quarter of the world's nations, or 45 of the 191 WHO member states (24 percent). These were mostly the affluent, Western nations that accounted for 91 percent of the world's gross domestic product.[52] By 2007, that number had expanded to nearly one third of the world's nations, or 59 of the 191

WHO member states (31 percent), including several nations in the global South.[53] But by 2010, when the IFFS survey was repeated for a fifth time, the survey team—headed by ninety-nine-year-old Dr. Howard W. Jones Jr., the man responsible for the birth of the first IVF baby in the United States in 1981—had some dramatic news to report: "There has . . . been an explosion in IVF in the developing world, with over 500 clinics in India. This globalisation of IVF has also seen a doubling in the number of countries included in the survey. Many developing world countries have only recently introduced IVF and were keen to be involved."[54] By 2010, more than half of the world's nations—105 of 191 WHO member states (55 percent)—had developed, or were on the cusp of developing, IVF services.[55] In that year, between 4,000 and 4,500 IVF clinics were estimated to exist. More than one-quarter of these clinics were located in just two countries, Japan (606–18 clinics) and India (500 clinics)—even though the population of India (1.28 billion) is one hundred times larger than that of the front-runner, Japan (128 million).[56] Other nations with large numbers of IVF clinics included the United States (450–80), Italy (360), Spain (177–203), Korea (142), Germany (120–21), and China (102–300), the latter offering the least precise estimate, but a burgeoning number of Chinese IVF megaclinics.[57]

Yet, according to the IFFS report, not all of the IVF clinic development between 2007 and 2010 had occurred in the West or in the "Asian tiger" nations.[58] By the mid-2000s, both the Middle East and Latin America had shown remarkable development of their IVF sectors, with widespread regional coverage and the existence of many clinics in some countries (for example, Argentina, Brazil, Egypt, and Turkey). Among the forty-eight countries performing the most ART cycles per million inhabitants, nine were in the Middle East. Israel ranked first in these nine and among all other nations, followed in the Middle East by Lebanon (sixth worldwide), Jordan (eighth), Tunisia (twenty-fifth), Bahrain (twenty-eighth), Saudi Arabia (thirty-first), Egypt (thirty-second), Libya (thirty-fourth), and the UAE (thirty-fifth).[59] Latin American nations were all in the bottom quartile. Nonetheless, as in the Middle East, nine countries—Argentina, Uruguay, Brazil, Chile, Peru, Mexico, Ecuador, Dominican Republic, and Guatemala—made the top-forty-eight list.[60]

The success of these three regions—Asia, the Middle East, and Latin America—stands in stark contrast to the absence of most sub-Saharan African nations in the surveillance report. As shown in table 2.1, as of 2010 only one-quarter of sub-Saharan African nations (fifteen of fifty-five,

Table 2.1. **IVF** A Regional Comparison

Sub-Saharan Africa		Asia		Latin America		Middle East and North Africa	
Country	No. of clinics	Country	No. of clinics	Country	No. of clinics	Country	No. of clinics
Burkina Faso	1	Bangladesh	10	Argentina	22–25	Algeria	7
Cameroon	2	China	102–300	Brazil	150	Egypt	52–55
Congo	0	Hong Kong	7	Chile	8–9	Iran	40
Democratic Republic of Congo	1	India	500	Colombia	19–21	Israel	24–30
Ethiopia	1	Indonesia	12	Cuba	1	Jordan	19
Ghana	7	Japan	606–18	Dominican Republic	4	Kuwait	12
Ivory Coast	3	Malaysia	26	Ecuador	6–8	Lebanon	20
Kenya	4	Nepal	3	El Salvador	1–4	Libya	9–10
Mali	1	Pakistan	10	Mexico	Unknown	Morocco	18
Namibia	0	Philippines	4	Panama	7	Saudi Arabia	24–40
Nigeria	16–20	Singapore	9	Paraguay	1–3	Tunisia	8
Senegal	2	Sri Lanka	5	Peru	5–7	Turkey	112–16
South Africa	12–15	Taiwan	72–78	Trinidad and Tobago	1–2	United Arab Emirates	10
Sudan	4	Thailand	35	Uruguay	4		
Swaziland	0	Vietnam	11–12	Venezuela	17–18		
Togo	1						
Uganda	1						
Zimbabwe	1						

Adapted from Jones et al. 2010.

or 27 percent) hosted an IVF clinic.[61] Of these fifteen nations, seven had just one IVF clinic. Three nations—Ghana (7 clinics), Nigeria (16–20), and South Africa (12–15 clinics)—could be considered comparative regional success stories. Nigeria led the way, opening its first clinic in 1984 and reporting its first IVF birth five years later.[62] But the vast majority of African nations had nothing to report to the IFFS surveillance team. In fact, Congo, Swaziland, and Namibia simply reported "0" on the IFFS survey, as shown in table 2.1. As summed up by the ESHRE task force, sub-Saharan Africa consists of "islands of high-tech infertility treatment in a sea of generalized poverty and medical neglect," a situation the members of the task force deemed "highly inappropriate."[63]

Although this tale of African absences is unacceptable given the high unmet need, Africa is by no means the only "global shadow" space in the uneven global topography of IVF. Several other regions of the world were missing altogether in the 2010 IFFS surveillance report. For example, none of the large Central Asian countries—Afghanistan, Kazakhstan, Kyrgyzstan, Mongolia, Tajikistan, Turkmenistan, and Uzbekistan—were included in the report (although Kazakhstan was said to offer IVF in one clinic in 2002 and in a dozen by 2013).[64] The absence of IVF in most of Central Asia is especially troubling, given that it has the world's highest rates of secondary infertility—probably due to unsafe abortions in this mostly resource-poor post-socialist region.[65]

Even in comparatively successful regions such as the Middle East, marked disparities can be detected as a result of political isolation and violence. To take two salient examples, Iraq and Syria were both in the early stages of IVF development when wars broke out in 2003 and 2011, respectively. Iraqis were said to be heading in large numbers to neighboring Iran, as only one IVF clinic existed in the city of Erbil, located in Iraqi Kurdistan.[66] Similarly, infertile Syrians crossed the borders into neighboring Lebanon or Jordan.[67] In the Arab Gulf, IVF disparities could be detected between more central, resource-rich nations and peripheral, resource-poor ones. For example, Saudi Arabia was one of the first three countries (along with Egypt and Jordan) to open an IVF clinic in 1986.[68] Yet Saudi Arabia's southern neighbors, Oman and Yemen, were more than two decades behind. Although both had opened at least one IVF center by the early 2000s, neither was included on the IFFS list of nations in 2010.[69] Yemen was also the only Gulf State excluded from the Gulf Cooperation Council, perhaps because of its lack of resources, large rural population, political isolation, and increasingly violent instability.

South Asia—the region of the world that now outstrips sub-Saharan Africa in terms of absolute numbers of infertility cases, with 14.4 million versus 10 million, respectively[70]—also showed pronounced regional disparities in IVF clinic development. Although India has become the new millennial "poster child" of IVF globalization—boasting approximately 500 IVF clinics and a growing industry of commercial gestational surrogacy—the neighboring South Asian states of Bangladesh and Pakistan, with populations of 161 million and 179 million, respectively, had opened only ten clinics each by 2010.[71] These two countries, therefore, were meeting less than 1 percent of their citizens' estimated needs for IVF services.[72]

Sadly, both Bangladesh and Pakistan slipped off the list—along with forty-three other nations—in the more recent 2013 IFFS surveillance report.[73] A new team of editors and the transition to a web-based survey meant that many nations—including those with less information technology (IT) infrastructure—were lost to follow-up. For example, only seven of the eighteen sub-Saharan Africa countries that reported in 2010 were included in the 2013 surveillance, and these seven nations (Cameroon, Democratic Republic of Congo, Ivory Coast, Senegal, South Africa, Togo, and Uganda) showed zero growth in their IVF sectors between 2010 and 2013. In fact, Ivory Coast reported the loss of one of its three IVF clinics, while Ghana and Nigeria, both IVF leaders in sub-Saharan Africa, were lost to follow-up in the 2013 survey. Only 60 of the WHO member nations reported in 2013, as opposed to 105 in 2010.[74] Thus, the actual number of IVF clinics around the globe—and the ongoing IVF absences in many resource-poor regions of the world—is even more obscure than before, a lacuna that the LCIVF movement hopes to rectify.

Stratified Reproscapes and Exodus of the Elites

Unmet need for IVF services across Africa, in parts of the Middle East, and in South and Central Asia is a major reason why people from these regions become reprotravelers. In my study at Conceive, I met many patients from these parts of the world with no IVF clinics, or with newly opened clinics that were seen as untrustworthy, unsuccessful, and thus best avoided. As mentioned in the last chapter, Conceive received reproflows from three distinct regions of the Muslim world: East Africa, South Asia, and elsewhere in the Middle East. Most of these reprotravelers viewed Dubai as a proximate regional hub, located in a Muslim-majority country, and thus an appropriate treatment destination. As I came to understand, Conceive was located in the center of a highly stratified regional reproscape, in which elites from resource-poor and IVF-poor nations such as Somalia, Djibouti, Kenya, Tanzania, Pakistan, Uzbekistan, Iraq, and Afghanistan were traveling to the Emirates to overcome their infertility. These reprotravelers were not just ordinary citizens, for most could afford IVF journeys generally costing in excess of $10,000. These elite reprotravelers had been pushed out of their home countries by the lack of IVF services. IVF absences at home had "forced" them to travel—*force* being the term they often used in their discussions. As a group, they were deeply critical of their own nations' failures to deliver appropriate infertility care. Furthermore, as elites, these couples viewed access to IVF as a basic reproductive right, and therefore something to which they should have access. Yet they found themselves in the difficult position of making uncertain and painful decisions about where and when to travel. This exodus of Muslim elites from resource-poor and IVF-poor nations to Dubai was an enduring theme of my study. On any given day, the waiting room at Conceive was filled with African, South Asian, and Middle Eastern couples, often dressed in exquisite fabrics and wearing generous amounts of gold, as they waited to be taken into the inner recesses of the clinic for their IVF and ICSI procedures.

Over the course of my study, I interviewed twenty African reprotravelers, including seven couples from the East African nations of Djibouti, Somalia, Sudan, Tanzania and others from South Africa and Nigeria. I also interviewed three reprotravelers from Afghanistan, Iraq, and Oman, all of which are "empty spaces" on the Middle Eastern IVF map. In addition, I interviewed twelve Pakistanis, including four couples who had left their country because they did not trust the fledgling IVF services there. As a group, they had much to say about Pakistan's relative dearth of IVF clinics, especially compared to the situation in neighboring India. I also met six Indian Muslim couples, who had come to Conceive because of perceived discrimination and the underdevelopment of IVF services in Muslim-majority regions of India.

Most of these Muslim reprotravelers were educated professionals and business elites. I interviewed a plethora of male and female physicians, professors, computer scientists, bankers, designers, urban planners, and construction contractors, as well as several men and women who owned their own businesses. This group contained an ambassador from an African nation and an extremely wealthy Somali businessman who, among other things, had a major supply contract with the United Nations. Interestingly, many of these elite individuals explained that, in the absence of children, they were expected to support other family members, and that these requests for support from family were both relentless and endless. This seemed especially true among the Sudanese professionals in my study, who lamented both the war-related political exile of the native population (including a growing Sudanese enclave in the Emirates) and the concomitant expectation for large-scale remittances from the more successful members of the family. Several infertile Sudanese couples in my study described the huge burden and "unlimited responsibility" they bore for their families back in Sudan, with some members expecting "100 percent support," even though life in Sudan was becoming increasingly expensive as a result of an impending oil boom and currency shortages. For example, Yusra, a Sudanese physician who was traveling to Conceive from Oman where she worked, had this to say about the state of affairs in her country:

Yusra: Sudan has so many problems. The economy is all bad. Still there is war—first the war between south and north, and now Darfur [as of 2007]. The war is affecting the economy. So now we have only two types of people—one group who is *so* rich, and another type who is *so* poor. All of us are working outside to make any money that we can. There is no middle class anymore in Sudan. All families have somebody who is working outside, sending back money to them, so that then they can live normally.

Marcia: Are you supporting your families?

Yusra: Yes, my husband, the reason he is not here with me today is that he has to work. He's a partner in a small factory. He *can't* leave his work, because his family is okay *only* because of his support. You see, his father had two wives. One is his—my husband's—mother, and another wife. And then his father died. So my husband is supporting both families. He's the eldest. And I'm the youngest, and I'm helping my family, too.

Marcia: So this must be difficult in terms of doing IVF. Did you consider doing it in Oman or Sudan?

Yusra: In Oman, I think there is only one clinic. I saw a center in Muscat. In Sudan, there are two IVF centers that I know of. I didn't visit, but I heard they are *very* nice, with a very nice doctor, in Khartoum. Two big centers in Khartoum. But they are *too* expensive. They are for rich people only. One day, I called one of them to see if they could make IVF for me, and I realized then that this is only for people with a lot of money. If you have money, then you can do it.

Even though Yusra did not consider herself rich enough to easily afford IVF, she had little choice: at the age of thirty-seven, she was facing declining fertility. She had waited seven years to marry so that she could finish medical school in the Ukraine and her husband could start his business and save some money. But after their marriage, they discovered that her egg quality was quite poor and that her husband suffered from obstructive azoospermia (no sperm were being released into his ejaculate). The obstruction was probably due to a prior STI and had to be overcome through delicate testicular sperm extraction techniques that were available at Conceive. Thus, Yusra had traveled alone to the clinic, at great expense, in the hope that her husband would soon join her to overcome their respective infertility problems.

Yusra was not alone in this regard. Of the twelve African couples in my study, five of the women, all professionals, suffered from age-related infertility, and six of the men suffered from male infertility. Only two cases involved tubal infertility, one following a miscarriage and the other a C-section. Overall, the African women in my study were highly educated professionals whose careers had pushed them into fertility postponement, age-related infertility, and eventual exodus to the Emirates in search of IVF.

Although Yusra felt excluded from the emerging Sudanese IVF sector, many of the other African women in my study were bitter about the total absence of IVF in their home countries. For example, Asma was a lawyer from Djibouti—a small coastal nation in the Horn of Africa, located in the midst of politically turbulent neighboring countries, including Somalia, Ethiopia, and Eritrea. Asma had been struggling with her infertility for over seven years of marriage. She told me how she finally made her way to Conceive:

> **Asma:** I started to see a doctor in my country, in Djibouti. For maybe two to three years, I went through too many exams, okay? The medicine, the injecting, was not working. Djibouti is not very developing. So, I went to Jeddah [in Saudi Arabia] first, because my aunt lived there. I saw a famous doctor in Jeddah, a gynecologist, who just did more exams. But he was not a fertility specialist. So I came back to my country, and I found a friend who had come from Djibouti and done IVF here [at Conceive]. And I asked her to refer me.
> **Marcia:** Was it far to come here?
> **Asma:** Farther than Saudi Arabia, which is two hours, but it's three hours to Dubai from my country by plane.

Marcia: Do they do IVF in your country?

Asma: No, no! They *don't* do IVF in Djibouti. They just do [hormonal] stimulations and normal exams, but no IVF. And every person who wants a family, who needs IVF, actually, they are going to France, because of the [postcolonial] connection between our two countries.

Marcia: Did you consider going there?

Asma: Yes, I thought about going to France. If I hadn't been referred here, I would *have* to go to France, because I didn't hear of even one IVF clinic, even in Ethiopia. So I learned about France from the Internet. And two of my best friends, they have the same problem, an infertility problem, and they took their treatment in France. And every day, I am going to the Internet. They have a forum—what do you call it? A chat room. It's a good, a very good French one, for information sharing and sharing personal experiences. I leave a message and people respond. People talk about their inseminations, their treatment, their IVFs. I *need* this for my psychology. It's better than a psychotherapist!

Marcia: Have you been feeling like you need a therapist?

Asma: Do you know how you feel after seven years? Desperate! Frustrated! Every cycle, every step of this process. But now that I've come here, I'm good. Since I'm in treatment, I feel like I'm *doing* something. Finally, I'm doing something that I could never do in Djibouti. Because there we have other problems, more important health problems. And we can't even talk about infertility and IVF.

Asma's and Yusra's belief that the problems of infertility and IVF were literally being overwhelmed in their African countries by war, poverty, poor medical infrastructure, and life-threatening diseases was shared by many other couples coming to Conceive from Africa. For example, Youssef and Khadijah, a couple from Tanzania, said they had "no confidence" in the "50 percent medicine" offered in their country. Khadijah had already suffered through a difficult first birth and C-section, which had resulted in a postpartum infection and blocked fallopian tubes. Khadijah had delivered a healthy daughter, Yasmine, through that C-section. However, she now felt forced to travel in order to build her family. As she explained, in Tanzania, most women in her social circle had four to five children. Thus, having only one daughter was simply not enough. Khadija desperately wanted IVF twins, while Youssef needed a son. Both of them hoped to provide at least one sibling for their lonely only daughter.

In their search for treatment, Khadijah and Youssef had started locally by visiting an Indian gynecologist in Dar as Salaam, Tanzania's capital. After discovering the tubal blockage, the physician they consulted told them matter-of-factly, "Your only solution is IVF. Go to India." As Muslims, Khadijah and Youssef were uncertain about their reception in a "Hindu nation." Accordingly, they considered South Africa, which they had heard was "technologically advanced," but they feared for their safety and security in a country with "a lot of crime." Eventually they settled on the Emirates, where Youssef had traveled many times during a decade for his construction business. He explained: "There is a common connection here. There is a communication between our two countries. We know people here, you know, from Tanzania. There are lots of Tanzanians here. We've seen the environment."

In addition, Youssef pointed to Dubai's favorable visa policies—especially important to sub-Saharan Africans, who are routinely turned down for visas when they apply to travel to the West. But despite their ease of entry into Dubai, Youssef and Khadijah found the cost of reprotravel to the Emirates to be quite burdensome. They had already spent an estimated $12,000–15,000 on three round-trips to Dubai—an amount that was two to three times the annual income of the "average" Tanzanian. IVF, they realized, was not an "average" affair. Although they were among the "lucky ones" who could access IVF through reprotravel, they still had no baby to show for their efforts. When all was said and done, their biggest hope was that their reprotravel to Dubai was not, after all, a costly and fruitless endeavor.

High-End IVF and Catastrophic Expenditure

As suggested in these African stories, IVF is an expensive technology, which is why the LCIVF movement has made the issue of cost its raison d'être, especially for Africa. The high cost of IVF has often been cited as the most fundamental arena of constraint, barring many infertile couples from trying the technology altogether, causing others to quit after a single cycle, and leading others to travel abroad in search of lower-cost IVF services. In the new millennium, cost has been deemed to be one of the most important factors fueling reprotravel, as infertile couples search for more affordable IVF services across regional, national, and international borders. The term "financial access" has been used to describe this problem of IVF affordability.[75] As noted by a prominent group of health economists, "ability to pay for treatment . . . plays a critical role in overall access to fertility treatment," and "choice to pursue expensive treatments, such as ART, [is] highly influenced by income."[76]

Why is IVF such an expensive reproductive technology in the first place? According to John Collins, who has undertaken the most extensive international survey of the health economics of IVF and ICSI, "IVF and ICSI treatments are costly technologies that involve several professions and expensive laboratory facilities. The direct costs of a cycle of IVF treatment arise from the medical consultation and visits, drugs, laboratory charges (general, hormone and embryology), ultrasound procedures, IVF procedures (oocyte retrieval and embryo transfer), hospital charges, nurse coordinator costs, administrative charges and fees for anaesthesia. Indirect costs include lost time from employment and travel costs, which are difficult to estimate."[77] Factoring in just the direct costs, Collins attempted to estimate the average price of an IVF cycle in twenty-six countries. Using data from 2002, he found that the United States was by far the most expensive country in the world in which to undertake IVF—at $9,547 for a single cycle of IVF and $11,818 for ICSI.[78] Outside of the United States, the average cost of a single IVF cycle was much lower—only $3,518, or about one-third of the American cost.[79] However, IVF prices varied quite widely around the globe, from a low of $1,272 in Iran and Pakistan to a non-U.S. high of $6,361 in Hong Kong.

Interestingly, the UAE was not included in this international comparison. However, when I arrived in the Emirates in January 2007, the going rate for a single cycle of IVF or ICSI was 20,000–25,000 dirhams ($5,500–$6,800), with ICSI cycles accounting for the higher figure. When I returned for a fourth time to the Emirates, in 2013, a newly opened private clinic in the exclusive Jumeirah Beach district of Dubai was charging American-level prices for a single IVF cycle at 45,000 dirhams ($12,000). Yet the waiting room was packed with infertile couples from around the globe, who were waiting to see the well-known Lebanese-American IVF physician who directed the clinic.

In short, in terms of global pricing, the Emirates was one of the most expensive countries in the world in which to undertake IVF—outstripping even neighboring Saudi Arabia, where a single IVF cycle cost approximately $5,000. Why was IVF in the Emirates so costly—especially in comparison to most other Middle Eastern countries, where a single cycle of IVF could be obtained for as little as $1,000–$2,000? As I would learn from Dr. Pankaj, the British practitioners who had opened the first IVF clinic in Dubai in 1991 had set their prices to match the rates at British private clinics. Thus, from the very beginning of IVF development in the Emirates, infertile couples were paying prices equivalent to those of the most exclusive IVF clinics on London's Harley Street. The stature of Dubai and Abu Dhabi as growing cosmopolitan hubs, with many British and other expatriate foreign workers, seemed to sustain these high fees. Thus, the Emirates' high-end IVF marketplace was, in some senses, the outgrowth of a British neocolonial pricing structure.

In addition, Dr. Pankaj explained how the high cost of living in the Emirates also played a role in costs in the IVF sector. Salaries for clinic staff exceeded those in any other Middle Eastern country, as did the costs of basic IVF supplies, such as culture media. Rents were also high. For example, the showroom in which Conceive was located had increased its annual rent from 250,000 dirhams in 2004 to 350,000 in 2007. Converted into dollars, the space alone cost $100,000 in 2007. This was inevitably passed onto patients.

Because of the high-end nature of IVF in the Emirates, I asked many couples at Conceive about cost considerations, and whether these had factored into their reprotravel decisions. Not surprisingly, very few couples—seven—had traveled to the Emirates in an attempt to access lower-cost IVF services than those found in private clinics in their European or American home countries (the United States, United Kingdom, Germany, and Sweden). In contrast, about one-fifth of the couples in my study had made the decision to travel to the Emirates, despite knowing that they could access IVF more cheaply back home. Leaving countries such as India, Lebanon, Nigeria, Pakistan, the Philippines, South Africa, and Sudan, they had decided to pursue IVF in the Emirates for reasons that outweighed the significant costs.

I asked couples if they could calculate how much they had spent so far in trying to make a baby. Fifty couples in my study, or nearly one-half, could provide me with fairly detailed financial information. Converting from rupees, dirhams, dinars, kroner, sterling, and other forms of currency into dollars,[80] we often sat together doing a kind of ethnographic arithmetic—recording figures in my notebook and adding them up together. Not surprisingly, cost estimates ranged widely, from a low of $762 for an Indian couple who had yet to try IVF to a high of almost $100,000 for an unfortunate Palestinian couple who had repeated ICSI nine times without success. Factoring in both the direct costs of the procedure (tests, ultrasounds, medications, anesthesia, oocyte retrieval, laboratory fertilization, embryo transfer, and so on) and the indirect costs of travel (airfare, ground transportation, accommodations, meals, and incidentals), the amount spent on IVF, ICSI, and related reprotravel among my group of fifty ethnographically calculating couples averaged $12,897.

This is an interesting figure in a number of ways. It is three times higher than the global average for a single cycle of IVF ($3,518). And it is a figure that nearly approximates the estimated cost for a single cycle of IVF in the United States ($12,513).[81] In other words, reprotravelers to the Emirates appear to spend as much as, if not slightly more than, they would for IVF in America, the costliest country in the world.

Most of the couples in my study could easily manage these out-of-pocket expenses. They often pointed to their good jobs, which sometimes included health insurance benefits to cover the costs of blood work, ultrasounds, and medications, if not the IVF and ICSI procedures themselves (which were rarely covered by health insurance). However, at least one-quarter of the couples in my study admitted that they were struggling to afford the treatment and travel. Some told me that they had saved up enough money for just one cycle, or two at most. Others said that they had already depleted their savings accounts. Some couples had borrowed money from a bank, employers, or family members. Others had charged part or all of their IVF and travel expenses on credit cards and viewed themselves as having accrued significant IVF debt. In one case, an infertile man had sold two trucks and taken out a bank loan in order to undergo two cycles of ICSI. In another case, a couple had sold their home to finance their IVF journey to the Emirates.

These kinds of tremendous financial sacrifices fall into a category that health economists call *catastrophic expenditure*—namely, any out-of-pocket payment that threatens household survival by exceeding 40 percent of annual nonfood expenditures. In general, infertile couples and particularly infertile women from resource-poor countries are at high risk of catastrophic spending.[82] To take but one example, a study in South Africa by the IVF physician-activist Silke Dyer and her colleagues found that 22 percent of infertile couples attending a public-sector IVF clinic had incurred catastrophic expenditures.[83] To cope with their IVF expenses, South African couples had reduced their expenditures on basic items such as food and clothing, depleted their savings, borrowed money, and taken on extra work. The poorest of the poor were the most likely to incur catastrophic expenditure, as were couples who had been infertile for longer periods. Extrapolating from this South African data, Dyer and her colleagues argued that the absence of any form of financial risk protection for IVF was likely to create similar financial burdens for households in other low-resource settings.[84]

This was certainly true for a significant number of the couples in my study. Nearly 20 percent of them had incurred catastrophic expenditures, in that they had depleted all of their cash reserves and gone into debt to have an IVF baby. Some were philosophical, saying that IVF was "very expensive, but worth every penny" if they could just make a child. Others injected sardonic humor into discussions of financial misfortune, saying that they could have "bought ten babies by now!" or "put a down payment on a Maserati!" Others were frankly bitter, describing the excessive costs as "ridiculous," "an extraordinary expenditure," like "shoveling money down a deep hole."

For example, Firas, a Syrian accountant, did not have the money to cover several cycles of ICSI in Dubai: "I've spent maybe 60,000 dirhams [$16,350]. I took out a loan and used credit cards. This is a lot of aggravation, a lot of debt. We tried to save something to do this, but we were forced to borrow. The part we couldn't cover is paid by a loan and credit cards, because we have no savings left." Borrowing money was a common strategy. Munira, a woman from the neighboring country of Bahrain, complained: "We had savings, but we had to take a loan from a bank in Bahrain. We couldn't ask our families, because they don't know that we're coming here. They think we're shopping!" Similarly, Samir, a well-to-do Somali businessman, had been forced to rely on credit cards when all of his savings ran out:

> I am a good businessman. In Somalia, I'm considered wealthy. But 20,000 dirhams [$5,445] is expensive. Last year, we spent here [in the Emirates] $10,000, on the x-rays, the testing, the eating. And now I am spending another $10,000 to stay, to do the IVF. It's totally expensive. Last year, we stayed in a hotel in Dubai for $80 a night. We stayed two months doing the tests, taking taxis to the clinic. It was too expensive. So now we have taken a [rental] house. Even though we're upper middle class in Somalia, we've used our savings and now we're using credit cards.

In short, some of the couples in my study could afford the costs of IVF and reprotravel, while others clearly could not. Those with the financial means often reflected on their good jobs and good fortune, while those who were struggling could only hope that the birth of a treasured child would be worth the significant financial sacrifice.

The Infertile Migrant Poor

Many of the couples I met at Conceive were from Pakistan, which, along with India, sends more migrants to the UAE than any other country. Umar was a Pakistani migrant and clearly a pious Muslim, given his long, untrimmed beard. He loved his infertile wife who still lived in Pakistan, and he had recently moved her to the UAE to undergo treatment. But the costs of IVF had worn him down: "IVF causes financial tension. Our finances are very difficult. I have my own business, a mobile phone and cargo registry business. But this market is very difficult; it's a very tough market. So the cost of IVF is very expensive for us. Local people can't afford the extraordinary expenditure. This IVF is not for all people. For example, back in Pakistan, some village people, mentally, they need a baby so much. But spending 24,000 dirhams [$6,540] for a baby, which is not even guaranteed, it's not a routine expense."

Umar's comment is very incisive. In his view, IVF is an "extraordinary expenditure," one that excludes the poor. Nonetheless, poor infertile people may strive for IVF, even presenting themselves at high-end clinics like Conceive and asking for help. In every IVF clinic at which I have ever worked across the Arab world, I have found poor infertile couples. Indeed, my initial research in Egypt was entirely devoted to poor urban infertile women, who were hoping to undertake IVF at a government maternity hospital in Alexandria.[85] Similarly, in private IVF clinics in both Lebanon and Arab America, I have found impoverished couples—including war refugees, urban slum dwellers, and poor rural farmers and bedouins—who were hoping to make a test-tube baby.[86] Their presence is indicative of a number of oft-ignored realities: that poor people want children just as much as elites do; that poor infertile couples may have enduring, committed relationships in the face of intractable infertility problems; and that poor couples may be willing to go to extraordinary measures to access IVF, even risking destitution in the process.

It was thus not surprising to me that poor infertile couples were coming to Conceive, and that, according to Dr. Pankaj's estimates, they constituted about 5 to 10 percent of the overall patient population. In my study, six couples (5 percent) fell into this category. But unlike in my previous research, these couples were not Arabs. Instead, they were Indians, Pakistanis, and Filipinos, and they were working in the Emirates in factories, construction sites, and other settings of unskilled labor (for example, they were taxi drivers, security guards, port workers, or hospital aides). Most of these couples lived in cramped apartments they rented with other couples from their home countries, and these apartments were generally located in outlying emirates such as Fujairah and Ajman. Thus, getting to work—or Conceive—often involved difficult travel on crowded buses and shared taxis in high heat and dense traffic jams.

When I asked what circumstances had brought these couples to the Emirates, the answer was always straightforward: money. Lacking well-remunerated jobs back home, these South and Southeast Asian couples had migrated to the Emirates in an attempt to make a better life for themselves. Actually, as married migrant couples, they were unusual; the majority of unskilled workers in the Emirates are single men who live together in squalid labor camps or in overcrowded apartment compounds, struggling to send remittances to their families back home. Had the couples in my study had children, such dual migration would have been less likely. But without children to tie them down, wives had migrated with their husbands, and most of the women had also begun to work in the Emirates in the low-wage factory or service sector. "Low wage," however, is a relative term. Combined household incomes in this group of six couples ranged from 3,000 to 5,700 dirhams per month ($817–$1,553), an amount that was two to five times what they could expect to make back in India, Pakistan, or the Philippines. Nonetheless, by UAE living standards, these wages were minimal. Renting a small apartment in Abu Dhabi, Dubai, or Sharjah, for example, cost no less than 4,500 dirhams a month ($1,226) at the time of my study.

During that same year, the UAE Ministry of Labor published its first reliable report on the scope of the country's imported foreign labor force.[87] Although Emiratis themselves numbered only 800,000, the country hosted 4.5 million foreigners—85 percent of the total population of slightly more than 5 million, and 99 percent of the private work force.[88] A full two-thirds of these foreigners were from South Asia, including more than a million Indians and nearly as many Pakistanis. In addition, workers were coming from other South and Southeast Asian countries, including Bangladesh, Indonesia, Malaysia, the Philippines, and Sri Lanka. Before the 2008–9 economic downturn brought the Dubai construction sector to a temporary but screeching halt, nearly one-quarter of the total foreign population was employed as construction workers, the vast majority of them South Asian men.[89] In addition, women constituted a significant part of the low-wage South and Southeast Asian labor force in the Emirates.

Many of these women were uneducated domestics who were employed in Emirati and expatriate homes as maids and nannies.[90]

These South Asian workers—who are referred to in the Emirates as "subcontinentals" or, more specifically, as "nonresident Indians" (NRIs) and "nonresident Pakistanis" (NRPs)—lack Emirati citizenship rights. They are sponsored by their employers on temporary, fixed-term work permits (that is, residence visas). They do not hold Emirati passports and often have their own passports kept by their employers until they complete their contracts. Because they do not have citizenship rights, they can be jailed or deported at will. And in general they are considered to be second-class "noncitizens"—the floating population of the Emirates who do all of the country's most undesirable, dirty jobs.[91]

For these legions of temporary workers, life in the Emirates could be quite difficult. For example, highways were often jammed with buses of exhausted, dust-covered South Asian construction workers, most of them painfully thin, who were being returned to remote desert labor camps after days spent toiling in the blazing sun on high-rise construction projects.[92] And in any mall or playground, Southeast Asian maids from Indonesia, Malaysia, and the Philippines sat watching their little charges or pushing baby strollers for their Emirati or expatriate employers. This massive South and Southeast Asian workforce could be found in almost every sector of Emirati life. For example, Conceive could not have functioned without its many care workers (nurses and aides), all of whom had come to work at the clinic from their home countries of India, Pakistan, and the Philippines.

Several of my South Asian informants at Conceive explained to me how the Emirates' labor force was affected by the country's unofficial but obvious national hierarchy of ethnic privilege. Local Emiratis were clearly on top, followed by other Gulf Arab nationals. Then came Americans and Europeans, most of whom were highly skilled professionals and constituted a privileged tier of expatriate workers. These were followed by other Middle Easterners, who were generally employed in the professional or business sectors. These included Levantine Arabs, Egyptians, and Iranians, in that order. South and Southeast Asians formed the bottom tier, with Indians generally ranking lower than Pakistanis based on religion (Indians are mostly Hindu, while Pakistanis are mostly Muslim).[93] Yet one's social class moderated the effects of one's position in the Emirates' ethnocracy.[94] Accordingly, a well-educated Indian doctor, pilot, or IT engineer or a wealthy Pakistani businessman would experience life quite differently in the Emirates, compared to a low-wage Indian or Pakistani laborer. Nonetheless, even Indian elites in my study sometimes complained to me of being treated like second-class citizens. Being forced to "swallow and suffer" the daily indignities of subtle and not-so-subtle discrimination, some of my Indian interlocutors said that they felt a "lack of ownership" in the country, even though in some cases their families had lived in the Emirates for generations.[95]

Some of the men and women who came to Conceive from other countries had noticed these local ethnic stratifications, and some expressed their concern about labor exploitation, especially of the South and Southeast Asian underclass. For example, Ziad was a Lebanese American man whose wife was Moroccan. They had started infertility treatment in the United States but then decided to travel to the Emirates, where IVF was considerably cheaper. In the UAE, Ziad found himself deeply troubled by his observations of the workforce:

> **Ziad:** It's unbearable to see the exploited labor here. If you're making only 2,000 dirhams a month [$545], that's low pay, and you can't find a place [to live] with this salary. So a lot of Indian employees send their families home and the men are sharing accommodations. All the Southeast Asian and Indian men live here and their families are back home. They see them one time a year, or every two years. They work and send money. Dubai is nice, but some are making so much, and some are like slaves—the maids and the construction workers. It's a rich country built on the back of poor, exploited people. It's modern-day slavery. There are advantages to being here, but at the same time, if you are a person who cares, it affects you knowing what you see around you.
>
> **Marcia:** But can't you find this kind of situation in Lebanon, too?
>
> **Ziad:** Lebanon is *not* as bad as this! There, it's maids only—although they treat them fairly, to a certain extent. But the issue of maids *is* a bad thing. I read that in Italy, maids are being treated like slaves, locked in. These things are happening everywhere, of course. But here in the UAE, it's obvious that the worst thing is the exploitation. These are my exact words: a rich country is being built on the backs of the exploited poor!

On the one hand, I found myself agreeing with Ziad's assessment. On the other hand, my interviews with the six poor, working-class couples in my study did not confirm the notion of exploitation, let alone slavery.

As I heard their stories, I came to think of these poor South and South-east Asian working-class couples as the *infertile migrant poor*. These men and women had been forced to leave their countries by poverty, unemployment, and living conditions that were far from hospitable. But all of them had come to the Emirates voluntarily, and most were satisfied with the idea of working hard there for some portion of their adult lives, simply to make money. Neither true "migrants" nor "economic refugees,"[96] they were not seeking permanent residence or citizenship in a country that rarely granted these statuses to foreigners. Rather, they were escaping to the Emirates for a temporary reprieve—to raise their standard of living from a baseline of poverty in their home countries, and to help their families back home through regular remittances. All of these poor couples could articulate quite clearly why they had come to the Emirates and why it was better than home. For example, as we sat by the bedside of his sleeping wife, a cargo worker from Pakistan named Latif had this to say:

> Right now and in the future, we're not interested in going back to Pakistan, because of the economy and lots of problems there. There are security problems and low job availability. Even the middle class. For Pakistanis, life there is *very* difficult, even for middle-class people. There you find only the very poor and the very rich. So being here is *much better*. The law and order, the regulation is better than in Pakistan. And the economy here is much better. I'm supporting my parents, my family back there. I haven't saved any money [for IVF] because of this. But I love them. They are old people, and I feel good when I am helping them. I'm happy with that.

Latif was very insistent in telling me that, despite all of the country's problems, Pakistanis were a "very loving" people, and that all Pakistanis loved children, including Pakistani men—who, like him, wanted to become fathers. However, he explained that infertile Pakistanis had little hope of receiving treatment in their home country, which had only four or five private IVF clinics serving a nation of 200 million. He quipped: "People in Pakistan are still bringing [having] twelve children! We, the infertile, are saving the population [from an explosion]! This is what Rashida and I have been doing for the last thirteen years—comically!" Fortunately for Latif and Rashida, who were pious Muslims, they had received a generous discount from Conceive's Emirati sponsor, who, as a wealthy Muslim, sometimes helped poor couples to pay for their IVF expenses.

Another poor couple, Angeline and Jerome, who were Filipino factory workers and practicing Catholics, still had to figure out how they would pay for IVF, for no such charity had been offered to them. They made a combined monthly income of 4,000 dirhams ($1,090), which they considered a "good income," considerably more than they could ever make in the Philippines. Angeline explained: "The Philippines is still a poor country. I might say that it is not a poor country, but it has a lot of corruption! And it's getting poorer because of this corruption." Angeline believed that the Philippine's corruption extended to health care. When she had spent her hard-earned cash on a gynecological consultation in her home country, "they could not find the exact problem about why we can't have babies." Thus, she had ruled out IVF in the Philippines, even though it was one-third the price of IVF in the Emirates. In fact, Angeline and Jerome were stunned to learn the prices of even the most basic diagnostic and treatment services at Conceive. Jerome lamented: "We had not planned for all of this treatment, and we cannot afford to get any savings because of the rent, paying our bills, and the money we send to both of our families. We haven't saved *any* money. It would be *very* hard. Dividing up our money between all of these things, there is no extra money to go for treatment."

Interestingly, Jerome and Angeline were sharing their apartment and pooling their expenses with another infertile Filipino couple. Their roommates were significantly older and were aging out of their fertility as the wife approached forty. Yet this other couple was waiting to see whether Jerome and Angeline obtained "good results" at Conceive. Fortunately for Angeline, she had a sympathetic factory boss, who had actually phoned the clinic on her behalf to obtain an appointment. Yet getting to Conceive was a struggle, as Jerome and Angeline had to travel by multiple vehicles across several Emirates to reach the clinic. When they arrived, Dr. Pankaj was made aware of their low income. Thus, he decided not to recommend IVF without first pursuing the much less costly route of intrauterine insemination. When that did not work, Angeline and Jerome scraped together just enough money to cover one heavily discounted ICSI cycle. Fortunately for them, their story ended happily, as Angeline became pregnant on the first try.

Without discounts and other acts of charity, most low-resource couples such as Angeline and Jerome have little chance of financing even one cycle of costly IVF unless they save strategically over many years. I met one low-resource couple who had done just this—and their story was most poignant. Beena and Atul were poor migrants from Tamil Nadu, India, who had managed after twelve years of marriage to save just enough money for one ICSI cycle, on which they pinned all of their hopes and dreams. The diminutive and lovely Beena was dressed in a colorful sari and covered in sacred marigold dust on the day that her pregnancy test proved that she had conceived. However, on the follow-up ultrasound visit, Beena and Atul were told the devastating news that the fetal heartbeat had stopped, with the ultrasound showing no signs of viable fetal life. Beena was in a state of shock, rendered speechless by the heartbreaking news. Atul, who was a low-wage pipe fitter for a construction company, immediately blamed himself for the fetal demise, as well as his severe case of male infertility, which was the cause of their childlessness. In Atul's view, he was being punished for a premarital sexual relationship with an "elderly" (that is, older) woman back in India. Although I tried to comfort Atul by suggesting that no one was to blame, it was truly difficult to find the right words of consolation. On that horrible day, Beena and Atul knew that they had lost almost everything—their one and only pregnancy, their life savings on a last-chance ICSI, and their decade-long dreams of parenthood.

Public Financing and the National Health Service (NHS) Refugees

Beena and Atul, Angeline and Jerome, and Latif and Rashida would all have benefitted immensely if they had been able access the free IVF provided by the Emirati government. To my knowledge, the UAE is the only Arab country that provides fully funded IVF and ICSI cycles for its citizens. But this state-subsidized IVF is a citizenship right—and expressly not a right for foreign workers.[97] As already noted, the UAE very rarely naturalizes non-Emiratis. Thus, the benefits of UAE citizenship, including state-subsidized health insurance and access to free IVF, apply only to Emirati nationals. Temporary foreign workers can access IVF at government clinics in the Emirates, but they must pay prices that, as already noted, are among the highest in the world.

Through interviews with eight infertile Emirati couples, as well as with Dr. Pankaj and his clinical staff, I was able to piece together the fragmented history of what I would characterize as the Emirates' brief experiment in IVF public financing. "Public financing" is the term used by health economists to signal the funding of health care by the state. In the case of assisted reproduction, public financing entails either direct payment by the state to IVF clinics, or state-funded health insurance plans that offer reimbursement for IVF to infertile couples.[98] As of 2010, thirty-two nations around the world reported some form of state-sponsored insurance coverage or direct funding for IVF. Most of them were located in Europe, and most justified their IVF coverage on one or more of five grounds: infertility is a disease (or is caused by a disease) to be treated; IVF is therefore a medical need; IVF should be a human (reproductive) right; IVF funding prevents health inequities; and IVF increases a country's total fertility rate and reduces population aging—a major concern in the so-called barren states of Europe.[99] However, many Middle Eastern nations do not share these concerns and thus do not offer any IVF health insurance to their citizens. In this regard, the UAE is unique: In 2010, it was the only Arab nation to provide full government funding of IVF for Emirati citizens through *daman* (the national health insurance system).[100]

Before 1991, when the first IVF clinic opened in the country, Emirati couples who were infertile could request public funding from the UAE Ministry of Health for reprotravel outside of the country. Many infertile Emirati couples took advantage of this early form of reprotravel, often heading to the United Kingdom or the United States for IVF procedures. Even after 1991, some Emiratis continued to travel outside of the country at the state's expense. For example, Khaled and Nura, a middle-aged Emirati couple in my study, had tried IVF when the government clinic in Dubai was first opened. Unfortunately, Nura experienced a series of serious medical mishaps and complications, which were caused by an overly aggressive hormonal stimulation protocol and the transfer of too many embryos. Nura spent a month in the hospital with life-threatening ovarian hyperstimulation syndrome, as well as an ectopic pregnancy. Determined never to return to the Dubai government clinic, Nura and Khaled applied to the UAE Ministry of Health for funds to travel to London for their second IVF cycle. Permission was granted, and the costs were covered by the ministry, with the exception of the couple's hotel expenses and a portion of their airfare.

Interestingly, however, the government did not cover Nura and Khaled's initial IVF cycle at the Dubai government hospital. There, IVF for Emiratis was never free. Like foreigners, Emiratis were expected to pay the high prices set by the clinic. Furthermore, both Emirati and foreign couples were put on long waiting lists, due to high demand for services at this single public clinic. Only with the opening of a second government IVF clinic, located in the more remote desert city of Al Ain, Abu Dhabi,[101] did the UAE government begin to experiment with public funding of IVF. From its inception, this IVF clinic was free for Emiratis through reimbursement by the national health insurance system. For a brief period in the early 2000s, the clinic also offered free IVF cycles to foreigners living in the country. However, the Emirati government had not realized that it had opened the floodgates of infertility in the country. Foreign workers—from elite European expatriates to lowly South Asian construction workers—began clamoring for treatment at the government clinic in Abu Dhabi. Soon there were long waiting lists, and because local Emiratis received priority scheduling, foreigners sometimes had to wait months, even years, to be granted an appointment.

Such "foreign flooding" of the "free" government IVF clinic quickly became unsustainable. By the time I reached the Emirates in 2007, this brief experiment with "IVF for all" through Emirati state largesse had ended. The state had returned to subsidizing only citizens, including providing them with the costly IVF medications for free at government hospitals. But even Emirati citizens were forced to travel to the remote government IVF clinic to access subsidized care. Occasionally, a free IVF cycle at the government clinic in Dubai would be granted after a request to the crown prince, especially for those Emiratis who had performed substantial government service. However, these were exceptional cases. On the whole, publicly financed IVF was exclusionary and restrictive for citizens and noncitizens alike. In retrospect, the brief experiment in IVF state subsidization in the Emirates could only be described as a half-hearted gesture, which lacked the necessary political will to sustain it.

Infertile Emiratis were not happy with this state of affairs. Even though basic health care was accessible to all people, Emiratis and foreigners alike, at the government hospitals scattered throughout the country, Emiratis in my study noted that health services that had once been free in government facilities were increasingly being billed to patients. Salman and Mounira, a young Emirati professional couple from Abu Dhabi, explained that their emirate had just implemented a new health insurance plan designed to address the needs of both local (Emirati) and nonlocal (foreign) residents. Yet they were upset that the new plan specifically excluded both dentistry and IVF, forms of health care that they deemed essential.

The UAE government's frankly retrogressive measures to publicly fund, and then defund, IVF services are, in retrospect, not surprising. Even though the UAE is a comparatively rich country, IVF is an expensive health technology, one that often requires repetition because of low success rates. The UAE thus made a strategic decision to fund IVF on a very limited basis for its citizens. In this respect, it is not alone. Only a handful of Middle Eastern nations provide public funding of IVF services, and even then the funding is only on a partial, limited basis. For example, Algeria reimburses citizens for the cost of IVF medications but not the procedures themselves.[102] Egypt and Iran both offer partially subsidized IVF cycles at a handful of government IVF facilities, but most IVF cycles in both countries are performed in the private sector.[103]

There are only two countries in the Middle East—neither of them Arab—that offer generous IVF funding for all citizens. As shown by the medical sociologist Zeynep Gürtin, Turkey began full funding of two IVF cycles for all Turkish citizens in 2005, when the Turkish Ministry of Health began to provide IVF health insurance redeemable at both state and private clinics.[104] Since then, the demand for IVF in Turkey has dramatically increased, causing a doubling in the number of IVF clinics in the country—from 66 in 2005 to more than 110 in 2013, the largest number in any single Middle Eastern country.[105] Israel, meanwhile, has earned the reputation as the world's most generous IVF funder.[106] As noted by the medical anthropologist Daphna Birenbaum-Carmeli, "publicly funded IVF is provided practically without limitations, for a wide range of indications, with minimal payment at the point of delivery. Women of all ages, marital status and sexual preference are entitled to treatment, until they have two children from the present relationship."[107] In both Israel and Turkey, pronatalism undergirds support for such generous public financing, with the state encouraging the birth of IVF babies for a host of religious, cultural, and political reasons.[108] In Israel, even Palestinian citizens of the country are entitled to a full suite of free IVF and ICSI services.[109]

These unprecedented levels of IVF support are quite unusual; indeed, very few other countries in the world are so generous. In Europe, Belgium and France are said to have the most "sophisticated coverage" of IVF, with Belgium's publicly funded program also tied to high standards of medical care.[110] Australia and the Scandinavian countries (Denmark, Finland, Iceland, Norway, and Sweden) are also notable for providing generous public funding—so much so that demand for IVF services closely approximates actual need.[111] Australia, in fact, provides such abundant federal funding that the cost of an IVF cycle there amounts to only 6 percent of the average annual disposable income,[112] compared to 50 percent in the United States.[113]

Although a variety of other Western and Eastern European nations subsidize IVF to some degree,[114] most do not meet the needs of their infertile citizens. The United Kingdom stands out in this regard as having a complicated, incomplete, and exclusionary system of public financing. According to recent estimates, only about one-quarter to one-third of IVF cycles in that country are publicly funded by the NHS, meaning that 60–85 percent of all IVF cycles are paid for by infertile couples themselves in private clinics.[115] The United Kingdom as a whole has no national IVF funding policy. Instead, NHS funding for IVF operates on a postal code lottery system, with each Local Health Authority deciding on the scope of its IVF funding and eligibility criteria.[116] These eligibility criteria are often quite strict and may include a woman's age (less than thirty-five), normal body mass index (BMI), no history of sterilization for either partner, a minimal period of infertility of two to three years, no existing children (thereby excluding cases of secondary infertility), and sometimes a normal sperm count (thereby excluding all cases of male infertility).[117] As noted by the medical sociologist Lorraine Culley and her British colleagues, in 2004 the United Kingdom's National Institute for Health and Clinical Excellence (NICE; in 2013 the agency changed its full name to the National Institute for Health and Care Excellence) set out guidelines for fertility treatment, recommending three cycles of free IVF for all of those deemed clinically suitable. "However, relatively few NHS commissioners have provided this level of treatment," Culley and her colleagues report, "and currently several are reducing the already limited access to public funding."[118] Given that only 12 percent of British citizens have private health insurance, most of which does not cover infertility treatment, the vast majority of British citizens who want IVF or ICSI must pay for it themselves in the private sector. Thus, the problem of public financing and the resultant high cost of care have been among the primary reasons for the flight of British IVF patients to clinics overseas.[119]

At Conceive, I met eight of these fleeing British couples. As a group, I came to think of them as the *NHS refugees*—British subjects who were seeking refuge in the Emirates after being deemed ineligible for publicly funded IVF; spending years on NHS waiting lists; or receiving ineffective, low-quality infertility treatment in overextended, public-sector IVF clinics. Some of these couples had been disqualified simply because they lived in the wrong postal code area, where local NHS authorities were unsympathetic to the plight of the infertile. The postal code lottery system was a particular grievance. A British teacher named Tracy described how "people are actually moving houses, like for schools, to get an IVF on the NHS." She described herself as "very lucky" in that she and her husband could afford to travel to the Emirates. She said, "We pay here, but what we do is easy in comparison."

A forty-two-year-old British lawyer, Kara, was facing the threat of age-related infertility. Calling British IVF "a bit of a palaver," she had much to say, in anger, about the inadequacies of IVF in the public sector:

Kara: Firstly, the National Health Services has an age cutoff of forty. This is a huge restriction. I'm pretty sure, in fact, that in some jurisdictions, it's earlier than that, younger than age forty. So women over forty definitely don't get IVF, but what about men? I doubt that it applies to men, so they are basically discriminating against women. Secondly, they give you two cycles, the NHS, but there is *a huge waiting list*, absolutely huge. So if you're thirty-nine, by the time you get around to getting off that list, you're too old. And then the cost of private IVF in England is insane. The NHS is a free service, but the private clinics cost the same as here, about £3,000, which is about 20,000 dirhams [$5,445], or closer to 21,000 dirhams [$5,717]. So the price is comparable, but you may end up waiting to get an appointment at a private UK clinic as well.

Marcia: Why do you think the waiting lists in the UK are so long?

Kara: Probably because the clinics are under so much demand pressure. Over there, they are just backed up because of all the demand. Here, you do not have to stand in any queue like you do in Britain. Over there, it's demand pressure, and so if you're the kind of person who has the money, you will go where you can to get better and quicker service.

I met several other British women in the Emirates who had fled the United Kingdom because long waiting lists were jeopardizing their chances for motherhood. Camilla, for example, was desperately trying to get pregnant at age forty-one after being successfully treated for thyroid cancer. She explained:

In the UK, I would *have* to do private IVF, because I'm old . . . er, at the end of my reproductive age. In the NHS, they have to say, first, "Try for three years before we'll take you." Second, "You have to be under age forty." And third, this is what I hear from my friends, "You have to be put on the waiting list." All in all, by that time, you're finished! There's no way for you to become pregnant. The NHS, they don't want to spend a lot of time and resources for people at the end of their fertility, or that's my opinion at least.

This maddening system of IVF inequity and long NHS waiting lists made the British couples in my study want to "jump the queue" by traveling abroad for IVF. Although a few had tried IVF in the United Kingdom's private sector, most couples had given up on the country altogether, saving their money for an IVF journey to Conceive. Some of these British couples had chosen the Emirates because of professional ties or friends who had moved there. Others were British citizens from immigrant backgrounds who viewed the Emirates as a sophisticated, cosmopolitan technohub, located relatively close to their nations of origin. In several of these latter cases, couples planned to finish their IVF cycles in the Emirates and then visit friends and family members living and working in nearby Gulf countries, other parts of the Middle East, South Asia, or East Africa.

Although British couples in my study unleashed the most vehement critiques of their nation's IVF system, they were not alone. I met infertile couples from Australia, Belarus, Bulgaria, Canada, Germany, the Netherlands, Romania, and Sweden—some of the most generous IVF subsidizers in the world—who complained bitterly about their frustrating and sometimes traumatic attempts to access publicly funded IVF care. Their list of complaints was substantial and included months of waiting to get an initial appointment; the need to get an initial referral from a reluctant primary care physician; public IVF clinics that were overflowing and disorganized; limits on the number of IVF attempts; and various exclusion criteria for couples living temporarily abroad or deemed to be too young or too old, to have too many infertility problems, and so on. These mostly European reprotravelers spoke of enduring "months of delays" and "harsh treatment" in overtaxed public IVF sectors. Some also felt that public clinics "cut corners" to save on costs, thereby reducing their chances of IVF and ICSI success.

The flight of the infertile from crowded public IVF clinics in Europe is not identical to the flight of infertile couples from countries that have no IVF clinics at all. Yet both of these forms of reprotravel speak to basic resource constraints. Whether resource-rich or resource-poor, few countries in the world, including the Emirates, have been able to provide enough IVF to meet the needs of infertile patients, especially those who are poor. Although the new global LCIVF initiative would seem to be a step in the right direction, it may take many years, even decades, to achieve the goal of "LCIVF for all." Thus, it would seem important to learn from reprotravelers' stories of IVF absences, inequities, and catastrophic expenditures. Their stories suggest that the provision of affordable IVF may be one of the most important issues of reproductive justice facing the world in the new millennium. Let's turn now to some of these stories of resource crisis.

ABSENCES: Reprotravel Stories

• Fleeing the NHS

Within my first few weeks at Conceive, I began to notice the significant numbers of patients coming to the Emirates from Great Britain, and I eventually commented on this to one of the female physicians at the clinic. She told me, "Many British citizens are fleeing their own medical system." When I asked her what she meant, she explained: "The UK medical system is supposed to be among the best in the world. But, at this point, I feel disillusioned by it. The way the NHS operates is *not* in the best interests of patients. So many infertile patients have gone five to ten years without proper diagnosis or treatment, which is unconscionable, in my opinion." When I asked Dr. Pankaj about this later, he stated pointedly: "The NHS is overworked and underfunded. Everyone is supposed to be entitled to two free IVF cycles, but there are age restrictions and a wait period even before you can apply for the waiting list!"

I stored these thoughts in my mind and in my field notes, and I remembered them when I was eventually introduced to Zahira and Naveed, a young British-Pakistani couple coming to Conceive from the United Kingdom. Perhaps to make a good impression on their first visit, Naveed was dressed formally in a Western shirt and tie, and Zahira wore a bright Pakistani *salwar kameez*, a long sheath over loosely fitted pants in a beautiful green fabric. They were a striking couple: Naveed was movie-star handsome, and Zahira had long, silky black hair, an attractive face, and expressive, kohl-rimmed eyes. However, it soon became evident that Zahira did not feel good about her appearance. Almost immediately, she apologized in her strong British accent for being "overweight"—a problem that was linked to her PCOS and infertility and that was shared by her older sister. Zahira told me:

> I was born and raised in the UK, but our families are from Pakistan, and we have a history of infertility in the family. My sister and aunts were not able to conceive easily, so they always told me, "Don't take birth control when you get married." My husband came to the UK from Pakistan in 1996. We had a brief courtship, and then we married. We were quite careful initially, because we were both quite young, but we always knew that we wanted a family. So one year after marriage, we decided to try. We had never, ever taken any con-

traception. Both of us had never been with anybody else, and so we didn't know if we had any fertility problems. But my older sister, she was infertile, and she went through a lot, the whole palaver—timed cycles, Clomid, Metformin, everything.[120] I suspected I might have the same problem, because we both have a weight issue. As of now, I am overweight, and she was, too. And we both have PCOS. I've gone through it with her, really.

Despite their similar diagnoses of PCOS-related infertility, the two sisters' experiences of infertility care in the NHS could not have been more dissimilar. Zahira's sister had been able to access "brilliant, absolutely brilliant" IVF services at Hull, the major government-sponsored IVF clinic serving the East Yorkshire region. "She is a doctor and so she has connections, medical connections," Zahira explained to me. "A lot of her friends helped push her there, and they told her what's going on. They gave her the time of day; actually, she got *more* than the time of day in Yorkshire. So, there *are* good places in the UK, where you won't pay. She was referred by other doctors, and she ended up having three children, all by IVF."

Zahira, on the other hand, had no such luck. It was Zahira who first explained to me the postal code lottery system in the United Kingdom—namely, that access to IVF depends on one's place of residence and the relative largesse of the local NHS health authorities. Although Zahira and Naveed were happy to own a small home outside of Windsor, the local NHS authorities in their area had not been generous in terms of IVF public financing. Thus, Zahira had never received any form of IVF assistance, even though she and Naveed had met the length of marriage requirement and Zahira had worked assiduously to reduce her BMI to the "acceptable band" for her age. After seven years of untreated infertility, Zahira was both frustrated and demoralized:

Everything is fine with me, apart from my PCOS. But the doctors are really not good at explaining. Only because my older sister is a doctor and I've been through it with her do I know what they're talking about. Trying to get any information is like getting information out of a stone! And I've had to move from one place to another to another, all within the NHS. One time, they lost my reports. They gave me the wrong appointments. Then one time I was told to turn up for an egg collection, and there was no doctor! They said, "Sorry, but first, we have to start a course of treatment before we can do an egg collection, and there's no doctor present." And this was a good hour's drive from where we were living. There were just so many issues. We were clearly living in the wrong place, but if we moved, we would still have had to wait a certain amount of time and begin again with a certain medical center. It's basically subsidized only if you're lucky and can meet all of the guidelines. Even though I was visiting NHS clinics, I still couldn't get into, or rather through, the system. I don't know why. But I didn't even get onto the ladder for IVF in the United Kingdom.

Eventually giving up on the public sector, Zahira and Naveed decided to make an appointment with a private clinic. Each consultation with the "pioneering" IVF doctor cost £200 (about $400 at the time), requiring Zahira and Naveed to save up between visits. Learning that one IVF cycle, including medication, would cost them £3,500 (about $7,000), Zahira and Naveed decided to sell their home—hoping that the proceeds would be "invested" in an IVF baby. But when their IVF cycle in the private clinic failed, Zahira's morale plummeted. Describing herself as "close to a breakdown," she lamented:

> I just couldn't take it any more with the medical services in the UK. I'd had seven years of issues with them. I don't know what the medicine is like in the rest of the world, but I was not getting anywhere. We had searched every-where, looking at success rates and trying to get answers. In the end, we just had enough. We thought maybe a change of air, a change of scenery, would do us good. So we came out to Dubai. We decided that if we came here, we'd definitely give IVF a try, because my friend had been here. He'd had treatment with Dr. Pankaj, and he definitely recommended him. So we moved, because infertility care in the UK was so poor. Given our experiences in the NHS, we had in mind that it would take us a long time to get an appointment here, but that wasn't true. We called in February, and now we're here in April.

In fact, at the time I interviewed them in the spring of 2007, Zahira and Naveed were living between the United Kingdom and the UAE. "We came over in December, and we're still not sure if we're staying here," Zahira told me. "We wanted to try the system here, but we have not yet moved officially." No longer anchored to the United Kingdom by home ownership, both Zahira and Naveed had quit their jobs, and they were now working in Dubai's business sector on two-month visitors' visas. If Naveed's real estate firm decided to sponsor him for a longer-term work permit, then their residence issue would be "settled," and they would remain in the country, Zahira told me. I asked Zahira if she considered herself to be a "reproductive tourist" or more like a migrant, and she responded: "It's more like 'migration' than medical 'tourism.' I think it's a very big issue in the UK, this tourism, because people are going to Spain and everywhere. That's because the guidelines are quite tough in the UK. The system is just so slow. It's a dinosaur system. And there are so many problems with the system—lost files, living in the wrong [postal] code, no doctors present, not getting answers. So people like us are just fleeing the NHS." Having fled but not yet resettled, Zahira and Naveed were living in a state of limbo. Seven years of ineptitude at the NHS had caused them to sell their home, give up their jobs, and flee to another country where they were living on visitors' visas. Yet Zahira and Naveed were not alone. Such NHS refugees were unfortunately common at Conceive—British citizens who felt like pawns in a place-based lottery system, the rewards of which they would never see.

• Pain, Poverty, and Persistence

Unfortunately, the NHS is not the only government health system that has failed to deliver on its IVF promises. Fatima and Mahmoud, who hailed from Kerala, India, were the victims of the Emirates' own shifting state subsidization system: they had lived in Abu Dhabi for six out of eight years of their marriage and had experienced the sudden withdrawal of state IVF support. As a religiously pious Muslim, Mahmoud wore an Islamic skullcap over his balding scalp and sported a calloused prayer spot on his forehead above his sparkling green eyes. Fatima was dressed completely in black, covering herself with an abaya and a facial veil, so that only her eyes—behind heavy glasses—could be seen. The couple was very poor. Mahmoud made only 3,000 dirhams a month (about $820) as an office clerical assistant, with half of his salary going toward the rental of their small apartment in Abu Dhabi.

Fatima had spent most of the past six years in that apartment, venturing out primarily for doctor's appointments. Unfortunately, she suffered from a painful condition called endometriosis, caused by the excess proliferation and sloughing of endometrial tissue into the pelvic cavity. Needing laparoscopic surgery to remove the excess tissue and relieve the unremitting pelvic pain, Fatima traveled with Mahmoud during his one-month annual leave back to Kerala, where they were hoping to obtain the surgery for one-fifth of what it would cost them in the Emirates. However, once in India, Fatima's case was determined to be severe. Her surgeon ended up removing both Fatima's right fallopian tube and ovary.

Demoralized by the outcome, Fatima returned with Mahmoud to Abu Dhabi, where they were referred by a kindly female gynecologist to the government IVF clinic in Al Ain. There, they were overjoyed to hear that IVF would be completely free to them. They accepted their place on the one- to two-year waiting list, believing that they were being tested by God for their faith and persistence. A full two years passed before an appointment was finally made. By this time, however, the Emirati government was no longer sponsoring IVF for non-Emiratis, news that came as a great blow to Fatima and Mahmoud. As Mahmoud lamented, "You know, we waited for two years like that—*two whole years*—before they started calling us for the initial checkups. But now, they tell us, you have to pay the full cost if you're an expat. That would be around 12,000 dirhams for IVF, excluding the medicine, or 20,000 dirhams altogether [$5,500]."

Feeling priced out of the high-end IVF sector in the Emirates, Mahmoud and Fatima traveled back to India on Mahmoud's next annual leave, checking on a "well-known" hospital in Karnataka. There, they were told that IVF was still in the "planning stages," and that they would have to wait another one to two years before a clinic would be opened. Fatima, meanwhile, was diagnosed with a cyst on her remaining ovary. The cyst had to be removed by a second laparoscopic surgery, and Fatima was instructed to return in another year once an IVF clinic had been established in Karnataka.

Upon their return to Abu Dhabi, Fatima became pregnant, but the pregnancy turned out to be an emergency ectopic, which was removed by medication. The same cycle—returning to India, being told that they had to wait for an IVF clinic to be opened, undergoing laparoscopic cyst removal, then becoming pregnant with an emergency ectopic—happened once again, although this time in their home state of Kerala. "After that, I was *so* depressed," Mahmoud explained, for he had come to realize that India's purported IVF boom had not yet reached the southern states—which he, Fatima, and the majority of Indians living in the Emirates considered to be their real home.

After returning to the Emirates from Kerala, Mahmoud and Fatima learned about Conceive, with its Indian clinical director. As pious Muslims, Fatima and Mahmoud would have preferred a female Muslim physician.[121] But they decided that the "quality of a doctor"—not the doctor's nationality, gender, or religion—were what really mattered to them in making a test-tube baby. Furthermore, once they met Dr. Pankaj, they were pleased with his demeanor and clinical competence. In fact, Dr. Pankaj was the first physician to diagnose Fatima's PCOS and insulin resistance, conditions that needed to be treated before she could safely embark on a round of IVF. Dr. Pankaj also determined that Mahmoud's sperm profile had been deteriorating over time, a finding that Mahmoud himself attributed to "all of the tension."

When I met Fatima and Mahmoud in the clinic, they had just undertaken their first cycle of IVF, and they laughed while telling me that it had taken them five full years to finally access this reproductive technology. Luckily for them, Fatima became pregnant on the first IVF cycle, which they attributed to the "great job" being done by Dr. Pankaj and his clinical staff. Nonetheless, as Indian Muslims, they did not plan on telling anyone about undertaking IVF at Conceive with a Hindu physician. As Mahmoud explained, "IVF is not accepted in our community. Actually, some people believe that what we're doing is against God's wishes. We don't believe this, but some people do. They don't agree with IVF." Mahmoud also stressed the need for absolute secrecy to prevent "family interference." Nonetheless, he had been forced to borrow money from his relatives, telling them only that Fatima was "receiving treatment." He explained: "For six years, I've been spending all my money on this. I don't have anything left. I've spent a *lot* of money over five to six years. So I took [out] a loan from my father and his relatives. They're helping, but I'll pay them back. It is my wish to pay for this from my own pocket. But it is *very* difficult to save for this. I brought her here only for this—to have a baby—nothing else. And a loan was necessary for that. And I've traveled a lot for this—two countries, two emirates!" Now $6,000 in debt to family members—an amount that would take them years to pay back—the couple was nonetheless ecstatic. Returning from her ultrasound scan, Fatima had the final word, which truly summarized their shared sentiments. "We were coming here from Abu Dhabi *very tense*," she emphasized. "But we reached here, and we became *very happy!*"

• **Crossing the Empty Quarter**

The term "cross-border reproductive care"—which is favored in the medical literature and which sounds so benign and compassionate—cannot begin to convey the difficulty of border crossings for infertile couples living in some of the most remote regions of the world. IVF patients sometimes relate harrowing stories of reprotravel under difficult, even dangerous conditions. The story of Aisha, an Omani woman who sought IVF in the neighboring countries of Saudi Arabia and the Emirates, exemplifies the complexities of reprotravel within the Arab Gulf. In this desert region, geographic isolation and the uncertainties of travel often pose significant obstacles to border crossing.

I interviewed Aisha as she lay in bed, having recently finished an egg collection procedure. I also met Aisha's husband, Sa'id, a short, smiling man, who spoke no English and who was identifiable as Omani by virtue of his *thawb* (a floor-length garment for men) and ornamented skullcap. Unlike other men who sat by their wives' bedsides, Sa'id appeared only briefly behind the curtained partition where Aisha rested, for reasons that would later become very clear.

I learned from Aisha that Sa'id was forty years old and an officer in the Omani defense forces. Aisha was thirty-seven, a nurse, and the mother of their two children, thirteen-year-old Hassan and six-year-old Laila. With only two children after a decade and a half of marriage, Aisha was under considerable pressure from Sa'id's family to have more children. Sa'id's mother—who had borne thirteen children and regretted that she did not have more—routinely patted Aisha's flat belly, asking, "Is there something inside?" Aisha said that she did not object to this behavior by her mother-in-law, who was otherwise kind to her. But she bemoaned the fact that Omani men's families took no pity on their infertile daughters-in-law, creating a kind of living hell for women:

Aisha: You know the Omani man, especially the traditional *gabali* man [from the mountains]. If a female has some fertility problem, he will divorce her, and he will marry maybe two, three, four, five times until he gets enough children. If there are no children from a woman, he'll go for another one. Even if he is an infertile male, that man will go to marry another. That's usually what happens. So you find one male with maybe three ladies, maybe four ladies. That means he'll get more children. In some families, the father doesn't even know the sons' names, because there are maybe forty to fifty children. From each woman, he gets ten children,[122] so how will he remember all of their names? And if they're a poor family with no money, how will they get all of those children to school? How will they take care of them? It's like this in Oman, and in Saudi [Arabia], the same thing. It's the same thinking. Even though things are changing, and people are going to study, it's still the same thinking.

Marcia: But what about your husband? He is here with you today.

Aisha: I don't know why, but he is different. Daily, they tell him to remarry— his brothers, his sisters, his father, who is now very sick. His family does pressure him, but he's not listening to them. He's not going along with them. He's playing along with them so that there won't be any trouble, because it is *haram* [sinful] to disrespect your parents. Especially my mother-in-law, my father-in-law, in front of me, they tell him, "Go and marry!" And I will tell them, "Okay, he can go and marry." But between me and my husband, no, he won't do this. My husband doesn't care about what other people think. He says that what we're deciding is for us, not for them. But in other families, the mother-in-law will even bring the lady to him and say, "Go and marry!" And maybe they will do this with my husband. Maybe they will bring a woman who has been pregnant before and has maybe five children and is divorced from her husband. They will consider her very nice because they know that she can have children. So there is real social pressure like this still going on in Oman. Even if the wife is a very nice lady, they will push the husband for children, to have *at least* eight, nine, or ten children. Less than that, and the lady will be in real trouble.

Marcia: So you are lucky that your husband isn't like this.

Aisha: Yes, my husband likes me.

Marcia: He loves you!

Aisha: Yes! That's why he's not going to marry another. He refused to do it! But I *need* another child. That's why he agreed to do this IVF with me.

For his part, Sa'id realized that Aisha was not to blame for their infertility problem. She had become pregnant easily during their first year of marriage but then experienced two ectopic pregnancies after the birth of their son, losing both fallopian tubes in the process. As a nurse, Aisha realized that IVF was her only solution. Yet Oman was without a single IVF clinic, making travel abroad the only possibility.

One evening while watching television, Aisha saw a program about Saudi Arabia, one of the first Middle Eastern countries to embrace IVF. With Sa'id's blessing, Aisha contacted a clinic in the western coastal city of Jeddah, where she made an appointment. Deciding that the 3,000-mile round trip would be too difficult by land, Sa'id, Aisha, and Aisha's mother and brother flew to Jeddah, spending approximately $8,200 on the air travel, hotel, and the IVF procedure itself. This was much more than the couple could easily afford, but Aisha's family lent their support and were rewarded with the birth of a baby girl, Laila, who was beloved by the entire family.

However, Aisha soon began to worry that Laila would grow up without a sister. As Aisha explained to me, every woman in Oman needs a sister for support in marriage, childbirth, and old age. Thus, Aisha was undertaking IVF at Conceive "for my daughter" and had even consulted a Muslim cleric to determine whether sex selection was permissible.[123] When she learned that it was not allowed, Aisha set a goal for herself of trying to bear IVF twins, hoping that at least one of them would become Laila's little sister.

I asked Aisha why she had traveled to Conceive rather than back to Saudi Arabia. Aisha explained that she had heard Dr. Pankaj give a lecture on IVF at her hospital in Salalah, and she was very impressed by his expertise. Although a new IVF center had opened up in Muscat, Oman's capital city, Aisha and Sa'id had no desire to try it, for fear of being seen and stigmatized by other Omani nationals. Aisha had heard that the Muscat IVF clinic was very poorly attended, probably for this reason. She also suspected that most infertile Omanis would try their best to travel to other parts of the Arab Gulf, where they were less likely to be recognized.

Yet leaving Oman, especially from the remote coastal city of Salalah, was not very easy. Flights were irregular, with the only major air carrier departing only once each weekend. To make their scheduled appointment at Conceive, Aisha and Sa'id were thus forced to take the bus—a twelve-hour journey across the notorious Rub' al Khali desert, translated as the "Empty Quarter" in English. The Rub' al Khali is the world's largest pure sand desert. Encompassing the southern third of the Arabian Peninsula, it has a uniquely harsh and unforgiving climate. Aisha enumerated for me the many dangers of crossing the Empty Quarter in any sort of vehicle. Sandstorms were common, bringing vehicular traffic to a complete halt. In addition, large herds of camels often obstructed the sole highway, which Aisha described as an "old, old road," filled with rocky, unpaved patches where the cement had eroded over time. Gas stations were located hundreds of miles apart, requiring every vehicle to have its own supply of gasoline. And, for much of the year, the heat was so intense that radiators often overheated, leading to dangerous breakdowns on the highway. Finally, because police stations were sparsely located in the Empty Quarter, the chances of being rescued were remote. Aisha claimed that deaths—some caused by heat stroke and dehydration, and others by reckless driving—occurred regularly on the desert road. Given these many risks, Aisha preferred to fly across the desert. But she learned that it was virtually impossible to coordinate air travel with timed treatment cycles. So she and Sa'id boarded the dawn bus for Dubai, crossing the Empty Quarter with a handful of other passengers and arriving in time for the evening prayer.

I asked Aisha if she would consider this dangerous journey to Dubai to be a form of "reproductive tourism"—especially if they could spend at least a little time enjoying the sights and sounds of the big city. Like so many others, Aisha was dismissive, rejecting the notion of tourism out of hand. For one thing, she said that she and Sa'id had no time to see the sights, given the intensity of the treatment cycle at Conceive. Furthermore, in Aisha's opinion, the term "tourism" could not begin to reflect the felt need for children, which is why Middle Eastern women like her would travel for IVF. As a mother of two, Aisha was in a privileged position compared to many other childless Arab women. Yet even as an educated nurse, Aisha still faced the everyday stigma and barrage of insults from her patients, who would ask about her children and then vociferously criticize her for having only two. Aisha told me that she loved her country—with its stunning mountains and fjords and oases of tropical vegetation. But she was nonetheless deeply critical of it, insisting that "family values" in Oman must change. This would not occur, she suspected, until more Omani men became like Sa'id— happy in a monogamous marriage, supportive of his wife, resisting his family's pressure, content with one or two children, and pleased with a daughter as well as a son.

Aisha knew that she was lucky to be married to a good man, one who loved her and their children, supported her career as a nurse, and traveled under difficult and costly conditions to make an IVF baby (or two). Yet all of this was not easy for Aisha's husband, Sa'id. In fact, on the day of Aisha's egg collection—when Sa'id's sperm were absolutely needed for the critical and precisely timed fertilization of her eggs—he was unable to produce a semen sample through masturbation, probably out of religious guilt and sheer, physical anxiety.[124] Although the Conceive staff gave Sa'id several hours to relax in a variety of "hidden" parts of the clinic, he was ultimately unable to produce the crucial cup of ejaculate. Thus, Sa'id was scheduled for surgery to aspirate sperm directly from his testicles. On his way to the operating theater, Sa'id peeked behind Aisha's curtained partition, dressed in a hospital gown and still smiling. Aisha wished him well as he left, then turned to me and said, "God help him. There is nothing I can do for him now."

I do not know if Aisha ever became pregnant, as she and Sa'id left Conceive shortly after their embryo transfer. Yet this couple's deep commitments to one another left a lasting impression on me. Aisha clearly believed that Sa'id was a new kind of Arab man, contradicting the many stereotypes that she held about her countrymen. Sa'id certainly proved this point through his embodied sacrifices. Having crossed the dangerous Empty Quarter with Aisha, he was about to put the most delicate part of his "manhood" on the line (or, rather, on the operating table)—all for the love of his infertile wife and her dream of a second IVF daughter.

• Love, Polygyny, and IVF

Part of the power of Aisha and Sa'id's story lies in its ability to debunk prevailing myths about polygyny in the Muslim Middle East. The common perception is that Muslim men will marry a second wife if the first wife is infertile. However, in my nearly thirty years of research in the Middle East, I have rarely encountered such cases. Instead, I have met hundreds of "new Arab men" like Sa'id who have refused to forsake their infertile wives, viewing infertility as a disease to be treated rather than as a failure of womanhood. Such men view polygyny as an outmoded solution to childlessness in the era of IVF and ICSI. Hence, polygyny in the Middle East is infrequent, occurring in less than 5 percent of marriages across the Arab world.[125]

Furthermore, polygyny's relationship to infertility appears counterintuitive. It is often presumed that an infertile first wife will be replaced by a second, but instead a second wife may be childless and be supported through IVF by her polygynous husband. This is especially true among middle-aged men and women who were once sweethearts, were prevented from marrying by their families, but were reunited in later life, rekindling their commitment through polygyny.

Having encountered these kinds of *infertile polygynous love marriages* in both Egypt and Lebanon, I was therefore not surprised to meet Nafisa and

Abdul-Rahman, a middle-aged Sudanese couple involved in a polygynous second union. Both Nafisa and Abdul-Rahman were physicians, and they had met during their medical school days in Khartoum. College sweethearts who were well matched in terms of intelligence, temperament, clan, and religion, Nafisa and Abdul-Rahman were nonetheless caught in the middle of family animosities. As they told me separately, their families never liked each other and were also from opposing political camps, of the kind that plunged the country into four decades of internecine civil war. Banned from ever seeing Nafisa again, Abdul-Rahman married another woman "out of obligation." She bore him two children, but over the years, she also lost four pregnancies due to diabetes-related complications. Nafisa remained a spinster for some time—entering the so-called "celibacy trap" that ensnares many Middle Eastern and African women when male-female ratios are disrupted by the deaths and exodus of a nation's young men as a result of civil war.[126] After an unhappy one-year marriage, Nafisa became a divorceé, effectively heaping one form of stigma on another.

Having few other options for family life, Nafisa moved by herself from Khartoum to Fujairah, one of the most remote and least developed of the seven UAE emirates. Working day and night as an on-call obstetrician and gynecologist, Nafisa's time was almost completely occupied by deliveries, which were frequent among Fujairah's Arab Bedouin population. Nonetheless, outside of work, Nafisa was very lonely—the emptiness of life as an aging female divorcee, constrained by the limited social opportunities in an unfamiliar and conservative Arab environment. Nafisa's single ray of hope was Abdul-Rahman: Without their families' knowledge, they had managed to maintain an ongoing "friendship"—occasional telephone calls and e-mail messages, which convinced Nafisa that "we still didn't lose our love."

Abdul-Rahman, for his part, was weighing his options. He had taken on a major university position in the city of Juba, which would eventually become the capital of the newly formed country of South Sudan. Living 1,200 miles from his wife and teenage children, and 2,200 miles from his college sweetheart, Abdul-Rahman had plenty of time to think about his current life and also about the future. Eventually, his path became clear. Following Islamic law, Abdul-Rahman informed his first wife that he intended to marry polygynously, and he asked Nafisa to become his second wife, an offer that she accepted without hesitation.

Embarking on their polygynous love marriage was a complicated and expensive proposition for the two middle-aged Sudanese physicians. Both of them were supporting their large, natal families; thus, neither could afford to give up their current stable, well-paying positions in Fujairah and Juba. As a result, the couple saw each other only twice during their first year of marriage, with Abdul-Rahman making the 2,200-mile flight from Juba to Dubai (via Khartoum) on Sudanese Air, each trip costing $1,200.

Despite the expense of travel, Abdul-Rahman was a "man on a mission"—namely, to impregnate Nafisa so that she could experience the "joys of mother-hood." At age forty-one, Nafisa was aware that she was facing serious age-related infertility, and she had already inquired about IVF in Khartoum. Although Sudan had had no IVF facilities when Nafisa had left the country in 1998, two clinics had recently been opened by Sudanese physicians who had trained in the United Kingdom and Saudi Arabia. Although Nafisa believed that these Sudanese IVF physicians were "well qualified," she doubted that she could successfully coordinate an IVF cycle in Khartoum, given her limited vacation time and Abdul-Rahman's residence so far away. Neither Juba nor Fujairah had any IVF facilities. Nafisa concluded that she must find an IVF clinic within easy driving distance from her workplace and close to the Dubai airport for her "traveling husband."

Because of Dr. Pankaj's fame in local gynecological circles, Nafisa decided to try IVF at Conceive, a choice that was enthusiastically endorsed by her physician supervisor. Yet reprotravel to Conceive was a major challenge, for it required Nafisa to drive several times each week to the clinic—a three-hour round-trip journey across emirates, which sometimes involved dense traffic. More important, Nafisa felt the absence of her husband acutely, especially in the couples-oriented environment of the clinic. She lamented:

> Not being together is one of the main problems. Maybe if we were together, maybe we would be successful getting a baby without this assistance. Another thing is that work is difficult. It is definitely a factor having to come here when I'm not living in the same emirate. And where I work, it is stressful, our department. We have twenty-four-hour continuous delivery duty, and the next day I feel exhausted, even though I have to drive here. Finally, the cost is a problem. I can manage, because I don't have so much pressure from my family. But most of Abdul-Rahman's money is going to support his family, so even though we are sharing the cost of IVF, it is very expensive for both of us, but especially me.

Given these various difficulties, Abdul-Rahman's two trips had been carefully planned to coincide with Nafisa's IVF cycles at Conceive. During the first cycle, Nafisa's "old eggs" were too few in number and too slow to mature, despite heavy application of hormonal medication. When Abdul-Rahman could no longer extend his work leave from Juba, the clinic asked him to leave a semen sample, which they froze until Nafisa's eggs were ready for fertilization. This less-than-ideal scenario left Nafisa alone during the surgical procedure of egg collection as well as the embryo transfer, points at which husbands are almost always present at their wives' bedsides. When the pregnancy test came back negative, Nafisa vowed that she would never again do an IVF cycle alone. She wanted Abdul-Rahman by her bedside, and Abdul-Rahman promised her that he would do everything in his power to achieve this on the second cycle.

I met Abdul-Rahman in the middle of that second cycle, while he was waiting for Nafisa to finish a scan. We spoke with each other while seated comfortably in the black leather recliners usually reserved for the clinic's female patients following their embryo transfers. At forty-seven, Abdul-Rahman looked old, even haggard, with thick glasses and an uneven complexion. He explained to me that it had been a full year since he had visited Conceive, because he had had to wait for his next annual leave and had successfully sought permission to extend it by an extra month. Furthermore, he and Nafisa had had to earn another 20,000 dirhams ($5,445) to undergo their second IVF cycle. Although they were part of the Sudanese elite, Abdul-Rahman explained why saving was so difficult. Their money simply evaporated via family expenditures in a poverty-stricken, postwar setting, he complained:

> Now, there is no war, as such. It is only normal conflict, the remainder of the war between militant groups. But the problem is the extended family. If you are a person responsible for a small, small family, then there is no problem. But if you are like me, or Nafisa living here [in the Emirates], then you are catering to everybody. Everyone says he needs some money, for school fees, for an operation. Even though we *have* money, this money cannot begin to meet all of their needs. It is like an open budget—to pay for their doctor, private clinics, medicine, food, travel. You cannot make excuses. Otherwise, they consider you a bad person. "You don't like your family! You don't like your people!" And even if you came to visit me, I would have to take care of you. We are expected to have "open hospitality." We are very friendly in Sudan, and we do not refuse to help other people. But sometimes this is a huge burden—sometimes at the expense of your own health and the education of your kids. You simply cannot save anything for yourself.

Although traveling to the Emirates was a considerable expense for Abdul-Rahman, he told me that he was "enjoying life" in Nafisa's presence, for the first time since college. Shy at first, he soon warmed up, professing his undying love for Nafisa and his willingness to undertake IVF "for her." He told me:

> I have two children, but I would like to have more for her. *This IVF is for her!* Because I love her, and I would like her to have a baby. If I get one more baby,

that's enough for me. But I know that she wants two or more, and that is no problem. *Alhamdulillah* [praise be to God]. This is a love marriage, and we are doing this IVF by ourselves. It's a personal thing. We are just doing it on our own, because we don't need their [family] help, and they have never helped us anyway.

Nafisa dreamed of becoming the mother of Abdul-Rahman's child—the proof of their abiding love, despite the opposition that had once prevented them from being together. However, as a gynecologist herself, Nafisa was also aware of the obstacles. "I'm facing my age, and so many factors," she concluded. "If I succeed in getting a healthy baby, maybe I will try one more time. But, then *khalas* [enough]! I will be elderly! To get the first child, this is my goal, *insha'Allah* [God willing]. *Insha'Allah*, in the near future, I can move back to Sudan with Abdul-Rahman and our baby. All of the time, this is what I'm thinking. *Insha'Allah*, this is my hope."

• **An African Woman's Duress**

These stories of four devoted couples—Nafisa and Abdul-Rahman from Sudan, Aisha and Sa'id from Oman, Fatima and Mahmoud from India, and Zahira and Naveed from Britain and Pakistan—are heartwarming and compelling, for they underscore the fact that reprotravel is usually undertaken out of marital love and commitment. However, it is important to bear in mind that reprotravel may be undertaken out of desperation, including as a last-ditch effort to save a troubled marriage. Usually, the desperate party is a woman, and depending on her geographical location and social position, she may face many forms of harm, including medical mistreatment, verbal abuse, social ostracism, divorce, economic abandonment, domestic violence, and even torture. Scholarship from around the world, but especially from sub-Saharan Africa, is replete with stories of women's suffering in cases of childlessness. This is why the LCIVF movement has focused so relentlessly on Africa. Getting low-cost IVF to African women may be a matter of life and death.

Joy was a young Nigerian woman in my study whose marriage was in crisis and who was living in harm's way by virtue of her childlessness. I found Joy sitting alone in the clinic one day and asked her if she would be willing to join my study. A little aloof at first, Joy required repeated reassurances that whatever she told me would be held in the strictest confidence—including from her husband, Kenneth, who would join us later, profoundly altering the quality of our conversation and noticeably subduing Joy's overall demeanor.

I learned from Joy that both she and Kenneth were Igbos who had moved from Lagos to Abuja, the capital of Nigeria. Although I had met several East African couples at Conceive, Joy and Kenneth were part of a West African vanguard, a new wave of reprotravelers flying across the African continent for IVF services in Dubai. Joy was quite young, only twenty-five when I met her. But she had already been married for five years and had yet to become pregnant. Joy told me a painful story of infertility and marital duress, which came pouring out as follows:

Joy: I didn't start trying to have children after marriage. I started trying to know if I could get pregnant when I was still dating Kenneth. I was eighteen years old, he was twenty-five, and nothing happened. He wanted to get married to me, and he didn't disclose if he wanted a baby right away. He wasn't thinking about this. He was only concerned about marriage. But I, myself, was trying to know if I could get pregnant. I wanted to get a baby before marriage. I didn't tell him this, because even if I was pregnant, he would still have married me.

Marcia: Were you trying to prove your fertility?

Joy: Yes, because I do have a problem of irregular menstruation. To come out, it takes maybe two to three months, sometimes six months before I see another one. I went to doctors there [in Nigeria]. But they would tell me that because I'm not married, they cannot take any action for my irregular menstruation. The last doctor I went to see told me, "Get married, and we'll discuss it." That's what the doctor said. But as of this day, I worry and worry and worry, because for up to one year, I would not see my period until I took some pills to force it out. I went to different hospitals. You can just walk into any hospital in Nigeria and see an ob-gyn. I was told that I could do IVF, but there were not many IVF hospitals, at least in Abuja where we are living. That was what I was told. But my husband didn't buy the idea of IVF. We didn't do IVF, actually, in Nigeria. The doctors were supposed to take us there, to an IVF center in Abuja. But they were asking for a big sum of money, and we had no guarantee that IVF would be successful. And if not successful, what will the doctor do? Repeat or refund? They were not giving us any assurance about that. So we didn't go.

Marcia: How did you get here to Dubai, then?

Joy: Well, my husband comes to Dubai to buy cars and other things here. He's a businessman. Sometimes when he comes for work, I come here on holiday with him. So we know Dubai. Actually, when I started coming on holiday, we looked for hospitals, different hospitals. We both did scans, and other things, and brought our reports. They gave me Clomid, but this still didn't work. And other drugs, too, I don't know their names. My period was still irregular.

Marcia: And what about your husband? Is he okay?

Joy: Yes, he's okay—very okay. He has no [sperm] problem. The problem is just from me.

Marcia: Is this a problem for your marriage—that you're the one with the fertility issue?

Joy: Yeah, not quite, but sometimes. . . . But I know he's not feeling the pain right now. Sometimes even, he will talk to me, telling me he's still by my side. He's trying to prove to me that he wants the baby, not that he wants to leave me. He mentions all the places we've gone for treatment when he talks to me. But the day we came here [to Conceive], he said that if he tries this [IVF] and it doesn't work out, maybe he will find a way to get a baby—not maybe, he's *going* to find a way to get a baby.

Marcia: Which means . . . ?

Joy: Meaning maybe he'll go for some other lady to have a baby, and that *hurts* a lot. I couldn't sleep. I wasn't myself the day he said it. It was the first day after we came here.

Marcia: How are you feeling now?

Joy: I feel abnormal, unsatisfied. I don't feel happy anymore. I don't feel satisfied. I'm feeling *very much worse* than I used to. And even if my husband does not pressure me, his family would like to do something like that. Some of the things that have been done to me have been done in his family. They *don't* listen to you, they *don't* even heed your opinion. Even when you say something [they reply], "You don't have a say. You don't have kids!" You will speak, but they will not regard it. They will speak to you badly. "You don't have a *stay* in your family yet!" In parts of Africa, that's the way it is. You *stay* in your home *if* you have babies.

Marcia: That's horrible social pressure.

Joy: It's incredible social pressure. And it's not just the family. It's friends. He's been under so much pressure for me to get pregnant because of his friends. His friends have babies now, and when they talk, they say to him, "You can't even get a woman pregnant! Why are you speaking?" So I know his feelings. That's why he said those bad things to me, even though he apologized. He said he was sorry. He didn't mean to say that to me. He was "hot" because of the way his friends talked. It's not easy to forget about, but you just have to forgive.

Marcia: Do you love him?

Joy: Yeah, we do—we do love each other. He just wants the noise of a baby in the house. To hear the noise. Someone to do this and that for. And when he's going out, he will take the baby with him. He *wants* the baby, that's what I feel. He sees other kids, and kids come to him and he wants his own.

Marcia: Has he ever threatened to divorce you?

Joy: No, no, because he's a Christian. But sometimes, I feel like divorcing him because of this problem—just letting him go so that he can find someone to get him kids. Then I could figure out my problem, and when it's time, I *will* get pregnant, when it's the right time for me. I don't want someone to be repeating this problem with me. That's what I feel. So I feel like letting him go. I've not said this to him, but, yes, I did say to him, I did get straight to the point, "I feel like divorcing you. I feel like letting you go, because I'm tired of all of these problems." But I just pray to God that I can manage and that it will be better if I have kids. If I did have kids from him, I'd be able to *control* those things. He wouldn't be happy to hear me say, "I'm going to leave you," because of the kids. Now if I said, "I'm going to leave you," he might say, "Okay, go ahead." But with kids, he wouldn't. He would actually plead with me, "Don't go! Don't leave the kids." He's going to feel it, feel the pain if I said, "I'm going to leave home." Like now, sometimes I do say, "I'm going to leave you."

Marcia: What does he say?

Joy: Well, he's said so many things to me, things that are hurtful. So I'm just not happy. When your friends say bad things to you, you don't go out with your friends anymore. So why am I still hanging around with him?

Marcia: Especially if he insults you.

Joy: Yeah, and he does. He does. And when he's angry, or maybe I provoke him when we argue—when I would argue with him, he might beat me. He hits me. He gets angry easily. After hitting me, or getting mad at me, or shouting at me, he still comes back and says, "I'm sorry." He's just hot-tempered.

Marcia: Is it common for him to beat you?

Joy: Yeah, it is common. There's a lot of wife beating in Nigeria.

Marcia: And you still love him?

Joy: He's okay, and this is why I like him—*he cares*. I know the only problem he has is a hot temper. He gets mad easily, so that's our problem, I think. But he cares. He takes care of me. If I have kids, he'll take good care of all of us, and this is not common in the country of Nigeria.

Marcia: It isn't?

Joy: No, less than 50 percent of men care for their wives. Only 20 percent are devoted to them.

Marcia: What's the difference?

Joy: The difference between caring and devoted is, if he's caring, he'll bring everything for her, everything she needs. But if he's devoted, he does not look at another woman—going somewhere else to satisfy himself. Only 20 percent of men are devoted to their wives, meaning they are not unfaithful.

Marcia: Is he faithful to you?

Joy: Yeah, he is faithful, and me, too. He did have other relationships, and I did, too—a lot. I have had different relationships I've passed through. And sometimes it hurts. Some of them [her old boyfriends] came to him and talked to him and said things that hurt. He came home with that anger, "Look at your boyfriend who talked to me!" It was a very hurtful remark. The friends he keeps, I think actually 50 percent of his problem is from his friends, reminding him, and telling him, "She was my former girlfriend. She cannot have a baby, or *you* cannot have a baby." They're teasing him.

Marcia: Do people taunt you?

Joy: No, maybe because of the way I act, maybe I don't give them a chance to talk to me. It's when you get so close to someone, someone who gets to know you very well. So I don't get so close to people, so that they won't hurt me. I only have a few friends, but we're not that intimate.

Marcia: So who do you confide in?

Joy: My *mom*, my *mom*—she's *intimate* to me. I tell her *everything*! All of my pains, I tell her. She just talks to me, "Oh, I pray to God, things will be better." But there was a time when she was so mad at my husband. I and my husband, we had a problem, and she called my husband and said, "I think this marriage will be over, and I'll take her back." My mom wasn't happy with him, so she told him, "We cannot continue with this relationship. She's got to come home."

Marcia: And what about your dad? Did he get involved?

Joy: Yeah, he is involved, but not too much. They're together [her parents], but they're not in peace. They're having problems, and she [her mom] does not want to see me go through that. Even before I got married, she refused the idea. She said, "No!" Even my dad said no, because my dad doesn't like him. So at first, neither of them wanted me to marry. My dad thought I was too young, and my mom didn't want me to pass through the same problems that she had. She wants me to feel loved and at peace in the house. She suspected there would be problems, because she told me that I was being "carried away by love." For my dad, it was about my age. For my mom, it was about me facing the same problems she had. She said, "At least get to know him very well before you marry." We dated two years at least, but she said that not enough time had passed.

When I asked Joy how she had met Kenneth, she told me she had seen him in a movie rental shop and had felt an overwhelming physical attraction to him. At that very moment, Kenneth opened the door to the interview room. He was a stocky, muscular man, which was apparent because both he and Joy were wearing Nike exercise clothes. The couple had joined a gym in Dubai after Dr. Pankaj had told Joy that she needed to lose some weight. Like so many other women in my study, Joy had PCOS, which was evident in her spotty complexion and facial hair. Yet Dr. Pankaj had been the first to make a medical diagnosis of her condition. The many doctors she had visited in Nigeria had never suspected PCOS.

Kenneth dominated the remainder of the interview. He had much to say about the poor quality of Nigerian medical care and why he had decided to pursue IVF in the Emirates:

Kenneth: According to my doctor in Nigeria, IVF sometimes fails. Is that true?
Marcia: Yes.
Kenneth: They do it in Nigeria, but I don't trust them. Why don't I trust them? Well, when it is your own country, you know how it is there. If there is no guarantee of success and if they are not giving you any guarantee that this IVF will work, they will definitely not tell you straight. Most of the Nigerian doctors are smart, but their problem is that they don't tell you, "This is what's wrong with you. This causes those things." This is wrong. Not enough information is given. There is no health education. They just place you on drugs. So I have no confidence there. It's better here, even though it's cheaper there. In Nigeria, IVF will cost a maximum of $3,000. But here, it's closer to $5,000. For someone to lose that kind of money if IVF fails, it's a big loss. It's one year of my salary! I make $5,000 and that is considered "very big money" in my country. So $5,000 can change somebody's life.

Another problem is that some professionals, some hospitals in Nigeria, are not honest. We Africans, we—sometimes in medical treatment, we use fake drugs, you know? Even if I am treated in a hospital and given a prescription, I will have no clue if it is a fake prescription drug or not. I cannot get the original brand. This is a complicated problem, and the government can't control it, because Nigeria is a big country. It's hard to fight. So that's why we travel. We have no trust in the medical system in Nigeria, including the drugs. That's the main problem. We don't know where they get these medicines. When you see the names on the bottles, you don't know. Somebody can enter his bedroom and manufacture drugs!
Marcia: So this is why you came to Dubai?

Kenneth: It's not only that. Dubai is also a place where you can get a visa easily. You can get it through an agency in Nigeria. Nigeria has a good relationship with the UAE, because Nigeria is the biggest, most populated country in Africa. If Nigerians need goods, they now come to Dubai to get their goods. We have a good business relationship here. So because of that, you can get a visa very easily. It's very hard to get a visa to Germany, Britain. Do you know, to get a European visa, it takes up to $5,000? They make papers at travel agencies. But to get a European visa in Nigeria, you can spend that amount and still not get a visa. This money goes to Nigerian agents and sub-agents, and they can scam you. But this country [the UAE] is a tourist country. They give tourist visas and visitors' visas, so there are many foreigners coming here. Some are medical foreigners like us. And there are medical professionals from many countries—India, America, Britain. We've seen them in the Indian hospital, the American hospital, the Canadian hospital. We've been to all those hospitals. Most of the hospitals in Dubai are not managed by Dubai citizens. They're foreign physicians, like Canadians and British, so we feel more trust over here. I don't play with my life! If I have any health problem, I have to go to the best place. Every person has health problems, and so now we come here for checkups. And if one of these hospitals sends an invitation letter to me in Nigeria, I'll be able to get a visa, maybe to the US! If my wife is pregnant, I would like my wife to deliver in the US. I want my child to be a US citizen. Most of my friends' wives delivered in the US for that reason.

Marcia: Really?

Kenneth: Yes, my friends got visas because they are connected. If I get an invitation letter from a US hospital, after getting an IVF pregnancy, or if she goes to London and gets a baby, and if we apply from there for a US visa, I think she can get it. I want the baby to be a British citizen or a US citizen. But you know, Canada, the US, Britain, it is difficult to get a visa from Nigeria, unless you have a contact or connection.

Marcia: Do you have a tourist or visitor's visa here?

Kenneth: It is not a tourist visa, because those are only two weeks. It's a visitor's visa for three months. We told Dr. Pankaj that we're under time pressure. I took a permission [leave] from work, and we came here on a three-month visa. So he's rushing a little bit just to help us.

Indeed, Dr. Pankaj was trying to do everything in his power to treat Joy's PCOS and undertake an IVF cycle within the duration of the couple's three-month visa. During those three months, I followed Joy's progress. Her diagnostic hysteroscopy had gone well, showing that a small, benign fibroid tumor was growing on the outside of her uterus and would not interfere with an IVF pregnancy. Dr. Pan-kaj was satisfied with their combined efforts—insulin medication and weight loss—to get Joy's PCOS under control. Thus, Joy was being prepared for her first IVF cycle. Happy with this turn of events, Joy underwent a makeover, having long, braided extensions added to her hair. Always happy to see me, she asked for me each time she entered the clinic.

My final visit with Joy occurred on the day of her egg collection. I stopped by her bedside several times to see how she was feeling. She had had fifteen eggs retrieved—a significant "harvest," because she was so young and had re-sponded well to the hormonal stimulation of her ovaries. I also saw Kenneth, who told me that they planned to remain in Dubai until they knew the results of Joy's pregnancy test.

I never saw Joy and Kenneth again, as I was about to leave for America. But I learned from the clinic that Joy was pregnant with twins—news that came as a relief but was also deeply unsettling. All I could hope for was that Joy's now high-risk twin pregnancy would go smoothly, that she would deliver healthy babies, and that those babies would somehow stabilize her troubled marriage—bringing to an end the anger, the social torment, and the physical abuse.

RESTRICTIONS
Religious Bans and Law Evasion

The Clinic Wars

When I arrived at Conceive in January 2007, I had no idea that 2006 had been a year of great turmoil and strife for the clinic. The trouble had actually begun at the end of 2005—on December 26, to be exact. A physician working at one of the Emirates' government in vitro fertilization (IVF) clinics had appeared as a guest on a local Arabic talk radio show. In response to a caller's question, the physician encouraged infertile Arab couples to attend only government IVF clinics, because the private sector, the physician claimed, was engaged in "foul play." In early 2006, the government's English-language newspaper followed up with an article, based on an interview with the same physician, who made very specific allegations. Dr. Pankaj and Conceive's staff were accused of engaging in illicit practices, primarily the unscrupulous "freezing and mixing" of gametes and embryos. The newspaper claimed that Conceive had been shut down by the Abu Dhabi Ministry of Health (MOH). Infertile couples were thus encouraged to seek treatment elsewhere, ideally in the public IVF sector.

None of these allegations were true, but the impact on Conceive was almost immediate. Worried patients began phoning the clinic, some canceling their appointments, but most simply wanting reassurance that the clinic was still open for business. The clinic never shut its doors, but it was prevented from accepting new patients until the MOH had assessed the situation. On March 8, 2006, a team of MOH personnel showed up on

Conceive's doorstep. For an entire day, they investigated the clinic, inspecting the ways in which gametes and embryos were handled in the IVF laboratory and scanning patients' medical files to look for signs of illicit gamete or embryo donation practices. Because no evidence of "foul play" could be detected, the government inspectors cleared Conceive of any wrongdoing and eventually allowed the clinic to take on new patients. By January 2007, when I arrived at the clinic, Conceive was back to normal and was busier than ever. Still, the clinic's staff members had been badly shaken by what they perceived as a vicious and premeditated attack on their professional ethics.

Conceive's chief embryologist at the time—a Sunni Muslim Palestinian woman, who was widely admired by patients of all faiths for playing a recording of soothing Qur'anic verses in the IVF laboratory—described the chain of events as "the war that was waged against us." Becoming tearful, she recounted her war story in this way:

> Last year was awful—*awful*! Our competitors gave us hell, or as we say in Arabic, "There can be no smoke without a fire." [The accusing physician] said that we were doing illegal things, and other clinics as well. She accused *all* the private centers of "foul play." But then came the personal attack. She attacked us and mentioned Dr. Pankaj by name. When they mention rapists and thieves in the newspapers here, they only use their initials! But *my name*, Dr. Pankaj's name, and the clinic were *named* in the newspaper! And they said the clinic was closed. People started calling and asking, "How do I know you didn't do anything wrong?" To be accused of something that you didn't do is so unfair. Especially this issue of freezing. They said something about us taking frozen embryos and giving them to someone else. This was *awful*! So evil. So the inspectors interrogated me about this for several hours, even though it was clear that they didn't understand everything I said. It was such a bad experience. You have no idea how much I cried last year. I was crying and telling the patients, "Okay, if you suspect us, do DNA testing! If you suspect us, do this testing to be clear. You don't have *anything* to worry about!" One of my patients came and said to me, "I heard Dr. Pankaj is using his own sperm." The poor guy—Dr. Pankaj. He doesn't even have time to scratch his own head! This horrible person [who launched the attack] is just trying to harm him, to put him in prison, or to get him kicked out of the country. And we couldn't do anything—we didn't even get the chance to hit back. We just had to

sit and wait until the government inspection was done. But after that, we got *more* patients coming, *more* business than before. And I think that God made this happen to us to fill *all* the gaps in our system. To make patients sign off on *everything*! We have to protect ourselves. We filled *all* the gaps to protect ourselves from this point on.

As suggested in this embryologist's recounting, the "clinic war" of 2006 had multiple motivations. On the one hand, public allegations made by one doctor against another suggest a lack of professional medical ethics in a country where competition between clinics can become quite aggressive, even malicious. Several private IVF clinicians I interviewed in 2007, including Dr. Pankaj, blamed the clinic war on a prevailing lack of medical ethics and "fear-mongering" in the country. Dr. Pankaj stated: "The kind of mentality and behavior here, well, there is very little ethical medicine in the UAE. I think powerful people in the country are misleading the authorities. 'We don't know what's happening in private clinics. We don't know if they're using donor sperm and donor eggs.' That sort of rubbish. People in positions who are not medically qualified to know, but have a vested interest, are spreading these kinds of rumors. Most physicians here are only out to make a fast buck."

What Dr. Pankaj left unspoken in his succinct assessment of the situation was that professional envy had also come into play. In Middle Eastern cultural terms, the personal accusations against Dr. Pankaj were a clear manifestation of *hasad*—the envy that is both powerful and inherently harmful.[1] Hasad, often translated as the "evil eye," is mentioned in the Qur'an as a source of great division and misfortune. Thus, protecting oneself against hasad, often by placing small amulets on one's person and possessions, is widely practiced across the Middle East, including among physicians, who often post protective amulets in their clinics.[2] Dr. Pankaj, of course, did not hail from the Middle East and clearly carried out his clinical duties with little concern about hasad. Yet, according to other clinicians, his success as an IVF physician in the Emirates was a source of great envy. Widely viewed as the "father of IVF" in the country and praised extensively by his patients in their global chat rooms, Dr. Pankaj had managed to build up the nation's busiest IVF private practice in only two years. Thus, the envy of a jealous competitor was likely behind the attack of hasad, which—had it played out differently—could have destroyed Dr. Pankaj's reputation, his clinical practice, and his livelihood, and even landed him in prison.

The clinic war, I argue, also involved other deep-seated cultural mores—namely, the belief in "rightful" and "wrongful" practices, which are a guide to daily living in Muslim societies. In the Islamic religious tradition, certain practices are *halal*—that is, morally acceptable and lawful. Practices that are *haram* are morally unacceptable, forbidden, and unlawful. The notion that some practices are haram carries great moral weight in the daily lives of practicing Muslims. For example, drinking alcohol, eating pork, and engaging in nonmarital sexual activity are all considered haram—acts or behaviors that are considered both sinful and un-Islamic.

The clinic war of 2006 involved an implicit accusation that something haram had taken place at Conceive and in other private IVF clinics in the country. Suggestions of "foul play" and "illegal practice"—especially the "freezing and mixing" of couples' gametes and embryos—were serious moral allegations. This is because IVF is allowed in the Sunni Islamic tradition only if it occurs between a husband and wife, using their own gametes. "Mixing" of gametes and embryos—either intentionally or by mistake—has thus been a major moral concern ever since the first IVF clinics opened in the Sunni-dominant countries of Egypt, Jordan, and Saudi Arabia. Ebrahim Moosa, an Islamic legal scholar, explains the concern over mixing in this way: "In terms of ethics, Muslim authorities consider the transmission of reproductive material between persons who are not legally married to be a major violation of Islamic law. This sensitivity stems from the fact that Islamic law has a strict taboo on sexual relations outside wedlock (*zina*). The taboo is designed to protect paternity (i.e., family), which is designated as one of the five goals of Islamic law, the others being the protection of religion, life, property, and reason."[3]

This concern over improper "transmission of reproductive material between persons who are not legally married" refers to what in Arabic is called *ikhtilat al-ansab* (mixture of genealogical relations). In my own discussions over the years with hundreds of Sunni Muslim IVF patients, such a mixture of relations is deemed to be haram, or morally unacceptable, for three important reasons. First, mixing gametes is seen as tantamount to adultery, by virtue of introducing the reproductive substance of another person into the sacred union between a husband and wife, even if no physical contact with the gamete donor has taken place. Second, mixing gametes creates the future potential for half-sibling incest, if the biological offspring of a single gamete donor should happen to meet and marry. Finally, mixing gametes confuses lines of kinship, descent, and inheritance. For Muslim men in particular, ensuring paternity and the "purity" of lineage through "known fathers" is of paramount concern, given that nearly all Muslim societies are organized patrilineally. Thus, preserving a child's genealogical origins (*nasab*) is considered not only an ideal in Islam, but also a moral imperative. The problem with gamete mixing is that it destroys a child's nasab, or known connection to its biological parents, which is considered immoral, in addition to being psychologically devastating for the child. Such a child would be deemed illegitimate and stigmatized in the wider society, and even its own parents might lack the appropriate parental sentiments toward it.[4]

Given this strong moral opposition to gamete mixing, all forms of third-party reproductive assistance—including sperm donation, egg donation, embryo donation, and surrogacy[5]—are considered haram, or explicitly forbidden in the dominant Sunni branch of Islam. This prohibition against third-party reproductive assistance has been carefully spelled out in numerous Sunni Muslim fatwas on IVF, including the initial, highly authoritative fatwa issued from Egypt's renowned religious university, Al Azhar, in 1980. This anti-donation position has been upheld repeatedly over the ensuing decades. For example, at the ninth Islamic law and medicine conference held in Casablanca, Morocco, in 1997 and sponsored by the Kuwait-based Islamic Organization for Medical Sciences, a landmark, five-point declaration prohibited all situations in which a third party invades a marital relationship through donation of reproductive material.[6] Coupled with numerous anti-donation fatwas, this bioethical declaration has served as a powerful ban on third-party reproductive assistance across the Sunni Muslim world, stretching from Morocco to Indonesia.[7] As a result, in Sunni-dominant countries such as Egypt, Saudi Arabia, Turkey, Pakistan, and Malaysia, IVF clinics simply do not offer third-party reproductive services to their patients. Furthermore, the vast majority of Sunni Muslims—who account for approximately 80–90 percent of the world's 1.6 billion Muslims—never consider undertaking such third-party donation practices, because they regard these practices as inherently haram.

Given the strength of this religious ban, the accusation that frozen embryos and gametes were being illegally mixed at Conceive and other private IVF centers in the Emirates was a particularly grave moral accusation. Not only is such mixing haram, but according to the accuser, in this case it was premeditated and allegedly taking place in private clinics without the prior knowledge or consent of patients. Children conceived through such ethical malfeasance would be *biotechnological bastards* of a sort—offspring of unknown parentage, conceived through technological misconduct. Intentional medical malpractice of this kind would be considered unethical in any part of the world, not only in the Sunni Muslim countries of the Middle East. This helps to explain why, during the midst of the clinic war, patients from many countries called Conceive, worried that something morally and ethically wrong had taken place in its IVF laboratory.

In the end, the moral battle subsided once the Abu Dhabi–based MOH cleared Conceive of any wrongdoing. The involvement of the MOH was critical, not only in settling the dispute but also in foreshadowing a new period of clinic regulation in the country. In the next section of this chapter, I examine the unique legal history of IVF in the Emirates—a country that slowly shifted from being the most "permissive" to the most "restrictive" country in the Arab world regarding IVF. This process, which I call *legal devolution*, took place over two decades and resulted in the passage of one of the world's strictest assisted reproduction laws. This law has forced some IVF patients to flee the Emirates, a form of law evasion that has reversed the normal pattern of incoming reproflows to Dubai. In addition, the law has led to a number of unforeseen gender consequences, including the fragmentation of women's medical care, increased physical risks for women, and a new pattern of gender selection involving clear-cut discrimination against daughters.

Legal Devolution in the Emirates

As should be apparent by now, the UAE is an exceptional nation on many levels. But in the world of assisted reproduction, it is unique: it is *the* only Sunni Muslim country in the world where sperm and egg donation were once regularly practiced. This little-known fact about the UAE makes it a true regional aberration. Furthermore, and quite ironically, third-party reproductive assistance services were offered at the main Emirati government IVF clinic! The question, of course, is how did this happen? How did the Emirates somehow fail to abide by the religious ban on reproductive assistance, and especially in a state-run IVF clinic? The answer lies in the medical cosmopolitanism of the Emirates and its neocolonial ties to the United Kingdom. As noted in chapter 1, a well-known and senior British IVF physician was imported by the UAE government to help found the first Emirati IVF clinic in Dubai's main government hospital. He did so by shuttling back and forth between Dubai and his bustling London IVF practice. He, in turn, convinced Dr. Pankaj to move from the United

Kingdom to the Emirates, along with an international team of nurses, embryologists, and clinic administrators. Once the team was established, the senior British physician ended his commuting relationship with the clinic, but Dr. Pankaj remained in Dubai, serving as the government clinic's deputy director from 1991 to 2004.

From the beginning, the government IVF clinic was a British import, practicing assisted reproduction according to British standards. As shown in chapter 2, it charged high prices, equivalent to those found in London's exclusive Harley Street. Given its location in Dubai, it served a cosmopolitan clientele, including many British and other European expatriate couples living in the Emirates. And, as one would expect in Britain, it offered a full range of IVF services, including third-party gamete donation. As a result, infertile male patients without viable sperm could import donor sperm via international couriers from sperm banks in London, Scandinavia, or India.[8] Infertile women—including many professional women who had aged out of their fertility—were allowed to bring their own "known donors" to the clinic, either family members or friends who were willing to undergo egg harvesting. Although surrogacy was rare, the Dubai government IVF clinic was otherwise the equivalent of a London IVF center. It served an international clientele, and it enjoyed a monopoly in Dubai because the local health authority, called the Dubai Department of Health (DOH), refused to grant licenses for non-Emirati IVF practitioners to open private clinics in the emirate.

At the outset, no one seemed to question what was going on in the government facility, which openly offered its third-party reproductive donation services to its non-Muslim patients. Hindu couples from South Asia and Christian couples from Europe and America freely requested sperm and egg donation services at the clinic. For the clinic's British team, such services were considered a routine part of IVF service. For Dr. Pankaj—who was trained in Britain, who routinely attended conferences in the United States, and who hailed from "donor-permissive" India—the use of donor technologies was a normal part of IVF practice, especially in a busy global reprohub. Furthermore, as a Hindu, Dr. Pankaj considered third-party reproductive assistance to be morally acceptable. As he explained, an ancient Hindu epic provided compelling religious justification for both reproductive donation and cloning. "Perhaps this is why *everything* is allowed in India," he said to me. "Surrogacy, egg donation, sperm donation, embryo donation—with absolutely no hang-ups! In fact, donor insemination is part of the Hindu tradition. There is a very nice movie playing now, in Hindi, about donor insemination. So, for Hindus, this is *not* an issue. Even Indian Muslims are more laid back. Some are actually doing it."

Having said this, Dr. Pankaj was quick to point out that the UAE was not the same as India, despite the Emirates' large South Asian population. While he was still working at the Dubai government's IVF clinic in the 1990s, Dr. Pankaj had observed the increasing "disquiet among the local population" regarding the use of donor technologies. Although all Muslim patients were deemed ineligible for third-party donation, many of the Emirati and other Arab patients coming to the clinic began to object to the third-party gamete donation services that were available, as did some of the clinic's Muslim staff members. As a result, by 1998, the DOH had effectively suspended third-party donation in the clinic, insisting that the clinic's bank of donor gametes and embryos be destroyed. This marked the end of Dubai's seven-year "permissive" period. From that point on, IVF in the Emirates would be conducted according to Sunni Islamic guidelines. These guidelines would be enforced through a new phase of government surveillance—not only in Dubai's government IVF clinic, but also in the private IVF sector that was now booming in the neighboring emirates of Abu Dhabi and Sharjah.

Dr. Pankaj was a part of the changes taking place. In 2004, he left the government clinic to open Conceive, locating it 50 meters across the Dubai border in order to avoid Dubai's ban on private IVF clinic construction. Sensitive to neighboring Sharjah's more conservative religious environment, Dr. Pankaj was careful to avoid offering any IVF services that would be considered haram by Muslims.[9] Most importantly, Conceive never offered third-party reproductive assistance. In addition, a form of selective abortion called multifetal pregnancy reduction (MFPR), which is used to "reduce" high-risk IVF pregnancies with three or more fetuses, was never offered at Conceive, as I will discuss below.

With the move over the border to Sharjah, Conceive was under different government jurisdiction. Dubai had its own DOH, but the Abu Dhabi–based MOH was charged with overseeing clinic licensing and policy in the other six emirates. By the time I arrived at Conceive in January 2007, the MOH was in high gear. A national MOH committee had been formed to develop federal guidelines on IVF in the Emirates. The committee consisted of politicians from the UAE's Federal National Council; Muslim clerics from the UAE's main fatwa-granting institution; lawyers from the UAE Court of Justice; two IVF physicians, one of whom was Arab but practiced in the United States; and a representative from Dubai's DOH. By the time I left Conceive in July 2007, the committee had already drafted a federal law on IVF, which was being vociferously debated in the Federal National Council (FNC), one of the UAE's main governing bodies. Two key points of disagreement involved whether to allow embryo freezing, and whether all IVF clinics must include Muslim physicians on their staffs. In a heated debate on the floor of the FNC, the UAE's minister of health argued that science and medicine "have no religion."[10] As he put it, "IVF centres were set up and excelled in non-Muslim countries. The UAE constitution does not discriminate against any citizen on religious grounds."[11] Similarly, the UAE's minister of state criticized the requirement for Muslim physicians as "uncivilized and not keeping in line with the UAE's progress in all fields."[12] This "progressive" viewpoint was not shared by most FNC members, who nonetheless agreed that the MOH should be left to deal with this matter during clinic licensing.

As a non-Muslim IVF practitioner, Dr. Pankaj might have been expected to be offended by this attempt to discriminate on religious grounds. Instead, he was both sanguine and relieved that a law was finally being passed. As he explained to me in mid-2007: "At the moment, there are zero regulations. But the Ministry of Health is developing guidelines, and they're approaching a very advanced stage in the cabinet. Actually, this is being *legislated*, and the reason why this is happening is me! Last year, they were here, and they came to shut me down. But once they found nothing wrong, the ministry said that they would draw up guidelines. I am *very* happy about this, because I think these guidelines will be good."

Over a three-year period, from 2007 to 2009, the MOH worked out its comprehensive IVF legislation. Drafted in 2008 and amended through a cabinet resolution in 2009, Federal Law No. 11—"in connection with the fertilization centers in the State"—was officially enacted in early 2010,[13] and was signed by all seven emirs of the confederation.[14] Most importantly, Federal Law No. 11 is one of very few assisted reproduction laws in the Middle East. Of the twenty-two Middle Eastern nations, only six—Algeria, Iran, Israel, Tunisia, Turkey, and the UAE—have enacted such legislation.[15] Three of these countries (Iran, Israel, and Turkey) are not Arab, and two of the Arab countries (Algeria and Tunisia) are in North Africa. Thus, the UAE is the sole Arab nation in the heart of the Middle Eastern region to pass an assisted reproduction law. Egypt, Jordan, and Saudi Arabia—the first three Sunni Muslim countries to open IVF clinics—have never passed such legislation,[16] relying instead on fatwa guidelines, which, although religiously authoritative, are not legally binding.[17]

Quite significantly, the UAE's Federal Law No. 11 can be described as one of the most comprehensive, but also one of the most draconian, assisted reproduction laws in the world. It describes how IVF clinics are to be set up, licensed, and staffed. It provides details about how medical records are to be kept, lab data entered, and pregnancies monitored to determine clinical success rates. Prices are to be displayed clearly in both English and Arabic. Waiting rooms and bathrooms are to be clearly marked and segregated by gender, with no pornography (which is illegal in most Arab countries) to be placed in the men's bathrooms where semen collection takes place. Couples coming to a clinic for treatment must bring valid passports or identity cards, a marriage license, and a photo of each spouse and must submit to testing for both hepatitis and HIV.

Beyond these general requirements of clinic comportment, Federal Law No. 11 is very specific about which assisted reproduction practices are legally allowed and which are illegal (see table 3.1).[18] Of twenty-two different assisted reproduction procedures, only seven, or approximately one-third, are allowed in the Emirates. Fifteen others are prohibited, including, most notably, cryopreservation (freezing) of embryos; gamete and embryo donation; surrogacy (including by a co-wife within a polygynous union); or any kind of assisted reproduction outside of heterosexual marriage. In addition, embryos are not to be transported across national borders by people employed as embryo couriers.

These prohibitions are completely understandable within the religious and moral environment described above. However, what is highly unusual for the Muslim world is the prohibition against embryo cryopreservation, with the concomitant ban on embryo banking. In no other part of the Sunni Muslim world is it illegal to freeze embryos, assuming that those embryos are legally created using the gametes of a married couple. Cryopreservation of embryos is considered a halal practice, and it is clearly designated as such in a variety of Sunni fatwas on assisted reproduction.[19] Hence, the UAE law prohibiting embryo freezing is particularly restrictive, comparable only to the Vatican-inspired ban on the practice in Italy.[20]

Similar to the Italian law, the UAE law specifies that only "the required number of eggs as necessary for implantation" should be fertilized, to avoid the presence of excess fertilized eggs (that is, embryos).[21] If any

Table 3.1. **The UAE's Assisted Reproduction Law** Permissions and Prohibitions

Procedure	Permitted (halal)	Prohibited (haram)	Comments
Anonymous third-party reproductive assistance		x	
Cryopreservation (freezing) of embryos		x	Only the "required number of eggs" are to be fertilized, but any excess embryos must be left to expire "in a natural manner"; this part of the law is being challenged by physicians and patients as "antiwoman" and thus is being applied differently across the emirates
Cryopreservation of sperm and egg	x		With annual written consent of both husband and wife, for a maximum of 5 years
Donation of embryos		x	
Donation of sperm and egg		x	
Embryo banks		x	The prohibition on cryopreservation of embryos (above) is being applied differently across the emirates
Embryo couriers		x	No frozen embryos delivered to or from the country
Embryo transfers	x		Maximum of 3 embryos into women ≤ 35 and 4 embryos into women > 35
Experimentation on the embryo		x	
Gender selection	x		Purportedly only for sex-linked genetic disorders
Intracytoplasmic sperm injection	x		Using only a married couple's egg and sperm
Intrauterine insemination	x		Same as above
In vitro fertilization (IVF)	x		Same as above
Multifetal pregnancy reduction		x	Not explicitly mentioned in the law, but not practiced in most of the emirates, where abortion is illegal
Polygynous gestational surrogacy		x	With a wife in a polygynous marriage serving as a surrogate for her co-wife
Posthumous insemination		x	After death of a husband or divorce, using cryopreserved sperm

(continued)

Table 3.1. (*continued*)

Procedure	Permitted (halal)	Prohibited (haram)	Comments
Preimplantation genetic diagnosis	x		For genetic screening and "family balancing"
Reproductive cloning		x	Part of a universal ban on this procedure
Same-sex couples using assisted reproductive technology (ART)		x	Marriage of a heterosexual couple is required, with three forms of identification (passport or ID, marriage license, and photos of both spouses)
Single women using ART		x	Same as above
Surrogacy via IVF		x	
Therapeutic stem cell cloning		x	Using stem cells derived from human embryos

Categories of procedures adapted from Jones et al. 2010.

excess fertilized eggs are created, then "the Center shall leave such fertilized eggs without any medical care to terminate the life of such extra eggs in a natural manner."[22] The use of the term "life" in this context is both interesting and important. Whereas the Italian law banning embryo cryopreservation stems from the Catholic belief in "life from the moment of conception," this is not an Islamic viewpoint. Instead, according to the four Islamic *madhabs*, or legal schools, life—that is, ensoulment, or the point at which a conceptus becomes a human person—begins at 40–120 days of gestation.[23] Like Saudi Arabia, the UAE follows the Maliki legal school, which defines ensoulment as occurring at 40 days.[24] Thus, even within the strictest interpretation of Islamic law found in the Arab Gulf, life is not considered to exist in embryos before 40 days. Therefore, freezing embryos has never been a point of moral contestation for Islamic religious authorities in either the Gulf or other parts of the Muslim world.

Given that embryo freezing is considered halal, the UAE's legal prohibition on this practice seems to have arisen from a different motivation—namely, the 2006 allegation that frozen embryos were being "mixed" without patients' prior knowledge or consent. Outlawing embryo freezing, then, was the UAE's attempt to prevent embryo and gamete mixing, which could be viewed as a positive step for patients' rights. However, what was not considered in the legal ban on embryo freezing was the detrimental effect on women's health. If a woman has excess frozen embryos, she can use them in a future "frozen cycle," which involves the simple transfer of the embryos back into her uterus via a catheter inserted through the vagina.[25] If there are no frozen embryos in storage, then a woman must repeat an entire IVF cycle each time she hopes to conceive—either because her previous IVF cycles have failed, or because she hopes to have another child. Repeating a full cycle of IVF includes costly and potentially risky hormonal stimulation, ultrasound scanning of the ovaries, egg harvesting under general anesthesia, and embryo transfer, which together costs at least $5,000. A ban on embryo freezing, then, effectively increases the cost to patients, increases the risk to women's health, and primitivizes the assisted reproduction process overall by disallowing an important health practice that is widely permitted around the world, including the rest of the Muslim world.

In a follow-up interview on June 9, 2012, I asked Dr. Pankaj how the embryo freezing ban was playing out in his clinic, and he replied:

> This is a big headache for us. When the law came out, the ban on embryo freezing was justified by a "mix-up of lineages." We stopped freezing but were given six months to dispose of embryos in storage. Then there was another six-month extension, and a third extension of six months. Meanwhile, I was aware that there was some lobbying among the senior ruling family members in the Ministry of Health in Abu Dhabi. They were considering whether this law is "anti-woman." If we are not able to freeze embryos, then men with poor semen samples can just give another sample on the second cycle. But a woman has to go through the entire IVF procedure again. Honestly, for us, it was more lucrative, because we had to do more cycles and no freezing. But it was heartbreaking to have to dispose of wonderful, five-day blastocysts [highly developed embryos] that couldn't be frozen. These ruling family members must have had some influence, because in August 2011 the ministry told all clinics that we could start freezing again.

For now, the MOH has imposed a legal moratorium of sorts; thus, the twelve IVF clinics operating in Sharjah and Abu Dhabi are still allowed to freeze embryos. In Dubai, however, the DOH strongly upholds the ban on embryo freezing in both its public and private IVF clinics. This apparent divergence in law enforcement between the MOH and DOH is a manifestation of *legal devolution*, a process of decentralization that is a regular feature of statecraft in the Emirates.

In legal theory, devolution refers to the statutory transfer of legal authority, power, or duties from the central government of a sovereign state to the regional, state, or local level.[26] Sometimes called *devolution of authority* or *devolution of power*, this process allows territories (in this case, emirates) to make national legislation relevant to their own areas. Legal devolution is regularly practiced in the UAE, with each emirate retaining a significant degree of control over its own internal affairs. Thus, enactments of national legislation can take quite different forms.

Although Federal Law No. 11 was intended for all seven emirates, legal devolution has diversified the law's effects, which have played out quite differently in the hands of different local health authorities. Whereas the DOH continues to prohibit embryo freezing in Dubai, the MOH has allowed freezing for emirates under its jurisdiction. Having dealt with both health authorities, Dr. Pankaj summed up the differences between the two in this way, "The Ministry of Health assumes people are good, whereas the Dubai Department of Health assumes that people are not to be trusted. They are two different bodies."

Although legal devolution has traditionally referred to the transfer of state power "down" to the local level—for example, to two different Emirati health authorities—the downward trajectory of legal devolution could also be viewed in terms of retrogression, or of things getting worse over time. I suggest that this kind of retrogressive legal devolution has occurred in the Emirates over the past twenty years.[27] Practices that were once openly offered and desperately desired by a globally diverse group of infertile patients have gradually been delegitimized, controlled, and then banished in the Emirates, sometimes with little moral (that is, Islamic) justification. Retrogressive legal devolution of this kind has proved extremely difficult for the thousands of non-Muslim IVF patients living in or traveling to the Emirates in the hope of obtaining the IVF services they need. Once they arrive, they discover a legal environment in which many potential assisted reproductive choices are greatly constrained. For many such repro-travelers, this conservative reproductive regime is oddly out of sync with the Emirates' progressive image, including its attempt to attract a globally sophisticated and cosmopolitan clientele to a bustling medical hub.

The Prohibitive Approach

Because of retrogressive legal devolution, the Emirates must now be described as having a *prohibitive approach* to assisted reproduction.[28] According to the IVF legal scholar Richard Storrow, countries may adopt one of four possible legal approaches to assisted reproduction, including *laissez-faire* (as in the United States), *liberal regulatory* (as in the United Kingdom, Spain, and the Netherlands), *cautious regulatory* (as in Denmark, Sweden, Norway, and France), or *prohibitive* (as in Italy, Germany, and Austria).[29] The UAE clearly falls into this latter category and shares its status with Italy, which is widely considered to be the most restrictive reproductive regime in Europe.[30] Storrow notes that prohibitive countries are characterized by bans—for example, on gamete donation, preimplantation genetic diagnosis (PGD), or embryo cryopreservation.[31] As shown in table 3.1, the UAE not only bans two of these three procedures, but many other practices as well. In short, what was once the most IVF-permissive nation in the Middle East has now become one of the most IVF-restrictive nations in the world—making it a kind of legal outlier within the region.

Nonetheless, the UAE is not alone; many other nations have also enacted restrictive IVF legislation. As of 2010, 43 of the 107 countries (42 percent) surveyed by the International Federation of Fertility Societies had passed assisted reproduction laws.[32] Twenty-seven of these 43 countries (56 percent) were in Europe. Among the large group of European nations, no two were exactly alike in the scope or character of their legal statutes. As the Belgian bioethicist Guido Pennings observed, "the most noticeable characteristic of the legal situation in Europe regarding medically assisted reproduction is the enormous variety of rules. It is hard to find two countries with the same rules regarding a topic like embryo research or donor insemination. Moreover, there has been a rapid evolution of the law and regulation of medically assisted reproduction in the last 15 years."[33] As a result, neighboring European countries have different laws regarding, inter alia, age cutoffs (an issue especially relevant to older women); patients' freedom from diseases and disabilities (for example, HIV infection); whether people using assisted reproduction must be married and cannot be gay; third-party reproductive assistance, including whether gamete donation, embryo donation, and surrogacy can be practiced and whether it can be anonymous; the maximum number of embryos that can be fertilized and/or transferred to a woman's uterus, and whether any excess embryos can be frozen; whether PGD can be used for genetic screening, gender selection of embryos, or both; whether embryos can be used for research and/or therapeutic stem cell cloning; and whether selective abortion can be performed in high-order IVF pregnancies with multiple fetuses.[34]

Given the great variability that exists within Europe, the IVF landscape there is said to be a *legal mosaic*, or a "patchwork" of "restrictive" and "permissive" countries.[35] For example, in Northern Europe, Austria, France, Germany, Great Britain, Norway,[36] Sweden, and Switzerland have enacted strict legislation prohibiting some or all forms of gamete donation, especially anonymous gamete donation, and surrogacy.[37] In Southern Europe, Spain prohibits surrogacy, although it actively promotes gamete donation; Italy prohibits surrogacy and embryo cryopreservation; and France allows anonymous gamete donation but prohibits gay couples and single men and women from accessing assisted reproduction.[38] Such restrictions have triggered European reprotravel on a massive scale, with patients from more restrictive countries traveling to more permissive countries.[39] In Western Europe, more liberal reproductive regimes exist in Belgium, Cyprus, Denmark, Greece, the Netherlands, and Spain. In Eastern Europe, countries such as Belarus, the Czech Republic, Romania, Slovenia, and Ukraine have either less restrictive guidelines or no relevant laws at all. Thus, as noted by Storrow, clinics in the former Soviet bloc can "employ the Internet to attract fertility tourists with promises of cut-rate in vitro fertilization, high success rates, liberal reproductive policies and little administrative oversight."[40]

In an attempt to ameliorate this situation, calls have been made in the European Union (EU) for so-called *legal harmonization* of assisted reproduction across the continent.[41] However, given the different religious and moral valences underlying individual countries' IVF laws, such harmonization is extremely unlikely. Pennings, who has written prolifically and persuasively on this topic, argues that attempts at harmonization might end up leading to more restrictive legislation, with majority blocs imposing their wishes on minority EU members.[42] In his view, the easiest way to eliminate a substantial portion of reprotravel within Europe would be to abolish all forms of restrictive and coercive legislation and to adopt a "soft law" approach, which would focus on issues of safety and good clinical practice. The latter approach, sometimes called *harm reduction*, appears to be gaining ground. For example, in 2010 an International Forum on Cross-Border Reproductive Care was held, emphasizing that quality and safety should be the key considerations among IVF physicians serving patients who travel for treatment.[43] A year later, the European Society for Human Reproduction and Embryology Cross-Border Reproductive Care Taskforce issued a "good practice guide" for IVF clinicians, with recommendations on how to care for patients seeking IVF across borders.[44]

Law Evasion: The Reproductive Outlaws

Despite these efforts to "soften" the law and increase safety, countries are still free to regulate assisted reproduction as they see fit. In such an inconsistent legal environment, reprotravel across borders is said to function as a "moral safety valve," allowing IVF patients to "evade" or "circumvent" the law.[45] The legal scholar Glenn Cohen calls this kind of law evasion "circumvention tourism," which he defines as "patients who travel abroad for services that are legal in the patient's destination country but illegal in the patient's home country—that is, travel to circumvent domestic prohibitions on accessing certain medical services."[46] According to Cohen, circumventing assisted reproduction laws is one of four main types of cross-border travel, along with circumventing laws that prohibit abortion, prohibit assisted suicide, and accept female genital cutting.

Many scholars have deemed restrictive assisted reproduction laws— and subsequent *law evasion*—to be the single most important factor pushing infertile couples across borders in the world today.[47] Infertile couples who are forced to flee a country, sometimes during difficult moments in an IVF cycle, become *reproductive outlaws*—literally navigating outside of the law to procure the prohibited reproductive procedures that they feel they need and that may also be medically indicated to produce or save an IVF pregnancy.

At Conceive, I met a significant number of reproductive outlaws who were evading various laws. These law evaders fell into three categories, which I will characterize as the *European outlaws*, the *third-party users*, and the *fetal reducers*. In addition, a fourth group, whom I will call the *sex selectors*, were not evading the law per se but were disobeying a religious ban. It is important to note that all of these groups were relatively small in number, but their presence was still noticeable. It is also important to emphasize that these reproductive outlaws considered themselves to be law-abiding citizens. Yet they had been forced to travel, either into or out of the Emirates, to bypass restrictive reproductive legislation or religious bans that they viewed as unjust and even punitive. In some cases, these reproductive outlaws had entered and exited the Emirates several times, while attempting to navigate restrictive laws in more than one country.

EUROPEAN OUTLAWS

Given the great legal variability in Europe described above, it is perhaps not surprising that six couples in my study were traveling to Conceive to bypass particular reproductive restrictions in their home countries. Two couples were German, two were Swedish, and two were from the United Kingdom. They faced four particular legal restrictions back home—age cutoffs, restrictions on how many embryos could be transferred, prohibitions on sperm aspiration, and bans on people with infectious diseases—that did not apply in the Emirates. As shown in table 3.1, UAE's Federal Law No. 11 does not prohibit assisted reproduction for older women, nor does it restrict to one or two the number of embryos to be transferred to a woman's womb. Women over the age of 35 may have four embryos transferred, while younger women may have three. Thus, the law is relatively generous for women facing age-related infertility, who might want to transfer higher numbers of lower-quality embryos to increase their chances of conception. Furthermore, the law does not prohibit azoospermic men (who produce no sperm in the ejaculate) from using intracytoplasmic sperm injection (ICSI). In such cases, sperm can be withdrawn directly from the testicles through two sperm aspiration techniques known as testicular sperm aspiration (TESA) and percutaneous epididymal sperm aspiration (PESA). Both are legal in the Emirates, although they have been outlawed in some Northern European countries (for example, Germany and, formerly, the Netherlands). Finally, some European countries will not permit doctors to perform IVF or ICSI on individuals with serious illnesses or disabilities. In the Emirates, hepatitis (B and C) and HIV are the only two diseases for which screening is required prior to IVF. People who test positive for HIV will not be allowed to undergo assisted reproduction (and, in fact, will quickly be deported back to their home countries).[48] However, hepatitis carriers are not banished and are allowed to undergo IVF and ICSI. Still, for the purposes of infectious disease control, they are not allowed to cryopreserve their embryos.

The story of Ebba, a petite blonde artist from Sweden, illustrates two of these four issues. Ebba was only thirty-two when I met her, and she had been married to her pilot husband, Lars, for five years. Yet during this brief time span, she had endured a host of serious medical problems, including a benign throat tumor; melanoma, which is the most serious form of skin cancer; and a painful case of endometriosis, which had become so severe that she had required emergency laparoscopic surgery in Sweden. Following the operation, the surgeon told Ebba, "In all my life, I don't think I've seen a more difficult case of endometriosis. How could you even stand up with so much pain?" The endometriosis had destroyed Ebba's appendix, and sections of her ovaries had to be removed. Furthermore, at the time of the surgery, blood tests indicated that Ebba was carrying the hepatitis B virus in her body. Having hepatitis made Ebba feel profoundly stigmatized, although Lars tried to lighten her mood by joking, "You never get normal diseases, like the common cold! Each year there is something new, which makes you exciting!" Ebba described to me what it meant to have hepatitis B in Sweden:

I have hepatitis B, probably since birth [through maternal transmission], but you never actually know with chronic hepatitis B. All my blood tests are otherwise good. But that's why I can't do IVF in Sweden. If they see you, they will send you immediately to the infection clinic! It's *very* unusual there, hepatitis B. But here [in the Emirates], it's common. In Sweden, with hepatitis B, they will put me in a special room with special cleaners and five pairs of gloves. They will treat me like I'm coming in with something, I don't know, in a bad way—like you're sharing needles with somebody, even though I did nothing to get this. So this is part of the reason I decided not to have IVF done in Sweden. They *would* do IVF for me [with hepatitis B] in Sweden, but they can't freeze any of my embryos because of the hepatitis. Furthermore, if I have three embryos and all are very good and I want to have them all put back [in my uterus], they wouldn't do it. They can only put one back, by law. It's a new law, and it's very strict. In *very* unusual and difficult cases, they might sometimes put in two, but it's difficult to get that, legally. In my case, I can't really afford to throw away any embryos. Whatever I can get, I don't have the luxury to throw away. I never produce five embryos, and so if I produce three, it's like "Wow! Let's have some champagne!"

Ebba's concern over the fate of her embryos was linked to yet another serious medical condition. When she arrived at Conceive and underwent a thorough evaluation, she learned that she was facing premature menopause, news that she also found devastating. Lars, who had become a "frequent flyer" to Conceive, often could not accompany Ebba to her clinic appointments. Thus, she found herself alone, racing against time, and needing to preserve every viable embryo. Dr. Pankaj supported Ebba's efforts to move quickly. Yet two cycles of ICSI had ended quite badly, as Ebba described to me:

I came here, like two years ago, maybe one and a half years ago. [Dr. Pankaj] examined me, he checked me, and he didn't want me to lose any time by just doing [intrauterine] insemination. I'm *way past that*! I did an ova test, an FSH [follicle stimulating hormone] test, and I'm 11.9 on the scale. I'm like forty to forty-five years old inside. So he said that we need to "get with it; don't lose any time." So I did two trials here with microinjection [ICSI]. I had success on the second trial, but then I had a very early miscarriage—a miscarriage here in the clinic. I had a funny dream the night before that my baby was crawling, looking back at me, and I couldn't get him. He was running away and laughing at me. And then I woke up, very sweaty, and went to the bathroom, and I knew it had happened. I had extra bad pain, and so I came here, and I was sitting in a pool of blood. This much blood [putting her arms out to show me].

Ebba was not the only European woman with a complex medical and reproductive history who believed that legal barriers were preventing her from accessing IVF services back home. For example, Sigrid, a thirty-nine-year-old German schoolteacher, had undergone surgical removal of an ectopic pregnancy three years earlier. Since then, she had not been able to conceive, even with five rounds of IVF. Sigrid and her husband, Thomas, now considered Germany to be out of the question, given that IVF in their country was strictly regulated. So, like many other Germans, they fled to the neighboring Czech Republic, where the assisted reproduction law was "very flexible," according to Sigrid. Yet repeated IVF failures in the Czech Republic made Sigrid and Thomas reconsider their options. Like Ebba, Sigrid's main concern was her advancing age, and the need to use every single viable embryo, as she explained:

It's not so easy in Germany. To prevent any kind of eugenics, they're not allowed to choose which embryos to transfer, and they're not allowed to let the embryos develop for more than two days. So all of the women like me with this problem of age should be allowed to wait a bit longer until their embryos are mature. But they can't. There's a big discussion in Germany right now, with some people arguing that it wouldn't be such a big change to modify this rule. But it's the law in Germany, and it's quite strict, very conservative. Egg donation is also not allowed, even though it could be very helpful for older women. So *a lot* of people like us are going from Germany to other countries.

Among these Germans were infertile men, two of whom I met at Conceive. Both men were azoospermic. In Germany, they were not legally allowed to undergo testicular sperm aspiration. Thus, both men had searched the Internet and had found Dr. Pankaj, who had developed PESA and had written several scholarly articles about this particular sperm aspiration technique. Both men made their way to the Emirates, where they expressed their frustration with Germany and the legal inconsistency of the EU overall. Gottfried, an engineer, complained: "They regulate the size of strawberries in the EU! 'This is the EU standard strawberry.' They regulate how much saturated fat and antibiotics are allowed in meat. And then there's nothing for this! There's no standardization, which is very strange. It's funny considering how liberal they are in Holland, where drugs and prostitution are apparently okay, but not TESA or PESA—at least until about two years ago. In Germany, it's still not allowed, because they worry about using 'immature sperm' [possibly genetically defective] and what this will mean for future generations."[49]

Gottfried had decided to undergo PESA and then store his excess aspirated sperm in a "sperm bank" at Conceive. In actuality, Conceive could not be classified as having a sperm bank. Rather, the clinic was legally allowed under Federal Law No. 11 to cryopreserve semen samples from men such as Gottfried—those facing complex male infertility problems, or those facing cancer who had been advised by their physicians to undergo sperm banking prior to chemotherapy.[50] At the time of my study, embryo freezing was allowed in the Emirates and was being performed regularly at Conceive. Even after the controversial embryo freezing law came into effect in 2010, Conceive and many other IVF clinics under MOH jurisdiction were able to retain their embryo banks. Thus, many European couples who had left their frozen embryos behind at Conceive still had the chance to retrieve them for future frozen cycles.

Nonetheless, issues of embryo disposition—what to do with these excess embryos, left in cold storage in a Muslim country—troubled some of the European couples in my study. Worrying out loud about the fate of their embryos, Jenny and Giles, a British couple, shared their feelings about what Jenny called "those seven little things that belong to me sitting in a lab":

Jenny: I find it very difficult, as an ethical, emotional issue. I don't find it easy. I don't think it's normal. It's a "mind trip" to have seven fertilized eggs. They're a precious thing, life. At the same time, I wouldn't have to go through the process again because they are frozen. But I find it very difficult, I must say, the whole concept of freezing them and leaving them here. They are embryos, and there is no home for them. I don't know.

Giles: We'll take that decision when it happens. I feel pragmatic about the whole thing. It's just science, as far as I'm concerned at this stage. Science and statistics.

Jenny: The statistics are definitely against us at this moment!

Giles: No! Don't be so pessimistic.

A German physicist, Viktor, and his Swedish wife, Annika, who worked in the tourism industry, were about to return to their home in Zurich, Switzerland. Both Viktor and Annika were in their early forties, but they had managed to have only one child, a son, after many years of marriage and five cycles of intrauterine insemination in Munich, Germany. Wanting to make "one last try" for a second child, Viktor and Annika had traveled to Conceive on a friend's recommendation. "We came here to see if something would happen," Annika explained. "But now we're concerned, because we'll be freezing our embryos and then moving back in two weeks. Will it be possible for us to come down [to the Emirates] and do it again? We don't know."

Perhaps the most interesting reflections on embryo disposition came from a Dutch couple, Amalia and Manfred, whose concerns about the fate of their embryos stemmed in part from their experiences in the 2006 clinic war. As a cystic fibrosis carrier, Manfred was born with a congenital absence of the vas deferens, one of the genital vessels required to transport sperm out of the body.[51] Although he produced sperm in his testicles, Manfred definitely needed either TESA or PESA, both of which were legally prohibited in the Netherlands at the time of his diagnosis. Through the Internet, Manfred and Amalia found their way to Conceive. There, Dr. Pankaj performed PESA, and the couple soon became the happy parents of an ICSI daughter. I met Manfred and Amalia at the clinic on their second ICSI attempt. In a vibrant couple's interview, they shared their feelings about the Netherlands versus the Emirates, as well as what it would mean to leave their embryos behind in cold storage:

Marcia: What will happen to your embryos?

Amalia: They will be in the freezer, so that I don't have to go through injections again. I listen to Dr. Pankaj. He is a great and very wise man, and very experienced.

Manfred: And he knows the two of us.

Amalia: We listen to his advice.

Marcia: So what if you still have embryos in the freezer when you go back home?

Amalia: We don't think about that. But they are potentially also children.

Manfred: That's an ethical thing. It will be very hard to decide.

Amalia: We would have to be given a choice.

Manfred: I can already see where your next question is coming [from]! If your embryo is in the freezer, what will you do? Will you donate it?

Amalia: It's illegal. From here, it wouldn't be possible, so they would let it die.

Manfred: I think it will be destroyed.

Amalia: Sperm and egg donation are illegal here. We know that, because that was going to be our only option in Holland. The urologist told us, "You will never be able to conceive. So you only have two options." Actually, *he* didn't spell out these options, but that was our conclusion—adoption or sperm donation.

Manfred: What he *did* do, to give him some credit, was to say, "This is how I diagnosed you now, but this is just a physical inspection. There are ways to inject fluid and do other things to check you, but we don't do them here [in the Netherlands]."

Amalia: But that statement which they made was kind of devastating in our lives.

Manfred: So we began seriously thinking about all those things, adoption or donation. But then we came here, and we learned that donation is illegal.

Amalia: Already, there were rumors. Somebody had been saying that they might have been doing this, and the whole thing would shut down.

Marcia: How did you learn about the rumors?

Amalia: Last year, we read it in the newspaper. It was in the [she named a newspaper].

Manfred: Which is *not* a newspaper! It's just full of happy news, or at least that is how I experience it. So this was very surprising. And then [another newspaper], the daily free newspaper, which takes anonymous complaints, said that Conceive was operating "on the edge of what is allowed here." I can't recall exactly how we saw this, but I think Amalia's obstetrician pointed it out. She told us, "The clinic is fiddling about with the rules. Doing abortions, and such." And she said that all the clinics maybe will be shut down.

Amalia: That was just before I delivered [our daughter]. But I knew that this would *never* happen here! My obstetrician was sure that she was right, and she asked if I had spoken to the doctor [Dr. Pankaj] recently.

Manfred: She said, "There is a big thing going on, and they are shutting down because of rumors."

Amalia: I told my mother, because it could have really affected us. I really believe that this is a *really* good clinic. I'm *really* impressed.

Manfred: We really believed that this was not going to happen, because if it was, we would have expected a phone call [from Conceive]. My stuff [sperm] is still in the freezer! What do you do with it? If they were closing down, it could really hurt everybody.

Fortunately for Manfred and Amalia, who had lived through the unsettling turmoil of 2006, Conceive never shut its doors. Thus, the couple was able to return for a second ICSI attempt in 2007. However, Manfred and Amalia were right in identifying gamete donation and abortion as two illegal procedures in the Emirates. Although they were lucky enough to conceive without third-party assistance—which, in their case, would have involved donor sperm—many other couples may have no other choice but to use donor gametes to achieve an IVF or ICSI pregnancy. When third-party reproductive assistance is needed, couples in the Emirates must make difficult decisions about their next steps.

THIRD-PARTY USERS

In some cases, couples must leave the Emirates to access third-party reproductive assistance. Because of the UAE's Sunni-inspired legal prohibition on third-party gamete donation and surrogacy, a "reverse traffic"—or outbound reproflow of third-party users—has been created. In my study, I met six infertile couples who found themselves on this outbound path. Half of these couples were European or American, and the other half were Indian. All of the European or American couples were in need of donor eggs, because wives in their forties had aged out of their fertility. The Indian couples, in contrast, had a diverse set of infertility problems requiring different solutions—donor eggs for premature menopause, donor sperm for atrophied testicles, lack of spermatogenesis, and resultant azoospermia, and surrogacy for a previously ruptured uterus. Two of the couples requiring donor eggs and donor sperm had already left the country to acquire donor gametes and then had returned to Conceive, where I met them. The rest were in the process of sorting out where to go and what to do—situations that were quite stressful, as will be shown in some of the reprotravel stories that follow the chapter.

For these third-party users, decision making about donors was complicated by being in the Emirates and having to orchestrate outbound reprotravel without any guidance. Following the clinic war of 2006, the staff at Conceive was extremely reluctant to assist reprotravelers who needed gamete donation, for they did not want to appear to be aiding and abetting an illegal process. Indeed, when I asked Dr. Pankaj about donation, he exclaimed, "Donation—we don't even think about it!" Then he added: "It will never happen here. Patients come and ask us, and we say, 'No.' So they ask, 'Where can I do it?' Europeans tend to go to London. Indians go to India. But I don't suggest names, so people have to figure this out on their own."

Interestingly and importantly, only one European in my study, a British lawyer married to a much younger Pakistani Muslim man, said that she was opposed to gamete donation, perhaps out of respect for her husband and his religion. All of the other Europeans, North Americans, and Australians in my study supported the option of third-party reproductive assistance, although most of them had come to Conceive to try IVF or ICSI using their own gametes. For example, Silvija, a Bulgarian woman who was facing premature menopause, was clearly a candidate for egg donation. During our interview, she surprised her husband, Grigor, by bringing up the subject:

Silvija: It was like a joke, but I recently asked my friend, "Why don't you give me a few eggs?" She said, "Of course!" But I don't know if they do it in Dubai.
Marcia: Would you consider it?
Silvija: Yeah. That's the thing. If nothing happened [to get pregnant], I'll ask my sister to give me some eggs, and she would.
Marcia [to Grigor]: Would that be okay by you?
Grigor: This is the first time I heard her say this!
Silvija: Sometimes, there are things you can't discuss easily. But this morning, I was actually thinking about this.
Marcia: Do they do donation in Bulgaria?
Silvija: I know that they do sperm donation in Bulgaria, because I finished medical college, and they used to have this practice in the hospital. So I've seen it, and that was, like, ten years ago. But I wasn't much interested at the time. It was just like blood donation. There was a sperm donation clinic.

Grigor: Everything is common in Bulgaria, just like everywhere else in Europe.

Marcia: And the church doesn't get involved?

Silvija: Still, we're Orthodox, but the church in our country doesn't control much, including people's minds. As far as I know, every time you have a reproductive problem, you'll get support from the church, and they'll tell you that it's your decision at the end of the day. The Catholics are more guided, so it's really difficult for them to take a decision, or they have to go and consult a priest first.

Grigor: Or it could be that the Orthodox church has some views, but we Bulgarians are just not that religious. If we want to do something, we do it!

Despite Silvija's and Grigor's conviction that Catholics were "more guided" by their religion in decisions about IVF and gamete donation, the Catholic couples in my study—who came from a number of European countries, as well as India and the Philippines—had chosen to ignore the Vatican's rulings against assisted reproduction.[52] They were eager to undertake IVF, were supportive of gamete donation, and sometimes noted that religion would have "no effect" on their decisions about assisted reproduction. As one Dutch Catholic man summed it up, "even if the church doesn't approve, we would still go for it. It's our lives."

Like the Europeans and Americans, Indian couples in my study, most of whom were Hindu, also supported gamete donation and surrogacy, often pointing to the rich panoply of third-party services now widely available in India. Only one Hindu woman, an artist in her early forties, said that she was opposed to donation for reasons that were more personal than religious. Most interestingly, several Indian Muslim couples in my study also said that they approved of third-party donation. One of these couples had already tried sperm donation in India several times. These pro-donation stances on the part of Indian couples in my study were widespread. For example, Darpak, an infertile Indian man who had traveled for ICSI to Dubai, said that he was willing to consider sperm donation: "With Hindus, it's no problem! We accept [it] nowadays. So back in India, *many, many* people go for sperm banks. Sperm banks are available there. So if we had needed that, we would *have* to go back to India." Similarly, Anandi, who had come to Dubai with her infertile husband, was proud of India's openness about both sperm and egg donation:

Quite a lot is being done in India. It depends on what kind of situation you are in, but if there is a problem, you *can* use eggs or sperm. There *are* sperm donation and egg donation clinics there, and everything is *very* confidential. It's done in a very high level, and it depends on what is necessary, what kind of treatment is needed. So, in India, we see on TV channels that they're doing this. They're quite open about it. In this country [the UAE], neither can I do gamete donation or adoption. So if we think this is what we need, then we have to go back to our country. We would have to see what is easier and more practical. Here it is *not* done, but both *are* socially acceptable in India.

Another Indian woman, Ekta, had already contemplated becoming an egg donor:

For us, or if somebody else needs, we don't mind donating, not at all. We've heard a lot about this in India, and the surrogacy method is happening as well. So once God will give you children, then, yes, why not give to somebody else who could benefit? Absolutely! It would be like a lift. People who can't afford to go through that, or if there are any problems or infertility issues, like no eggs or what not, then why not? But I would want it to be anonymous from my side, for the mental health of both parties. So they would not feel, "Stay away from her!" "She'll take the baby away from me!" So for the donor to be contacted is really not fair.

Whereas virtually all of the Hindu couples in my study approved of third-party donation and surrogacy, most of the Indian Muslim couples, all of whom were Sunni, disapproved of third-party donation, considering it to be haram. When I asked Muslim couples their views on third-party donation, statements of opposition were often fervent: "I would *never* consider it" and "it is *totally* haram!" For example, Malik, an Indian Muslim man, explained the Sunni opposition to donation in this way:

I don't think these things were there when the Prophet Muhammad was alive 1,400 years ago. So now there are debates on, say, giving blood or not. But both of us feel the same thing. You should *not* take from "outside." There should be *no* artificial donor. The donation is haram. Both donors and surrogate mothers. There was one case where they planted it [the embryo] in the mother-in-law, because they wanted the child to be very closely related. But *not* among Muslims. Muslims in India don't prefer even IUI [intrauterine insemination] or IVF. They're scared, because they think that Islam doesn't allow you to do these things.

Along with the South Asian couples in my study, most of the Middle Eastern and African couples were opposed to donation. For example, a Sudanese man, Karim, had been rendered infertile by cancer chemotherapy. He was coming to Conceive in the hope that a few viable spermatozoa could be retrieved from his testicles. When I asked him whether he would consider sperm donation, he replied: "For I myself, even if it was approved from my religion, I would *not* do it. It won't be my baby. It would be someone else's baby. Sperm donation, this would be like haram. So we don't even think about it! Maybe I would have done some other things, like a testicular biopsy. But to think about other [men's] sperm is prohibited completely. We do not feel optimistic about either sperm or ova donation because of our religion." Similarly, an infertile man from Syria, Firas, had gone to great lengths to ensure that no third-party donation practices were being carried out in Conceive's laboratory:

> I agree with this—no donation in Islam. I'm *sure* they will not use other than my sperm and her egg here. I'm *sure* about this, because I checked, of course. I checked with the [Muslim female] doctor. "What's the environment for the egg after the injection?" What she told me made me more satisfied: "We will keep it in a suitable environment, under the best conditions, and we'll turn on the Qur'an." For me, I just asked about the environment, and this made me have more faith. So I have no doubt. They do not take eggs or sperm from another [person]. And this is logical. How can you take some egg from somebody unless she is your wife? Or the other way. For me, I cannot imagine it. It will not be my son! Not from the husband, the generations. I don't know, but this is my opinion. I will never, never, never, completely never receive or give [our gametes]. This is my own point of view, and my wife's point of view. We cannot share.

Most Muslim women at Conceive were equally adamant in their objections to third-party donation. For example, Hajira, who had debated about whether to pursue IVF in Dubai or in her home country of Pakistan, responded to my question about third-party reproductive assistance in this way:

> That is why we chose Pakistan at first. It's more safe there, because they don't do this "mixing" there. Muslim people are very much worried. That's why most Muslims in Pakistan are not doing IVF. They don't have any knowledge, and on this point, they say, "Maybe the doctor

mixes our sperm or our eggs." And if that happens, it's *totally* haram in Islam! So it's a huge concern. Even when I was going for IVF or for ICSI, I first went to a mullah and asked, "Do we have permission in Islam to do this treatment and take this treatment for our child?" They said, "Yes, no problem, as far as your egg and your sperm will be taken. If it's your husband's sperm, it is permitted. You have permission." So in Islam, it is permitted, but if I take donor sperm or a donor egg, it is *totally* haram. If you talk about haram and halal, there is a big difference.

These Sunni Muslim patients' objections to third-party donation were also clearly linked to the legal and cultural prohibitions against adoption found throughout the Sunni Muslim world.[53] Few of the Sunni Muslim couples in my study would contemplate adopting an orphan, stating with conviction that it is "against the religion." Adopted children and donor children were considered by them to be of the same strange ilk—basically, "somebody else's baby," a "stranger" who "won't be my son."[54] Although adoption was considered to be a viable next step for many of the infertile European and American couples in my study, it was not a popular option among Hindus,[55] and it was rejected out of hand by most of the Muslim couples in my study.

Adoption in the Muslim world is a complex matter, which deserves its own extended discussion.[56] Suffice it to say here that I have spent many hundreds of hours discussing Muslim couples' attitudes toward adoption, including at Conceive. Over the years, I have met only four couples—two Egyptian, one Palestinian, and one Pakistani—who have actually taken legal steps to permanently foster an orphaned child. In the Palestinian case, the child was the husband's infant niece, whose parents had been killed in an auto accident. But the adoptive uncle did not consider the little girl to be his own child, and was therefore seeking ICSI in Beirut in an attempt to overcome his male infertility problem. In short, adoption—as a form of "third-party assistance"—is not a socially, religiously, or legally sanctioned strategy to overcome childlessness in the Muslim world.

Nonetheless, the growing numbers of infertile couples whom I would call *Muslim religious resisters* suggests that the landscape of reproductive donation in the Muslim world may be slowly shifting in the twenty-first century, as more and more infertile Muslims decide to go against the religion in seeking third-party reproductive assistance.[57] For example, in my previous study in Lebanon, I met Muslim religious resisters from several Arab countries who were secretly crossing the border into "liberal" Lebanon to access donor gametes, especially donor eggs.[58] As I noted in the introduction, Iran and Lebanon are the only two Muslim-majority countries in the world that allow third-party reproductive assistance, because of influential Shia fatwas that have condoned both gamete donation and surrogacy. Iran and Lebanon are now receiving inbound reproflows of couples from Arab countries such as the UAE, as well as from the wider Muslim world.

At Conceive, I also met a small group of Muslim religious resisters who were calling into question the dominant Islamic religious narrative that disallows any form of third-party reproductive assistance. Third-party donation, they argued, could be justified on both medical and moral grounds, especially in Muslim societies where childbearing is expected and infertility is thus invariably stigmatized. Most of these Muslim religious resisters were from South Asia, either India or Pakistan. The comments of Ekbal, a Muslim Indian man, were typical of these new sentiments:

> We are Sunni Muslim, but we are very broad-minded, educated. So we have heard of donation. Still, they don't take it in the religion as something acceptable. But, again, this is an emotional, psychological issue, rather than a religious problem. Because you are accepting somebody else's egg, a "stranger's egg." So it's more of a psychological stigma. But it's being done in India. The procedures in India are not as tough as here [legally and religiously]. And in Western developed countries, there are legalities surrounding donation, but less so in India. So if I had a problem with my sperm, I would have this done in India. They do *everything* now in India—or maybe 96 percent, actually. So, I want to have a baby with our "eggs," and I don't mind attempting many times, whatever amount of attempts it takes. But if her egg fails, *only* if her egg fails, then if she likes to do egg donation, I don't want to superimpose [my values].

Firdous, a woman from Pakistan, compared third-party donation to adoption. Although she knew that both paths to parenthood are considered haram in Sunni Islam, she was open to both of these possibilities: "Especially in our culture, your need for children is so much. If they had—if there were donors and surrogacy was allowed in our religion, people would be resorting to it! In Islam, adoption is a big, bad taboo. 'You're adopting? How could you do this?!' So, yes, it's a big taboo. But it hit me, four to five years ago, 'Why not adopt a child?' It started from [my] thinking, 'Why not?'"

Opposition to adoption in the Muslim world may be quite surprising to Westerners, especially when juxtaposed with Muslim attitudes toward abortion. Whereas Westerners seem to accept adoption as a highly valued act of altruism and beneficence, many Christians oppose abortion on deeply felt moral grounds. In the Middle East, however, the opposite could be said to be true: Adoption is automatically rejected as haram, while attitudes toward abortion are far less morally contentious. As noted above, the four Islamic legal schools consider fetal ensoulment to occur at 40–120 days of gestation. Thus, abortion—especially if induced early in a pregnancy—is not considered by many Muslims to be morally repugnant, because abortion does not result in a human life being taken and is therefore not a grave sin.

In this moral milieu, abortions are widely practiced in the Middle East, with one in every ten pregnancies ending in this way.[59] For example, between 1995 and 2000, more than 2 million abortions and approximately 2,500 abortion-related deaths occurred in Egypt alone; nearly 700,000 abortions and 1,000 deaths in Saudi Arabia; and nearly 80,000 abortions and 50 deaths in the UAE.[60] Furthermore, Iran outpaced all of the Arab nations, with its nearly 2.5 million abortions during this five-year period.[61] Despite these high numbers, abortion was illegal in all of these countries. Only Tunisia, Turkey, and Kuwait allow full legal access to abortion.[62] In all other Middle Eastern countries, abortion is criminalized to varying degrees, with the region's abortion laws largely based on outdated, colonial-era, civil codes rather than the moral precepts of Islamic jurisprudence.[63] As a result, thirteen Middle Eastern countries have abortion laws that have been described as "very restrictive"; in these countries, abortion is allowed only in cases in which a pregnant woman's life is in jeopardy.[64]

The UAE's abortion law falls into this "very restrictive" category. Adopted on December 20, 1987, as part of the country's penal code, the law permits abortion to save a woman's life but grants no other exceptions, such as abortion for the purposes of physical or mental health, after rape or incest, because of fetal impairment, or for economic or social reasons.[65] A person who induces an abortion is subject to imprisonment for five years, or for a maximum of seven years if the abortion is performed without the woman's consent. The UAE's approach to abortion, which some reproductive health experts have characterized as "punitive,"[66] poses real problems for IVF clinics in the Emirates. This is because the country's very stringent abortion law conflicts with its assisted reproduction law, the latter of which creates the need for a form of selective abortion known as fetal reduction.

How has this happened? As shown in table 3.1, Federal Law No. 11 allows three or four embryos to be transferred into a woman's uterus depending on a woman's age. According to international experts, the number of embryos transferred is "the principal contributor to the multiple pregnancy rate."[67] Thus, the legally sanctioned transfer of three to four embryos means that many women undergoing IVF in the Emirates end up with multiple-gestation pregnancies. Multiples, especially twins, are often thrilling to IVF patients, who have waited for years to have a baby and desperately desire twins in order to "complete" their families in a single IVF attempt. However, the joy of a multiple pregnancy is often overshadowed by its significant complications. Maternal risks include gestational diabetes, hypertension (including the life-threatening hypertensive condition known as preeclampsia), and postpartum hemorrhage.[68] Infants born as part of a multiple pregnancy are at a greater risk of prematurity, low birth weight, chronic lung disease, cerebral palsy, a range of cognitive delays, and higher rates of perinatal death.[69] The financial costs associated with multiple births escalate with each additional fetus.[70] A 2013 report by the American College of Obstetricians and Gynecologists estimated that health care expenditures "are quadrupled for twins and are 10 times higher for triplets."[71]

Given these various untoward outcomes, women with high-order multiple pregnancies (HOMPs)—those involving three or more fetuses—are often medically advised to undergo MFPR, a form of selective abortion discussed above. In MFPR, a potassium chloride solution is injected under ultrasound guidance into one or more of the fetal hearts, causing the heart to stop beating and leading to fetal demise. Fetal reduction is generally used to "reduce" quadruplet and triplet pregnancies "down" to twins. Without such "fetal reduction," a HOMP is, by definition, a very high-risk pregnancy. From a medical standpoint, then, fetal reduction is a way to diminish that risk, by "reducing" a HOMP to a more manageable pregnancy with one or two fetuses.

Whereas current international standards advise the transfer of only one or two embryos for women under thirty-five,[72] the higher embryo transfer rate legally allowed in the Emirates produces many multiple pregnancies, which must then be "reduced" to ensure their medical safety. However, given the strict Emirati abortion law, fetal reductions are technically illegal in the Emirates, unless a woman's life is in danger. This *HOMP–fetal reduction nexus* is a very twenty-first-century dilemma in the Emirates. In the early "progressive period" of IVF in Dubai, fetal reductions were regularly performed on patients with HOMPs and, in fact, were approved by formal request to a DOH committee consisting of seven government physicians. However, over time, as the IVF legal environment in the country became more restrictive, fetal reduction, like gamete donation, was called into question. This was because fetal reduction could rarely be justified on the grounds required by the UAE's strict abortion law (that is, to save the mother's life).

The subsequent decline in fetal reduction in the Emirates does not appear to be occurring in other Middle Eastern countries, which share this HOMP–fetal reduction nexus. Because of the widespread use of ovarian stimulant medications, as well as the transfer of high numbers of embryos in IVF clinics across the region, multiple pregnancies are a frequent occurrence in the Middle East—estimated to account for one-quarter to one-third of all IVF pregnancies.[73] Accordingly, fetal reductions are widely practiced in many Middle Eastern IVF clinics, including in countries with otherwise restrictive abortion laws.[74] Fetal reduction is accorded a kind of "exceptional" status—it has become a "legitimate" form of abortion that is necessitated, quite paradoxically, by women's desperate desires to become pregnant, especially with twins.

Whereas fetal reduction was practiced quite regularly in both Cairo and Beirut where I conducted my previous research, fetal reduction was never practiced at Conceive. Dr. Pankaj himself had no moral qualms about abortion, which was legally available in both India and the United Kingdom, the two countries in which he had trained. But because of the combined force of the UAE's assisted reproduction and abortion laws, Dr. Pankaj was loath to offer this procedure to his patients. For his patients who were morally opposed to abortion, he attempted to prevent the need for fetal reduction by transferring only one or two embryos. Most patients, however, desired three or even four embryos—particularly the older women, who were hoping to increase their chances of conception.

When triplet or quadruplet pregnancies occurred, women were faced with difficult decisions about what to do—either to maintain the pregnancy and face the many risks, or to travel abroad to reduce the pregnancy to twins. I met six of these women, who had already grappled with or were in the midst of making this excruciating decision. Not all of these women had become pregnant at Conceive, but they were seeking Dr. Pankaj's expert advice on how to proceed with their risky pregnancies. For those women choosing reduction, Dr. Pankaj generally directed them to London or Mumbai, where he maintained strong professional connections and could refer them to well-qualified maternal-fetal health specialists. South and Southeast Asian couples thus tended to head east to Mumbai, while Middle Eastern and European patients tended to head west, often to London.

These back-and-forth reproflows for fetal reduction were difficult for all six couples in my study. The need to leave the country for fetal reduction led to the *fragmentation of pregnancy care*: IVF was started in a clinic in one country, fetal reduction was undertaken in another country by a completely different set of practitioners, and then follow-up care of the reduced but still risky pregnancy took place back in the starting country, but usually with a different set of providers specializing in high-risk pregnancies. This fragmentation of pregnancy care was much more of a burden on wives than on husbands. Although husbands were often sympathetic and supportive of their "multiply pregnant" wives, it was women who underwent the embodied disruptions of reprotravel during high-risk pregnancies, and tended to feel great moral angst engendered by the "selection" of some fetuses over others.

I met several of these women who had become fetal reducers, returning to Conceive only after their fetal reductions had been undertaken in another country. In most cases, they described the actual fetal reduction as a form of trauma, accompanied by significant emotional anguish. For example, Adiva, a thirty-year-old Indian specialist in information technology, had undergone fetal reduction in Mumbai two weeks before I met her. Adiva had clearly been shaken, and she poured out her story to me:

Adiva: We did three IUIs, and they were unsuccessful. Then we did an IVF, and it was unsuccessful. Finally, we had some frozen embryos, so one month after the IVF, we used them, and it worked. I got pregnant with triplets. But then I had to have an embryo reduction,[75] which was very, very traumatic. They reduced to twins. I had identical twins, and in the same sac. They did the embryo reduction with one twin, but we lost both of them. So the reduction was on one, but we lost both. So now, it's a singleton, rather than twins.

Marcia: That must have been very difficult.

Adiva: Well, it was Dr. Pankaj's advice, and also the radiologist we visited in Bombay, and the gynecologist, plus my family doctor. They were also suggesting the same thing. They said there could be complications with twins in the same sac. We definitely couldn't keep triplets; that was too much of a risk. And we didn't want to gamble with the whole pregnancy. So lots of people were saying the same thing. "It's best that you do this, and not get all emotional." But it *is traumatic*! *I would have kept all three*. That would have been totally fine. And my husband was the same as me. We were both *very emotional* about it. But, in the end, however, it was obviously our decision. After all this treatment, this [single] baby, *it's precious*. I feel blessed to be having this one.

Marcia: Might I ask, were there any religious issues with doing this reduction?

Adiva: We're Hindu, so it doesn't matter. In India, it's fine to do this. I think here in the Middle East, they don't consider it good to reduce. I think there is a law that you can't, maybe in Sharjah, but I don't think such a law exists in Dubai. At any rate, they don't do it here, which is why we went to India.

Marcia: And where exactly did you go?

Adiva: We're from Delhi, but we did the reduction in Bombay. We have lots of family there, but we didn't tell them anything. I decided to keep it quiet. They didn't even know about the pregnancy, because I don't think I would have been in the mood to make any small talk after this! "What did you do?" The inertia, the trauma! I wouldn't want to explain. So we decided to do it very quietly. Only my family knows and his family knows. Our nuclear families, but not the aunts and uncles. There's no need for it. Because if I tell them, then they'll all know.

Marcia: So you've been through quite a lot recently.

Adiva: I've had so many things done! I don't even remember. But it's a small price to pay for something so precious.

In her brief narrative, Adiva describes the many issues at the heart of the HOMP–fetal reduction nexus. These include the conflicting desires and clinical risks accompanying a multiple pregnancy; the weight of a couple's decision making amid practitioners' recommendations for fetal reduction; the emotional trauma of undertaking this procedure; the illegality of abortion in the UAE, making reprotravel for fetal reduction a necessity; and the desire to keep the fetal reduction secret, including from family members and friends. Given these many issues, fetal reduction was one of the most challenging forms of law evasion that I encountered in the Emirates. Women who were already quite pregnant and often quite nauseous were forced to travel abroad to eliminate one or more of their cherished IVF fetuses. Not always sure that they had done the right thing, these women returned to Conceive, praying that the remaining fetus or fetuses would "hold" inside their wombs, lest they be faced with an unbearable pregnancy loss.

SEX SELECTORS

Fetal reduction was one of the most clandestine forms of law evasion that I encountered in the Emirates. But I also encountered a perfectly legal procedure, *sex selection*, that was beginning to occur in the country under a shroud of secrecy. Sex selection against girls—including female infanticide—has a long history of moral opprobrium in Islam, with the Prophet Muhammad specifically condemning this pre-Islamic practice.[76] However, the preference for sons, with the accompanying discrimination against daughters, continues to occur across the Muslim world for reasons having to do with patrilineal continuity, the ongoing existence of patriarchy, and the lack of a social safety net, which means that sons are expected to contribute their labor to the family and to support their aging parents.[77]

Studies from across the Middle East have shown that son preference is diminishing over time.[78] In my research during the past twenty-five years, I have found that both men and women are increasingly likely to express their desires for daughters, often finding them superior to sons in many ways. However, even if Arab parents say they *love* their daughters and prefer them as lifelong companions, they still *need* sons in order to complete their families. This belief that sons are socially mandatory within family life is still widespread; thus, ensuring the birth of at least one son is vitally important. Furthermore, creating a "balanced family" of both sons and daughters is considered more difficult nowadays, because smaller families of only two to three children have become the new social norm. Couples wanting to "plan" their small families—which includes ensuring the birth of a son—are turning to new sex-selective technologies, which are making their way into the Middle East's IVF clinics.

Until the early 2000s, the only available sex-selective technology was called "sperm sorting," a technique intended to divide the spermatozoa into two groups—those bearing X (female) chromosomes and those bearing Y (male) ones. Only 85 percent effective in ensuring the desired outcome, sperm sorting was quickly replaced by the more costly, but much more foolproof, technique known as PGD, originally invented to identify genetic defects in embryos created in IVF laboratories. Before transferring these embryos back into a woman's uterus, PGD could be performed on each embryo to determine whether it carried a genetic defect. Those embryos with defects would be culled and discarded, so that only disease-free embryos would be transferred as part of an IVF cycle. PGD could also be used to determine the sex of each embryo, an important diagnostic tool for a number of sex-linked genetic disorders.

However, by the mid-2000s, at least nine Middle Eastern countries were performing PGD primarily for the purposes of sex selection.[79] The UAE was one of these countries. PGD was introduced there in 2007, had become widely available to patients by 2008, and was formally legalized in 2010 with the enactment of the UAE's assisted reproduction law. Indeed, PGD was one of only seven halal procedures sanctioned by Federal Law No. 11 for the purposes of sex-linked genetic screening.

In the Emirates, such genetic screening is clearly important, because the country has one of the highest frequencies of genetic disease in the world.[80] Genetic problems in the UAE are clearly tied to consanguineous unions (inbreeding). More than half of all marriages in the Emirates are between cousins, with first-cousin marriages being the most common type and accounting for one-quarter of the total. Furthermore, because cousin marriages occur within small tribal groups, the risk of genetic diseases within tribes and families is significantly heightened. Although consanguineous marriage is widely practiced across the Muslim world,[81] its particularly high frequency in the Emirates has led to serious genetic disease problems, and PGD can play a vital role in screening for those diseases.

However, the increasing demand for PGD among Emiratis has little to do with genetic disease screening. In an interview I conducted with Dr. Pankaj on June 9, 2012, he reported an alarming new trend of sex selection, which he had observed among Emiratis and his South Asian patients:

> There is a lot of demand among "locals" and Indians, and the Indians more than among the Emiratis. They seem even more interested in getting a boy! [Another IVF physician] offers it to *all* of his patients, and 60–70 percent of them do PGD. Here, if the couple brings it up, then we have a discussion. The only times I recommend PGD are for recurrent miscarriages, where there could actually be some genetic translocations, and then this is the correct thing to do. Also for repeated, unexplained IVF failures, we offer it then. But some couples ask for sex selection.

We're not doing PGS [preimplantation genetic selection] often, maybe only five to six cycles a month. But [my colleague] is doing 40–50 cycles of PGS a month, and then you could really start running into problems of gender imbalance. Ninety percent will want to select for boys, and only 10 percent for girls. Among Arabs and Indians, all will want a boy, I'm afraid.

As the proud father of two teenage daughters, Dr. Pankaj did not condone gender discrimination. Furthermore, he worried about future gender imbalances, particularly among the indigenous Emirati population of just 800,000 tribally organized people. His concerns were reflected in my study, which was undertaken at the very beginning of PGD's introduction at Conceive. Two of the eight Emirati couples I met at the clinic were seeking sex selection; having produced only girl children, they wanted at least one boy. One couple, Samya and Najib, were high-powered Emirati professionals. Samya worked as a senior broker in an Emirati investment firm, while Najib was employed as a hydraulic engineer in the government's agricultural ministry. Married for eleven years and the parents of a six-year-old daughter, Samya and Najeeb were careful planners who wished for only one more child in the context of their busy careers. But to ensure the birth of a son, they traveled to Conceive, where I met them on their first IVF cycle. With her shoulder-length dyed brown hair and stylish glasses, Samya did not look like a "typical" Emirati woman. Nonetheless, she told me that she was deeply embedded in her Emirati community, and that she had specifically chosen reprotravel to Conceive to avoid the possibility of seeing other Emiratis in a public IVF clinic in her home emirate. Samya was most worried about running into several physician relatives, who might learn of her IVF and sex selection and would view both procedures as morally dubious from an Islamic perspective.

Samya was not alone in her desire for secrecy. Virtually all of the Emirati couples in my study had come from other emirates in an attempt to avoid their friends and relatives. Once at Conceive, they were taken to the special "VIP room" at the back of the clinic, where they could wait for their appointments in privacy. It was there that I met Huda and Adnan, a "traditional" Emirati couple who had secretly traveled to Conceive from the neighboring emirate of Ajman. Huda never removed her black facial veil during the course of our interview, but from behind it, she engaged in jovial banter with both me and Adnan, lightly slapping his knee when the jokes were particularly funny. As I did my best to follow their particular dialect of Emirati Arabic, Huda and Adnan explained that they already had four daughters, ages ten to three. The family of six was living in two rooms of Adnan's family compound, but they were planning to move to their own larger "villa," which was currently under construction next to his parents' home. Adnan joked that he hoped to fill the villa with many children—including male *quadruplets* (using the English word with emphasis). When I asked why they needed four sons, Huda answered immediately: "*Laazim* [I must] have a boy! If no boy, maybe my husband will leave me!" Chuckling at Huda's half-humorous, half-serious remark, Adnan elaborated that he needed sons to carry his family name, to help him with his "showroom," and to inherit the proceeds of his business. Furthermore, he worried about his four daughters, who would need at least one brother to help them solve life's problems, including any future difficulties with their Emirati husbands. After a brief discussion of the mechanics of PGD, Huda and Adnan left the clinic, and I never saw the couple again.

I never knew if Samya and Najib or Huda and Adnan were successful in "selecting" their sought-after Emirati sons. These couples pursued their sex selection in secrecy, largely to avoid moral condemnation in their Muslim local worlds.[82] Yet my brief encounters with these Emirati sex selectors made me realize that technologically and legally assisted gender discrimination has found a new home in the Emirates, with the restrictive assisted reproduction law paradoxically upholding one of the acts most regarded with opprobrium by Islam. This new sex selection in the Emirates provides yet another example of how law and religion are having very unpredictable effects in a country whose history of IVF has been marked by openings and closures, permissions and prohibitions, allegations and interrogations, resistances and evasions. This intersection of law and religion in the Emirates has created clandestine flows of reprotravelers, many of whom are morally anxious women. Their stories highlight the untold difficulties of law evasion and religious resistance—or what it means to become a reproductive outlaw.

RESTRICTIONS: Reprotravel Stories

• The Price of Privacy

Reem was the first reprotraveler I met at Conceive. Half-Lebanese and half-Egyptian, with curly honey-colored hair and sparkling green eyes, Reem looked much younger than her thirty-four years. Yet she felt that she had aged dramatically as a result of recent physical and emotional traumas. As it soon became clear to me, Reem was in the midst of a serious medical crisis, the story of which she told me as it unfolded over several weeks at the clinic.

Reem and her Egyptian husband, Amr, were a successful Arab business couple who had met and married in Dubai while pursuing high-powered careers. Reem was the public relations manager of a luxury car company, and her job involved frequent travel to seventeen different sales regions. Amr—a tall, distinguished man with a full head of salt-and-pepper hair—had a major media position in the Emirates. Somewhat exempt from the parenthood mandate by virtue of their successful careers and cosmopolitan lifestyles, Reem and Amr were nonetheless hiding a shameful secret—namely, that Amr was azoospermic and had been considered by both his Egyptian physicians and his former Egyptian wife to be a "hopeless case" of male infertility.

When Amr first met Reem, he assumed that she would have no interest in marrying an infertile divorcé. But as they began to fall in love with each other, Amr decided that he must tell Reem about his medical condition. Reem decided "not to take this into consideration." She explained to me: "Yes, it's a *very* important factor. But I know there is treatment and medical enhancements and everything's possible now. And even if it didn't work, it is *Rabbina* [our lord] who decides."

Following their marriage, Reem began searching for a solution to Amr's condition on the Internet, describing the process as "actual, pure research." She realized that ICSI with sperm aspiration might be the answer to Amr's azoospermia, and she surveyed the global reproscape of IVF centers to find the right clinic. According to Reem, her search was guided by seven major factors. First, she wanted a clinic that was not commercially driven to inflate its success rates. "You can tell this by the language they use," she explained. "Not all the websites are the same. Some exaggerate their success rates and are *not* credible. Thirty-five percent is reasonable. But 80 percent success, even 50 percent, you never know if they're being honest." Second, Reem desired personalized service. "It's whether you feel comfortable or not," she claimed. "For example, I looked at clinics in London. But in London, they are so busy that there is no personalized service. They just refer you and treat you as another case." Third, Reem was sensitive to cost. "The rates and the costs of traveling are important," she explained. "For example, is it going to cost 2,500 euros [$3,200] with or without injections? With or without airline tickets and hotel?" Fourth, given Amr's severe infertility problem, which was probably of genetic origin, Reem wanted the option of genetic testing through PGD. "I read a lot about it," Reem said. "They do it as a precautionary treatment—*if* there are lots of IVF failures or abnormalities of the process. Even though everything looked really good in my case, I've researched male infertility, and we wanted to have this option." The fifth factor was the country. "We don't want to have to travel twelve hours," she explained. "We thought about other parts of Europe—for example, France and Spain. But because of the language difference, I wasn't convinced. I want to understand what they're telling me." As a result, Reem and Amr contemplated ICSI in Lebanon, but a sixth factor, their desire for privacy, intervened. "Even though my family lives in Lebanon, we decided *not* to try in Lebanon," Reem told me. "You know, with these things, it's a *very* sensitive subject. We're known in Lebanon. I'm known there, and he's from Egypt, and he's known there. And he's very well known *here*, also. So he's very concerned about privacy." The final factor in the couple's decision was clinic responsiveness. "I sent lots and lots of e-mails here and there," Reem said, "but no one responded. In fact, only one person responded to me in a very professional manner, and that is how we ended up going to the island of Crete."

At the time I met Reem, she and Amr had just completed a "fertility tourism package" on Crete, one of the scenic Greek islands. The Greek clinic had made all of the arrangements, including hotel accommodations and airport transportation, and in general had offered "very personalized" service, which was important to Reem. Amr was eager to leave the Middle East for ICSI, so that the secret of his azoospermia could be kept from both sides of the family. Furthermore, as Sunni Muslims, Reem and Amr did not want to raise any suspicions about third-party donation in their social circles. Yet, secretly, Reem had contemplated the option of sperm donation, which was offered in the Greek clinic. Rationalizing her opinion, she told me: "I'm Sunni Muslim, and they [the Sunni Muslim religious authorities] don't accept sperm and egg donation. But, personally, I *would* consider it. I'm a very religious person. I pray, I practice the religion. But I think this thing is purely medical. It has nothing to do with halal or haram, because it's not doing an act of *zina* [illicit sex]." On the other hand, Reem realized that Amr would probably reject the idea of sperm donation out of hand, so she had placed all of her hopes on ICSI with sperm aspiration, both of which were fully legally available under Greece's permissive assisted reproduction law.

Before heading to Greece, Reem and Amr had been given two major options— to undertake the entire treatment cycle in Greece, including three weeks of hormonal injections, or to begin the hormonal injections in Dubai and then travel to Crete for only the brief period of egg collection, sperm aspiration, and embryo transfer (approximately two to four days). Given the demands of Reem's busy job, she chose the second option. However, this meant finding an IVF physician in Dubai who would be willing to collaborate with the Greek physicians. To that end, the clinic in Crete highly recommended Dr. Pankaj, who had a global clinical reputation. Thus, Reem came to Dr. Pankaj to receive the hormonal injections prescribed by her Greek physicians.

On December 20, 2006, Reem and Amr were on a plane to Greece. When they arrived, "the physicians in Crete were very happy about the way Dr. Pankaj prepared me," Reem told me. "They said it was perfect! They collected fourteen eggs, all very good." On December 22, Amr underwent a painful process of repeated testicular biopsies to find a small number of viable spermatozoa, which could be used to fertilize Reem's eggs. Four days later, on December 26, the embryo transfer took place, as Reem recounted:

> I met with a very scientific embryologist at the clinic. He gave me the option to transfer four. He asked us: "Are you ready to have twins? Do you want one, two, three, or four embryos? You never know if you'll become pregnant, because at your age and with his problem, the chances are less than 5 percent." Even though it seemed like I was very fertile, he recommended four.[83] He told us that because of the 5 percent chance we have, it was unlikely that the four embryos would work. But even if they did, then two could be removed without affecting the other two. So, you know, we just went with the doctor's recommendation. We put back four, and kept another four frozen there in Crete. They gave me free freezing for one year—even though it usually costs 400 euros [$513] for each frozen embryo—because they saw that we are suffering.

Little did Reem realize that incredible physical suffering was yet to come. Amr flew back to Dubai, while Reem headed to Beirut to be taken care of by her mother. But a mother's care was not enough to head off the medical crisis that was about to ensue. As Reem recalled:

> I started coughing. I thought it was just a cough, maybe something I had picked up in Greece. But it wasn't. It turned out that water was building up around my lungs and tummy. I was having hyperstimulation [a life-threatening complication of IVF]. I was vomiting and having feelings of being out of breath. The problem is that my IVF doctor was in Greece, and with that Greek doctor, everything was "over the phone." I told him that I'm having trouble breathing, and he said, "It's normal. But how much out of breath?" I don't want to make a problem for the doctor, *but maybe* he gave me too many hormones. Or maybe my body is releasing lots of hormones. Maybe I'm a bit weak, body wise. I don't know how many embryos are alive inside of me, and I was really suffering, with lots of water around my lungs. I was suffering. I couldn't breathe, couldn't sit, couldn't sleep. I was really suffering.

Not knowing what to do, and without adequate follow-up care by the Greek clinic, Reem decided to head to Dubai to be seen by her regular gynecologist. Blaming herself, Reem described how she had "waited too long" to reach the doctor:

When he saw me, he said he couldn't take me. "I don't specialize in these things," he said. He said I should go immediately to the American Hospital [in Dubai] emergency room, where they would have to accept me [as an inpatient]. My husband was panicking. I was really in pain. My colors were changing. I couldn't breathe. And, on top of it, Dr. Pankaj was in a conference in London. So at the hospital, they tapped me and removed 2.8 liters of water from my abdomen. After that, I stayed at home for two days, but I still didn't feel well. I was coughing, and I couldn't breathe well. I couldn't speak, eat, sit—anything. So, when Dr. Pankaj returned from London, he saw me at 8:00 AM on Saturday morning, his first appointment of the week. He saw that my lungs had lots of water surrounding them, and he referred me immediately to [another] hospital, to a doctor who was specializing in the chest. I was admitted on that same day, Saturday. They tapped my left side, 750 milliliters, and still there were 250 milliliters more. Then, the next morning, they tapped the right side, and removed 700 milliliters. My concern the whole time was the effect on the fetus. So that same day, they did a pregnancy test. The numbers were very high, suggesting that I was definitely pregnant, maybe with more than one. So I called a doctor back home in Lebanon to ask his opinion. He said, "This is the 'big if.' If God wants all four to be alive, with your 5 percent chance, would you keep all four?" The answer was no! I cannot take care of four at once. I cannot take care of three. Two is okay, because I have a history of twins in my family. My mom is a twin with her brother, so the daughter has a higher chance of twins. But if all four are alive . . .

As Reem contemplated the likelihood of quadruplets, a HOMP remained a major concern during the next six weeks. Reem visited Conceive many times during the cool winter months of January and February along with her worried mother, who had flown in from Beirut to care for her daughter. During the entire period, Reem continued to suffer the effects of severe ovarian hyperstimulation syndrome, an uncommon but life-threatening condition resulting from an overly aggressive hormonal stimulation regime—in this case, the one prescribed by the Greek clinic. One February morning, I found Reem lying on a hospital bed as her mother, distraught, cried into her cell phone. Reem was definitely pregnant with twins but required another procedure to drain excess fluid from her abdominal cavity. A week later, another abdominal tap was required, at which point a third fetus was detected through ultrasound. By Valentine's Day, the number of fetuses had increased to four, turning the purported "5 percent pregnancy" into a HOMP nightmare.

Dr. Pankaj highly recommended a fetal reduction, especially given Reem's unstable medical condition. Reem asked him to perform the reduction, but she was told that "they don't do it here. It's considered abortion and not right." She lamented: "So I have to travel three and a half hours to Lebanon. In Lebanon, they *do* do it. But they don't advertise it. It's not on the Internet. They never declare it, because it's illegal. But that's the Lebanese way. In Lebanon, it's a very complicated issue because of the different religions. The Muslims will say one thing, and the Christians will say something else. But in Islam, abortion is okay *if* for the sake of the mother's health, and so the Muslim doctors will do it."

In the second half of February, still sick from hyperstimulation, Reem was forced to become a law evader. She flew to Beirut, where she underwent a fetal reduction that she could only describe later as "awful." She was wide awake during the entire procedure and thus watched the ultrasound screen as potassium chloride was injected into two out of four of the fetal hearts, making them stop beating. Looking back, Reem admitted to having profound regrets about ever having traveled to Greece:

> If I had done everything here [at Conceive], I think it would have been perfect. I probably wouldn't have had hyperstimulation and quadruplets and a fetal reduction. But how was I to know? You feel like you're in a vacuum, and you don't know what to do. My husband wanted his privacy, and I thought this was a simple thing, doing ICSI. I had no way of knowing that I would come back from Greece with all of these symptoms, or with four [fetuses] still alive. As much as I tried to find out, you can't ask people about these kinds of things, especially when your husband is very, very worried about his privacy. But when you go through all this, you can sometimes lose hope.

Reem had truly paid the price for her husband's privacy—ending up with a complicated, high-risk pregnancy that had to be dealt with by medical staff in several countries. Yet all of Reem's suffering was not in vain. By mid-March, she was declared medically stable, and her care was subsequently transferred from Conceive to a high-risk obstetrics practice in Dubai. And by the end of summer, Reem and Amr became the proud parents of healthy ICSI twins.

• Seeking Eggs and the Sound of Music

Just as Reem was being transferred out of Conceive, Dr. Pankaj introduced me to another woman, Elaine, who was on a quest to become pregnant at the age of forty-five.[84] Elaine told me that she had always imagined herself as the mother of many children, much like Maria in *The Sound of Music*. That particular story, featuring a family's escape from Nazi-controlled Austria largely through the efforts of a singing nun who became the stepmother of seven children, was significant to Elaine. For Elaine was Jewish—one of only two Jews whom I encountered during my many years of working as an anthropologist in the Arab world.

Elaine explained to me that she had been born in the United States, raised in France, and had lived in Israel for the previous eighteen years, until she and her husband, Leib, moved their family to Dubai in the previous year. They had come for Leib's work, the details of which Elaine could not share with me.[85] Furthermore, they had used their American passports to gain residence in Dubai, since Israelis are prevented from traveling to most Middle Eastern countries, including the UAE.

During our first conversation, Elaine proudly showed me the photographs of her seven-year-old IVF twins, Elly and David, who were wearing their private school uniforms and had sandy blonde hair like their mother's. Elaine was a thin, light-skinned woman who could easily blend into Dubai's European-American community as the trailing spouse of a professional husband. These so-called "Jumeirah Janes"—the pampered, stay-at-home wives of European or American executives—live in posh residential areas such as Dubai's famous beachfront. They are the subject of both envy and local derision because of their high-end lifestyles. Yet, as I was to learn from Elaine, she was no ordinary Jumeirah Jane. Instead, she had been on a secret mission to obtain donor eggs in Cyprus, through a complicated story of reprotravel and accompanying law evasion.

Elaine's reproductive path was being blocked by two countries, the UAE and Israel. In Israel, Elaine had undergone seven cycles of IVF, producing large numbers of eggs that were generally of poor quality. Although she had conceived and delivered her IVF twins in Tel Aviv, none of her other IVF cycles in Israel had been successful. She had also undertaken two fruitless rounds of IVF at Conceive during the year prior to our meeting. After a total of nine IVF failures, Elaine regretted that she had not gone "the donor route" several years earlier. With egg donation entirely off-limits in the Emirates and exceedingly difficult to obtain in Israel because of donor shortages, Elaine headed to Cyprus, a common destination for Jewish women from both the United States and Israel. There, an American IVF physician of Russian-Jewish origin was partnering with a Cypriot clinic to recruit anonymous egg donors from Russia. According to Elaine, Israeli women were particularly attracted to this program because they could obtain "white" Russian eggs in a nearby "offshore" clinic (that is, only forty minutes from Tel Aviv by airplane). Thus, in Elaine's view, the Cypriot program was a "win-win" for both donors and recipients:

I don't know any of their details. The women who are chosen are all previously married, and all have at least one child, so they have proven their fertility. I don't know how often they use these women as donors. But all the ladies are from Russia, and they're not Jewish. I was told at the clinic that they rely only on Russian donors, as opposed to Polish or anything else. It was easier in terms of getting the thing organized, because Russians who want to come to Cyprus on vacation don't need visas. So one of the two doctors who organized the program is Russian, and he got Russian ladies who would do it [egg donation]. They get paid, of course, though not nearly enough, because I pay a lot more than they get [paid]. But they can combine it with a vacation. They fly them to Cyprus. They do the [egg] aspiration, and they put them up in a hotel. They get a one- to two-week paid vacation. So after they are done with the aspiration, they can continue with their vacation, you see. They come with their husbands and with their kids, and then the whole beach is full of beautiful-looking Russian ladies. This is because, at present, it's a bit of a hard life in Russia, and so they do this for a vacation. Other than being egg donors, these women have other professions, like being nurses or teachers.

Although the Russian-Cypriot program was based on donor anonymity, the clinic claimed to carefully "match" the phenotypes of the donors with potential recipients. For Elaine, the donor's "white" phenotype was what mattered most:

At my age—I'm forty-five—I can still say that it's mine, precisely because there *could have been* a good egg. I can still get away with it. So I need a *white* person. I need an Ashkenazi-looking person, not a dark-skinned person. In Israel, the donor would have to have been another Ashkenazi Jew, because an Arab-looking person is not my thing. So in Cyprus, I told the doctor that I just want her [the donor] to look like me—not like with a big nose or something protruding! He said to me, "These Russian ladies are all pretty! All the donors are pretty ladies."

Despite the purported physical attractiveness of the Russian donors, the eggs of Elaine's first Russian donor did not yield "beautiful embryos." Thus, on the second attempt, a donor with a slightly different physical profile was used:

I think [the doctor] told me that she's married and has a child. The details I know are her age, her weight, her height, the color of her hair, and the color of her eyes, which are like mine. Luckily for me, I'm Ashkenazi. I'm pale like all of the Russian ladies. So, you know, they have my look. But she's much shorter than I am, 160 centimeters [5'2"], and I'm 167–68 [5'6"]. The first one was more my height, like 165 [5'5"]. The first one was maybe twenty-eight [years old], and the second one was maybe thirty.

By the time I met Elaine at Conceive, she had just completed her second donor cycle, using the shorter donor's eggs and the frozen sperm of her husband, Leib. Leib was largely absent from the process. He had flown to Cyprus on only one occasion, to deposit his sperm; his only other role was to pay the $8,000 needed to cover the two donor cycles. After Elaine returned to Dubai for follow-up care at Conceive, Leib never set foot in the clinic, including on the anxiety-provoking day of Elaine's first pregnancy test. Instead, Dr. Pankaj appeared to be Elaine's main moral support. Having seen her through two failed IVF cycles, he did not judge Elaine for her middle-aged desires to have more children via egg donation, and he was willing to provide follow-up care when Elaine returned from her law-evading reprotravel to Cyprus.

When I asked Elaine why she still wanted more children at the age of forty-five, she responded in a way that reflected her view of herself as a sophisticated, cosmopolitan mother with much to offer to her children:

Well, it's true that this is a good question. Already some people say, when people look at me, they say, "You did it all! A boy and a girl." I don't know. I'm not certain why. But I'd like to have more children. I like the idea of having lots of children. I see myself, you know, kind of like Julie Andrews in *The Sound of Music*, with eight kids behind me.[86] I'm an educated person. I speak a lot of languages. I'm a native French speaker, and I speak French to my children. I speak Hebrew fluently. I studied German and Spanish and a little Italian. I'm taking Arabic. My children are trilingual in French, English, and Hebrew. My children know that I'd like to have more babies. I say to them, "I love you so much, I want to have more of you!" And I remember reading articles. A woman with six children wanted more, so she decided to adopt. They were saying, "Isn't six enough already? Do you really need to adopt?" But who is to say what's enough? If you have two children, and it's not enough, or no children, or five children—how can you say to someone, just because you have five and you desire to have more, it's not supportable? You don't have the right? If your desire is just as strong, then it's legitimate, I suppose. I have two children, but I always see myself with four. I'd like to have four children.

Even though she desired two more children, Elaine did not want to repeat the trials and tribulations of a twin pregnancy. Indeed, Elaine was one of the very few women in my study who did *not* want twins. Thus, as her pregnancy hormone levels began to rise,[87] she began to fret:

I'm already feeling physically terrible. My breasts, also—I feel I'm bursting with milk! I'm very nervous. I don't know what's going on in there. But we'll know in ten days [at the first ultrasound] and take it from there, one step at a time. But it's keeping me up at night. I'm really worried. The difference between one and two babies isn't even close. It's not like, "Oh, it's one more." The difference is between one and five hundred! You know what I'm saying? It's a million things. We're talking breastfeeding, prams, the car—millions and millions of things. I was saying to my husband yesterday, "If I have two again, and I'm breastfeeding, it's so limiting. I could never go outside the home." You can't do two easily at the same time. We'll have to get a bigger place and hire a live-in maid, plus a part-time nanny so that she can get my kids from school and I can breastfeed. It's really important to me that the children's life—that they don't get less because of another child. You have to try to provide the child with attention and care. Look, if you can't afford it, that's one thing. But I want to bring nice people so that my children get more attention. I wouldn't want someone else to raise my child. But I do want *maximum assistance*. If I can't be there, then if I get a nice nanny, and the kids like her, I'm not just shoving them on her. That's why I need a live-in for the house and a part-time nanny. A maid can clean and cook and also watch the kids. But a nanny has to be a "proper" person, an educated, trained nanny, not just someone who I throw a few dollars at every month.

Like so many of the elite women I encountered in Dubai (as well as in my previous research in Egypt and Lebanon), Elaine deemed it necessary to rely on a small staff of nannies and maids, women who were "imported" into Dubai from foreign countries, mostly from South and Southeast Asia. Elaine justified her need for additional motherhood "assistance" based on the fact that Leib worked most of the time, and she did not expect him to be an active co-parent. As with her decision making about egg donation, Elaine had spent a great deal of time contemplating the kinds of women who would help her. The ideal nanny would be a Western-educated single woman, perhaps from India, while the live-in maid would be a low-cost and unobtrusive presence in the household, meaning that she would probably come from one of the poor South or Southeast Asian countries such as the Philippines or Sri Lanka.

Although Elaine could afford to hire these various assistants to help her take care of a new set of twins, she still longed for the simplicity of a singleton pregnancy. As we finished our first, lengthy interview at Conceive, Elaine told me frankly that she was "freaking out" over the possibility of multiples and the probable need for a fetal reduction:

It's a huge thing if I need to do a reduction. In Judaism, it's not a problem. I don't think so. I *can* be open about selective reduction. For me, personally, I feel that this shouldn't become a taboo, hidden, something to be ashamed of. I've read accounts where some women, to save one child, they have to reduce the rest of the children.[88] I've read that it takes five days. You get there a day and a half before, they do it, then you rest two days. But I don't know. I read that it can increase the risks if you travel too soon. But I don't know.

Unfortunately, Elaine's worries about fetal reduction were soon justified. She phoned me after her first ultrasound to say that she was pregnant with triplets. She had called her gynecologist in Israel, but he had informed her that fetal reduction in Israel was tightly controlled by medical ethics boards. Thus, she would have to wait at least two weeks for a committee to decide about her case. The thought of waiting for at least two weeks was unbearable to Elaine, even though she had already spent "three long years of trying" to become pregnant. "I'm already feeling terrible," she lamented. "I feel nauseous. I feel heavy. I'm going to the toilet all night. I have very, very sore breasts, like I'm engorged." Just about to vomit, she cut the conversation short.

The next morning I found Elaine lying on a clinic bed, undergoing intravenous rehydration. She had been vomiting all night and was pale and dehydrated. The next time I saw Elaine at the clinic, she was truly morose. She was feeling desperately ill with the triplet pregnancy but was now forced to decide between Mumbai and London for the fetal reduction. Angry with both the Israeli and Emirati abortion restrictions, Elaine had no choice but to head overseas, and she ultimately chose London, where Dr. Pankaj had given her the name of a good fetal reductionist.

Trying to imagine how Elaine could manage an eight-hour flight to London without retching, I also wondered whether her "missing" husband, Leib, would accompany her to London and whether the fetal reduction to a singleton pregnancy would be successful. But I never saw Elaine again. A few of the Conceive staff members who knew about Elaine's case were openly critical of her decision to reduce the pregnancy to one fetus. One of the Muslim physicians asked me, "Have you met the woman who had tried so many times to get pregnant by IVF, and when she finally got her wish, chose to eliminate not one but two of her fetuses?" In this clinician's view, Elaine had done something highly sinful, doubly haram, by taking the lives of two potential children. I imagined that, had she known that Elaine was a Jewish Israeli woman, pregnant with a Russian donor's eggs, this Muslim physician's moral outrage would have been even more intense. In short, Elaine would be not only a reproductive outlaw but also a true reproductive outcast—a woman whose reproductive rejection of her fetuses would be deemed unforgivable.

....

• Limited by Sharia Law

On a steamy day in late April, I met a delightful Indian American couple, Ramita and Karthik, who were waiting to be discharged from Conceive's recovery room. The petite Ramita, whose short, fashionable haircut and sleeveless shirt were designed for the heat outside, was sitting on her bed wearing jeans, with her knees tucked up to her chest. Karthik, who was born in upstate New York and was a proud graduate of the University of Michigan's School of Engineering,[89] also sported a fashionable pair of glasses. Of all the Indian couples I had met at Conceive, Karthik was the only one who was significantly lighter than his darker-skinned wife, a reversal of the usual racial profile that I had witnessed in Indian marriages.[90] As I was soon to discover, Karthik was devoted to Ramita, who had withstood two painful miscarriages and two job relocations during their six-year marriage, the first to London and the second to Dubai. Karthik had a successful career in the international division of an American engineering firm. But with the recent move to Dubai, Ramita had been forced to give up her job as a New York librarian and had planned to remain unemployed in the Emirates to pursue her difficult path to conception.

Ramita and Karthik had just completed their first cycle of ICSI, even though Karthik did not suffer from a male infertility problem. Following hormonal stimulation, Ramita had produced only two eggs, both of poor quality. Thus, Dr. Pankaj had urged them to consider ICSI, which might increase their otherwise slim chances of conception. Although Ramita was only thirty-two, she suffered from a difficult constellation of infertility problems, including a blocked fallopian tube, an inactive thyroid that required medication, and a hormonal imbalance problem that was not polycystic ovary syndrome (PCOS) but that had put her into a state of premature menopause. "Actually, I have subovarian function," she explained. "I have more testosterone and less estrogen than I'm supposed to. We were living in London, but I flew back to the [United] States to do the testing. I have a high FSH level.[91] I'm always below the cutoff, but that's when they started doing more testing."

When I asked Ramita why she had traveled from the United Kingdom to the United States for medical tests, she and Karthik described the poor quality of medical care that they had received under the National Health Service, which made them reluctant to seek care for Ramita's infertility problems in the United Kingdom. Thus, Ramita traveled by herself to New York City, where she sought the services of an infertility specialist. However, a minor scandal erupted when the seventy-year-old American IVF doctor "ran away with his thirty-year-old patient," according to Ramita. Fed up, Ramita hoped to find a trustworthy female IVF physician in Dubai, but instead she was referred to Conceive, where she began her treatment with Dr. Pankaj almost immediately.

From the beginning, Dr. Pankaj was honest with Ramita, telling her that her chances of conception were low because of her impaired ovarian function. They discussed the subject of egg donation, a technology that had been recommended to Ramita by her physicians in the United States. A willing subject, Ramita was dismayed to learn from Dr. Pankaj that egg donation was definitely not allowed in the Emirates. Ramita complained to me: "We didn't know about the sharia law! We only found out after we moved here. Originally, I called [one of the government clinics] to get into their donor program. But they said it wasn't allowed. And Dr. Pankaj said the same thing. So we'll probably have to go to India for an egg donor, because it's closer than the US." In fact, Ramita had already traveled on three separate occasions to access egg donation in India. Yet her reprotravel had been in vain:

In India they're very cautious, like in America. They have very nice centers, and you can even request their statistics. But I would have to be there the entire time, which means I would have to stay three months. They want to make sure to prevent miscarriage if you have a history like mine. And they don't want to lose sight of you! They want to make sure the patient returns to track their success rates. The place I went was in Bombay. It was a little nursing home [that is, a specialty clinic], with a lot more individual attention, no waiting list, with the donor acquired immediately and everything done for you. I had to pay the doctor a lump sum, and probably out of that, some goes to the donor. I had to pay in cash, and then the doctor pays the donor. And they are putting much stricter limits on the donors than in the US. The age cutoff for the donor is thirty. She has to be educated, with a college degree, in good health, nonsmoking, nondrinking, with a general health checkup, including an STD [sexually transmitted disease] check. They try to match the donor's appearance to [that of] either the husband or the wife. So I had to submit [Karthik's] photo, so that the donor will look like him or me, not too different when you have the baby. I didn't ask about caste or class. I wasn't bothered by this, as long as the donor is healthy.

Although Ramita had already paid for the donor cycle in advance, the Indian IVF physician postponed Ramita's donor-egg cycle on three separate occasions.

"I was coming all the way from Dubai," Ramita complained, "but she acted like I was just driving down from the Bombay suburbs! Each time, I thought I was going for the actual procedure. But I would get all ready, and then at the last minute, she would tell me to come back one more time. It was getting kind of expensive, and I kept having to wait it out. She was a very good doctor, but a little bit too casual."

When I asked Ramita how many times she had traveled altogether, she counted nine trips—six between London and New York, and three between Dubai to Mumbai. These trips were expensive and exhausting, and Karthik's work usually preventing him from accompanying Ramita. When I asked Ramita and Karthik whether they could call these trips "reproductive tourism," they responded:

Ramita: I *wish* I could get what I need here in Dubai! It would be a lot easier, with less travel, and I wouldn't have the stress. It would be quick and easy. We have family in the [United] States and in India, so I can combine seeing my friends, my family, and shopping. I try to enjoy my time while I'm there.

Karthik: The term "tourism" implies that we'll fly somewhere like to Paris or Tokyo, where we have no relatives. But we fly to places where we have a big network of physicians and family. We fly "home," so this is *not* tourism per se.

Karthik went on to explain that they planned to move back to America at the end of the year—although he was pleased to have received expatriate health insurance coverage for their entire ICSI cycle. Ramita could not wait to leave the Emirates. She said that she felt highly constrained by the religious ban on egg donation, and she planned to apply for egg donation as soon as she returned to New York.[92]

At this point, I asked Ramita and Karthik why they were still pursuing ICSI at Conceive, given that they could not access donor eggs there. Like so many couples with complicated infertility problems, they admitted that undergoing ICSI in the Emirates was "one last chance," and they wanted to "see what would happen here first," before abandoning the idea of biological conception altogether. Furthermore, as one of the only couples in the study to possess the privilege of comprehensive American health insurance coverage, they realized that conceiving and delivering an ICSI baby in the Emirates would be entirely "free." Thus, after an exhaustive Internet search, Ramita and Karthik decided to take the ICSI plunge at Conceive—holding onto the hope of a successful conception. At least until they returned home to New York, a last-chance ICSI was better than other less appealing options, including the exhaustion of further reprotravel, the burden of additional emotional and financial duress, and the necessity of circumventing the Emirati sharia law in the search for donor eggs for Ramita.

• A Sperm Donation Cover-Up

A month after my discussion with Ramita and Karthik, I met another Indian couple, Lamees and Najeeb, who were reclining in the large black leather chairs usually reserved for women following their embryo transfers. However, Lamees had not undergone an embryo transfer. Instead, she had come to Conceive after four frustrating visits to India—all of them involving a sperm donation cover-up.

Lamees and Najeeb were the only couple in my study who had tried sperm donation—which was particularly surprising, given that they were Muslim. Quietly, they shared their story of religious resistance to the Emirati sperm donation ban, their repeated law evasion to access donor sperm in India, the secrecy and dissimulation designed to hide their illicit reprotravel, and the frustrating medical malpractice, which had prevented Lamees from ever becoming pregnant.

Lamees and Najeeb were a middle-class professional couple, she an insurance company administrator and he a construction engineer. Lamees had grown up in southern India but had moved to Dubai after her marriage to Najeeb, who was part of a multigenerational, Dubai-based, Indian Muslim family. As the eldest son, Najeeb was expected to have children immediately following marriage, thereby setting an example for his younger siblings. After a long year of "trying to get pregnant," Lamees saw a gynecologist, who prescribed the overused fertility drug, Clomid, and folic acid, recommended for pregnancy. However, when pregnancy did not occur, Najeeb consulted a urologist. Following a semen analysis, a physical examination of his testicles, and a series of painful testicular biopsies, Najeeb was deemed azoospermic; his shrunken testicles were so atrophied that no sperm were being produced inside them.[93] Without viable sperm, Najeeb was not a candidate for ICSI and was permanently sterile.

Demoralized but not defeated, Lamees and Najeeb began to assess their options, quickly realizing that sperm donation was their only answer. As secular Muslims, they cared little about the religious rulings on sperm donation, but they were frustrated to learn that sperm donation was banned in Dubai, where they lived:

> **Lamees:** The only option for us is to go to India for ICSI with donor sperm, because this is not permitted by law in the UAE. There are no doctors doing it here, because of the religious law.

Najeeb: Before, we had no need to know about this. But when we found out that it was not possible here, we were *forced* to travel.

Lamees: We haven't done it here because we *cannot* do it here!

Najeeb: I mean, we're Sunni Muslims, but we're not much interested in this. It doesn't matter what the religion says, because we're not that religious. In fact, we have the plan that we want to go for some more [donor sperm] cycles. But if it doesn't work out, then we'll go for adoption. We know that that can be done in India as well, even though we would have to search for it.

Lamees and Najeeb told me how they had traveled to Mumbai on four separate occasions, finding an IVF clinic that was even more cosmopolitan than Conceive. "People from all around the world were traveling there," Najeeb exclaimed. "From Africa, the [United] States, the UK, Sri Lanka, the UAE, Oman, and all of the Middle East. *Many* people from *many* nations. If you visited the clinic, you'll know how crowded, how busy it was. And it felt even more international than here."

Over a series of visits, each involving ten days of unpaid leave from their jobs, Lamees and Najeeb underwent four cycles of donor ICSI. They were provided with no information about the donors but were told that these men were mostly medical students, selected only after "proper screening and regular checking." With the accompanying costs of round-trip travel and accommodation, each donor cycle cost roughly 20,000 dirhams ($5,500)—meaning that Lamees and Najeeb had spent at least 80,000 dirhams ($22,000) by the time they were done. Najeeb sighed, saying: "We took no loans, but we have no savings. *All* of our earnings have been going to this."

In addition to the economic hardship, the secrecy of the reprotravel had been difficult to maintain. Lamees had manufactured elaborate excuses about why they were traveling together to Mumbai "on business," even though they worked for different employers. She explained that her sperm donation cover-up stories had become more and more convoluted over time:

Everybody knows that we've been going to Mumbai, but for different purposes—artificial reasons. We can't say that we're going on holiday, because India is *our* place—not a place for vacation. So we had to say that we were traveling for work, on "official business." Since you [Marcia] are doing travel research, I'll tell you what we did. Once, we said we went to Qatar for a business trip, when we were actually in Mumbai. The second time, we said that we were going to Mumbai, but for something official, some training. The third time, it was just an embryo transfer, so I went alone. It was a total secret. No one knew that I was traveling. But the fourth time, I said we were going to Malaysia. And we actually *went* to Malaysia for four days, because I knew that they would be asking for pictures! Malaysia was actually a holiday, but we couldn't say that it was a holiday, so we told them that Malaysia was a business visit, then we secretly headed to Bombay. For us, we cannot tell our families what we're really doing. We have to have that much secrecy. Neither his brothers, nor the rest of our families and friends know what we're doing. Even if we're gone for a week, we always have to keep in touch with our families and friends. So it's difficult to keep a secret. But, if we didn't, there would be *so much* family interference. So it's important to us that we're traveling in secrecy.

Realizing then that I was the privileged recipient of the couple's confidences, I wanted to make sure that I understood why they were coming to Conceive, a clinic where sperm donation was definitely not available. It was then that I learned about their four donor ICSI failures in India. They were coming to Conceive to seek a second opinion, which they received on the very day I met them. In fact, Lamees was distraught, wiping back her tears as she spoke to me:

Lamees: For us, it was very difficult to travel there to India and come back. So I came here to see if Dr. Pankaj could help us. I came here, and I found out a new twist to the tale. He says that I've got PCOS, and this was not known earlier.

Najeeb: We've been consulting *so* many doctors over the past two years, and she's had many scans, and no one's ever told us this.

Lamees: But I have multiple signs of PCOS. Dr. Pankaj looked at my face [with mild acne], asked me to do an insulin test, and took a scan and confirmed this. He said that I won't become pregnant until I get my PCOS under control. This is definitely frustrating! It's not just the amount of money we've spent, but all that we've had to go through. I've been to so many different centers. Initially, I did an ovulation study, and before my initial cycle, I was going for IVF treatment where they would do scans from day three. If I had polycystic ovaries and they couldn't find this, then this is surprising! For almost eight months, I was on an ovulation study. But only at Conceive did he diagnose my PCOS from the very first visit. We can see it clearly on our scan today.

Fortunately for Lamees, Dr. Pankaj had been calm and reassuring. He promised Lamees that with weight reduction and medication, they would get her PCOS under control so that she could eventually become pregnant. Although Dr. Pankaj had nothing to offer Najeeb to overcome his testicular atrophy and nonexistent sperm production, he did tell the young couple—still in their late twenties and early thirties—that time was on their side. On their next visit to India, he promised to refer them to a reliable IVF center in Mumbai, where medical malpractice would no longer impede their quest for donor conception.

• Fifteen Failed ICSIs

The story of Lamees and Najeeb and their sperm donation cover-up is quite remarkable, in that the very thought of using donor sperm is extremely unacceptable to most Muslim men. In more than two decades of research with hundreds of Muslim men from many countries, I have met only one other man besides Najeeb who had actually undertaken sperm donation. In fact, of all the assisted reproductive technologies now available, sperm donation is the one least accepted by Muslims, who seem to view the procedure as tantamount to a wife's adultery and the child conceived through donor sperm as "someone else's son."[94] At Conceive, then, it came as no surprise to me that virtually all of the Muslim men in my study were adamantly opposed to sperm donation, including in cases of intractable male infertility.

Ibrahim was one of these intractably infertile Muslim men.[95] The carrier of a genetically based sperm defect, Ibrahim was a candidate for sperm donation, but he absolutely refused it on religious grounds. His story demonstrates the local moral religious norms that prevent the vast majority of Muslims from accepting third-party donation of either egg or sperm, as well as adoption. Yet it also highlights how difficult it can be, within this prohibitive moral environment, to find a solution for childlessness when one's genetically flawed gametes fail to produce a pregnancy.

I met Ibrahim and his wife Nura outside Conceive's ultrasound scanning suite, just as I was packing my bag to leave for the day. Ibrahim approached me, having read my study advertisement that was placed on the waiting room tables. We made a tentative appointment to meet later in the month. But as soon as I stepped into a waiting taxi, I received a call from Ibrahim on my cell phone, asking if we could meet sooner, ideally at his home. I agreed, and two days later, on Ibrahim's way home from work, he picked me up at the clinic for the short ride to his and Nura's spacious, high-rise apartment, overlooking an inland lake in Sharjah. I commented on the beauty of the couple's home and its surrounding view, and Ibrahim proceeded to give me a tour, showing me the second bedroom where he hoped there would soon be a child. We then sat down on the ornate, Louis XIV–style furniture in the living room to talk about Ibrahim's infertility problem and the couple's ICSI quest.

Married for thirteen years, Ibrahim and Nura were first cousins, the children of two Palestinian sisters. Although Ibrahim had grown up in Kuwait, it was when he visited his mother's family in Jineen (on the West Bank) that he met his beautiful cousin Nura, falling madly in love with her. They married "for love" in 1993, and by 1994 the questioning began about why Nura was not yet pregnant. "You know our traditions in the Middle East," Ibrahim said to me. "We get married, and after one year, everybody starts asking what's going on. If you go for more than one year [without a pregnancy], this comes to be seen as a problem."

Nura began the treatment quest by visiting a doctor in 1995. When the doctor told her that she was able to become pregnant, Ibrahim did his first "check-up," a semen analysis that proved to be "very bad." The physician advised Ibrahim to go to a "specialist." Ibrahim consulted a urologist and, in accordance with Middle Eastern medical tradition, he ended up undergoing a varicocelectomy—an unnecessary and usually ineffective form of genital surgery designed to remove varicoceles, or varicose veins, on the scrotum.[96] Not surprisingly, the varicocelectomy did nothing to improve Ibrahim's sperm count. "After that, I did many tests," Ibrahim told me. "And still the results turned out to be very bad." He then volunteered: "I have a copy of all my medical reports. I could show them to you on Sunday. Always, the semen count was 400,000–500,000—very, very weak.[97] And after one half hour, everything died. There was fragmentation, also."

"Our journey starts here," Ibrahim said, immediately launching into a story of thirteen failed ICSI attempts between 1995 and 2007, the last one conducted during the sacred month of Ramadan in 2006. In the early days of their ICSI quest, Ibrahim and Nura focused on Jordan, a country with a Palestinian majority, Palestinian-run IVF clinics, and a "famous" IVF hospital in Amman, one of the first to perform IVF in the Middle East. Traveling from their home in Kuwait to Jordan was financially, physically, and emotionally taxing. Nonetheless, Ibrahim and Nura attempted ICSI seven times in Jordan at three different IVF centers. At that time, the cost of one ICSI cycle was 1,500–2,000 Jordanian dinars (approximately $2,100–$2,800), but Ibrahim's monthly salary was only 200 Jordanian dinars, or one-tenth the cost of one ICSI cycle. In desperation, Nura contemplated selling her bridal gold. Fortunately, however, Ibrahim secured a good job in Dubai as an accountant, and the couple moved to the Emirates in 1999.

Within their first year in the UAE, Ibrahim and Nura underwent two ICSI cycles in Emirati government hospitals, when assisted reproductive technologies were still partially state subsidized. However, both ICSI cycles failed, and the couple became concerned about standards of cleanliness, having seen cockroaches on the hospital walls.

As the new millennium was fast approaching and their nine previous ICSI cycles had failed, Ibrahim decided to "stop searching in Arab countries." A Palestinian friend in France made an appointment for Ibrahim and Nura at an IVF clinic in

Rouen. There, a chromosome test of Ibrahim's sperm showed "fragmentation," an indication of a chromosomal defect. Reviewing Ibrahim's case, the French doctors told him bluntly: "We can't do anything for you. And since you did ICSI more than nine to ten times, we cannot do it again, because the French rules say that we cannot do ICSI after four times." They then suggested adoption, which shocked Ibrahim. "That's fine for you," Ibrahim told the French doctors. "But for us, as Muslims, we have a different tradition."

Demoralized but not destroyed, Ibrahim began his "research," drawing on his global network of relatives and acquaintances in the Palestinian diaspora. Fortunately, one of Ibrahim's Palestinian friends in Los Angeles told him that he would be willing to help with the ICSI quest. Despite the difficulty of obtaining visas for travel to the United States after 9/11, Ibrahim and Nura's patience paid off. They were eventually allowed to seek medical care in America. There, they visited IVF centers in both Las Vegas and Los Angeles, agreeing that their best chances for ICSI success were at the University of California, Los Angeles (UCLA), where, in the words of Ibrahim, a "master doctor" was in charge of the IVF clinic.

For the first time in a decade of ICSI seeking, Ibrahim and Nura were offered PGD. In Ibrahim and Nura's case, the UCLA physician wanted to determine whether the couple's ICSI embryos were carrying genetic defects that caused their repeated ICSI failures. After verifying that PGD was religiously acceptable, Ibrahim and Nura agreed to the procedure and learned that eight of their twenty embryos were free from obvious genetic disease. Defying the common stereotype that Arab men prefer sons, thus automatically desiring PGD-assisted sex selection, Ibrahim recalled: "He [the IVF doctor] told me something funny then. He said, 'You have seven girls and one boy.' I said, 'I don't give a damn shit for girls or boys, Doctor! All I want is a child!' So he returned back [to Nura's uterus] three girls and one boy."

Ibrahim and Nura were scheduled to return to Dubai a week after the embryo transfer, and Ibrahim carefully changed their tickets from economy to business class, so that Nura and the four ICSI embryos could "recline" in transit. After their return to Dubai, Nura underwent a pregnancy test—again negative. "My God, you cannot imagine how disappointed we were," Ibrahim exclaimed. Calling me by my first name, he continued:

In the US, Marcia, the trip cost me, with the travel, with everything, around $35,000. Maybe I've spent more than $100,000 in total for all of the [ICSI] trials. If somebody else had done this to Nura, I'm sure she couldn't stand it. Sometimes, I come back home, and I find her crying. The environment here in the Arab countries—I mean, her sister is getting pregnant, my brother's wife is getting pregnant, and sometimes they cannot stop it [their fertility]! Our family is not interfering, and it's a love marriage. But sometimes, you know—I told her, "All of the problem is because of me, not you. It's from my side. If you want, we can divorce." But she refused. She told me, "If there is going to be a baby, it has to come from you."

He then asked me, "It's *so* frustrating; I have to do ICSI. But how and where?" At this point, I broached the delicate topic of sperm donation:

Marcia: Would you ever consider sperm donation?

Ibrahim: Somebody suggested sperm donation, but we totally refused. For both of us, it's not in consideration.

Marcia: Why?

Ibrahim: Because I refuse it. If the sperm comes from somebody else, you know, inside your heart, you will know it is not yours. Not our color, not our eyes, different things will come out. That's why we refuse. *He will not be my son*. But maybe I will go for the other one, cloning, or how they did Dolly the sheep. This cloning I have no problem with.

Marcia: Even if Islam doesn't allow it?

Ibrahim: I'm sure they *will* allow it eventually. IVF started in the 1980s, and at first, the Islamic authorities didn't accept, but now they accept.[98] Maybe after five years, they will accept cloning. But using a donor, no. It's not from your back [where sperm are thought to be made]. It's not from you.

Nura, who had been quietly following the conversation, added: "It's like adoption. I wouldn't do it because I don't like the idea." Given their opposition to both adoption and gamete donation, Ibrahim and Nura explained to me that they must use their own gametes. According to Ibrahim, their reproductive fate was ultimately in God's hands:

I believe in science, but also God. I believe in science, but if God wants to give, he will. We have the same belief, that if God wants to get us something [a baby], he will give. One of my friends, he was having the same problem as me. Every year, he was going on a vacation with his wife to Jordan and doing ICSI, and it was not happening. Then two years ago, I got back in touch with him. He said, "You'll never believe what happened! I got fed up going to clinics here and there and just spending money. So my wife and I went to Saudi Arabia on the *umra* [a form of pilgrimage], and we were staying there and praying to God. And, yes, it happened." So you see, this is from God. You have to believe.

According to Ibrahim, he would be satisfied if God granted him one child: "One baby and that's it! Not more. I told Nura, 'If I get one baby, your ovary, I will remove it!' I don't want to think about it anymore! This is the only, and lonely, problem in my life. I don't have any other problem."

Ibrahim told me that he had contemplated going to Belgium, where ICSI was invented, but he had decided against it: "One doctor, he advised us to go to Belgium. But after we tried ICSI in America, I feel that what we do here [in the Middle East] is the same." At the time of our meeting, Ibrahim had placed his hopes in Conceive, where he found Dr. Pankaj "down to earth"—a physician who had still "found hope" in Ibrahim's poor sperm profile. Ibrahim continued:

> When I'm alone, I start thinking, "What's wrong with me?" I don't know how to explain it. Sometimes I think my problem was caused by the fear I faced in Kuwait in 1991. The Kuwaiti people came back to Kuwait [from Iraq], and I was there after the [First Gulf] war finished. They came back and caught all of the Palestinians they could find [whose leader, Yasser Arafat, had supported Saddam Hussein]. They caught me for one night and tortured me, blindfolding my eyes and beating and slapping me. They took me from my house, and I didn't know where I was going because they put a blindfold over my eyes. I was blindfolded, but I felt that there were about eight people there, in a building or a basement, and they tortured me. Then after that, they threw me out, and when the blindfold was removed from my eyes, my eyes opened, but I couldn't see anything for about one half hour. This happened two years before marriage, and the shock of that, of this happening in the place where I was born and lived for twenty-five years—I don't know, but I think this experience may have caused my problem.

After this sobering conclusion to our interview, Ibrahim and Nura drove me home, chatting amiably about how much they enjoyed the United States and the "friendliness" of Americans. I was able to show them around the pretty, American-affiliated desert campus where I lived with my family. I promised to keep in touch and to make a few inquiries on their behalf. I was heartened by the fact that Ibrahim and Nura still had three female embryos in frozen storage at UCLA. Ibrahim had told me that returning to America to try a so-called frozen cycle with these embryos was too difficult, financially and emotionally. "If it is guaranteed that I will 'catch' these three girls [as my children], I will go and put [in to Nura's uterus]!" he had exclaimed during our interview. But Ibrahim correctly realized that there were no such guarantees.

Several weeks after our interview, I inquired about whether it was possible to transport three viable embryos all the way from Los Angeles to Dubai. Because it was 2007, embryo transport was still allowed in the UAE, although the practice was later outlawed by Federal Law No. 11. When I met the short, talkative,

Australian-Greek embryo courier, he confirmed the possibility of transporting embryos from the United States to the UAE. Thus, I decided to introduce him to Ibrahim, a meeting that took place after Ibrahim and Nura had experienced their fourteenth ICSI failure at Conceive. Ibrahim was very excited about this prospect. When he was told by the courier that embryo transport would cost approximately $2,500, Ibrahim laughed: "What the hell! After all I've paid, this is nothing!"

I left the UAE in July 2007, several months before Ibrahim's and Nura's embryos finally arrived at Conceive. But I learned from the clinic's embryologist—a fellow Palestinian who had taken a special interest in Ibrahim and Nura's case—that the three embryos were flown from Los Angeles in a cryopreservation tank that was carried by hand all the way from the Los Angeles airport through customs at the Dubai airport. With the help of Dr. Pankaj, Ibrahim's and Nura's "three girl embryos," made in America and thawed in the Emirates, were transferred into Nura's uterus on Conceive's main operating table.

Unfortunately, God decided that the time was still not right for Ibrahim and Nura to become parents. On their fifteenth ICSI attempt, the three female embryos did not implant in Nura's womb, and Ibrahim's dreams of fathering three little "American-made" Palestinian daughters vanished.

DISCOMFORTS

Medical Harm and the Search for High-Quality IVF

An IVF Idol

Dr. Pankaj has made many appearances in this book so far, particularly in reprotravelers' stories and in the recounting of the 2006 clinic war. Dr. Pankaj emerged unscathed from that war and was viewed by his many patients as a kind of local hero. In all my years of studying in vitro fertilization (IVF) in the Middle East, I have never heard so much praise bestowed upon one doctor. I was not unfamiliar with Middle Eastern "doctor adulation." For example, during my previous research in Egypt, patients gushed over one beloved IVF physician, who was also a former movie star. In another IVF clinic there, women fawned over the "tall, dark, and handsome" IVF physician who was also a compassionate philanthropist, taking on many poor IVF charity cases. But physician adulation is not a given in the region. In Lebanon, I rarely heard praise for individual physicians. In that strife-weary country, IVF patients often complained about all that they had been through—in both war and assisted reproduction. In general, Lebanese patients viewed medicine as a mercenary profession, in which greedy physicians were "out to make a buck" at the expense of their patient-victims. This critique was not unfounded. For example, many of the men in my study, both fertile and infertile, had undergone senseless genital surgeries at the hands of unscrupulous urologists. Although a few of the IVF physicians in Lebanon were considered sympathetic by their patients, the IVF and intracytoplasmic sperm injection (ICSI) success rates in my study were so low that they fueled patients' skepticism about the overall quality of medicine in their country.[1]

When I arrived at Conceive, I had no idea about how Dr. Pankaj would be viewed by his patients. The quality of IVF care—delivered by particular physician specialists—was rarely mentioned in the literature as a primary motivating force in reprotravel, unlike legal or economic factors. However, when I arrived at Conceive, I soon came to realize the error of this view. At Conceive, men and women spent hours describing to me how they had searched the globe for a competent IVF physician, and how finding Dr. Pankaj was their good fortune and a huge relief. Patients had often learned about Dr. Pankaj through circuitous pathways involving extensive Internet research, patients' testimonials in online chat rooms, word-of-mouth referrals from fellow patients, and direct physician referrals across a wide reproscape encompassing five continents.

Over many months at Conceive, I heard a steady stream of praise for Dr. Pankaj, who was deemed by his patients to be a "pioneer," an "innovator," the "father of IVF," and the "magic man of Dubai in getting people pregnant." Such adulation came from both men and women and from patients of many nationalities, educational and professional levels, socioeconomic statuses, and religions. Their praise was lavish and unsolicited. I never once asked the question, "How do you like Dr. Pankaj?" Instead, men and women in my study offered their kudos and gratitude, many of them explaining to me that Dr. Pankaj himself was the main reason they had traveled across countries and continents. Dr. Pankaj, in short, was patients' IVF idol.[2] Although Dr. Pankaj never thought of himself in this way—and, in fact, was quite leery of advertising his services in the aftermath of the 2006 clinic war—he had nonetheless gained many devoted followers, who often referred to him as a "god," a "blessing," and a "savior."

Dr. Pankaj had unwittingly developed what I would describe as a *cult of clinical personality*, which was comprised of six important dimensions. First, Dr. Pankaj was highly respected for his *clinical acumen*. A stickler for obtaining detailed reproductive histories, Dr. Pankaj was considered an exceptional diagnostician, someone who invested the time and effort required to make a thorough clinical assessment instead of rushing patients into IVF. This was especially important to couples of lesser means, who could ill afford the costs of assisted conception. But it was also important to couples who had failed at IVF many times and were traveling to Dr. Pankaj to seek his opinion. At these appointments, many couples learned for the first time why they were not becoming pregnant.

Underlying infertility problems had often been overlooked or misdiagnosed, especially insidious cases of polycystic ovary syndrome (PCOS) or difficult cases of male infertility. Both men and women praised Dr. Pankaj for his superior diagnostic skills, as well as his up-to-date clinical knowledge, which he shared with patients in a non-patronizing manner. Repeatedly, I was told that Dr. Pankaj was "spot on" in his clinical assessments. For couples who had been searching many years for answers, the understandings they gained through their interactions with Dr. Pankaj could only be described as revelatory.

Second, Dr. Pankaj was widely extolled for his *clinical trustworthiness*. Patients repeatedly told me that Dr. Pankaj was honest and sincere. Such clinical honesty, I knew from my previous research, was rare in the Middle East. In Egypt and Lebanon, I learned that physicians often under-communicated relevant clinical details in their efforts to retain their authority or to soften the blow of particularly devastating diagnoses. Furthermore, because God is viewed as the ultimate arbiter in all matters of health and illness, many Muslim physicians see final clinical outcomes as beyond their individual control. Thus, they may engage in clinical evasiveness, in the hope that God might intervene. Dr. Pankaj's direct style, therefore, stood in stark contrast to this regional norm of under- or nondisclosure. He was considered highly communicative, taking the time to deliver decisive clinical information to patients about their cases. Patients lauded him for being "honest," "genuine," "sincere," "ethical," and "trustworthy." This was especially important to reprotravelers who felt that they had been deceived, or even injured, in their prior medical encounters. Moreover, those patients who received bad news from Dr. Pankaj came to appreciate his clinical candor. Although his frank interactional style and honesty about poor prognoses were described by a few patients as "abrupt," "brusque," and even "arrogant," all of them had remained as Dr. Pankaj's patients because they came to appreciate his no-nonsense approach. Dr. Pankaj, they explained, was not a physician to "waste time" with false hopes or to rush to judgment about IVF when it was unnecessary. In other words, Dr. Pankaj was seen as clinically trustworthy, a feature of his care that his patients viewed as beyond reproach.

Third, when Dr. Pankaj did advise couples to undergo IVF or ICSI, his recommendations often resulted in *clinical success*. Clinical success in IVF is a relative term, given that assisted reproduction fails much more often than it succeeds. Worldwide, only 25–30 percent of IVF and ICSI cycles lead to pregnancy.[3] However, some of these pregnancies are lost as miscarriages, making the overall success rates significantly lower. The so-called "take-home baby rate"—or the actual delivery rate per started cycle of IVF and ICSI—is 18–25 percent, according to three large European data collection studies.[4] For couples with the resources and willingness to repeat IVF and ICSI cycles multiple times, the so-called "cumulative live-birth rate" increases to nearly 50 percent.[5] But this rate diminishes with women's advancing age and the genetic problems found in their embryos, as well as in the embryos of men with genetically based infertility problems.

At Conceive, these two groups—older professional women and men with severe male infertility problems—were common in the clinical population, suggesting that pregnancy rates at Conceive would be much lower than the global averages. However, Dr. Pankaj was famous for producing viable pregnancies, even in the most recalcitrant infertility cases and without the benefit of donor gametes. In 2005, for example, 41.5 percent of all IVF and ICSI cycles initiated at Conceive resulted in a positive pregnancy test. Some of these pregnancies ended in early miscarriages, but 33 percent were considered "ongoing" and were transferred out of the clinic for obstetric care. Among the female patients under forty at the clinic, the statistics were even better—44 percent of these women got pregnant, and 36 percent had ongoing pregnancies. In other words, of all the patients who underwent IVF and ICSI at Conceive in 2005, about one-third would go on to deliver babies—a success rate substantially higher than the global average of 18–25 percent noted above.

In my study, 20 percent of the women were pregnant when I met them, including eleven women who were carrying twins. In addition, six couples in my study had already successfully delivered their IVF or ICSI children and were returning to Conceive in an attempt to create siblings for their sons and daughters.[6] Those who had achieved viable pregnancies at Conceive were often ecstatic, believing that Dr. Pankaj had performed some kind of miracle, especially in "last resort" cases of assisted reproduction. This happy pregnant patient population would eventually scatter to other clinics. Although many patients wished that Dr. Pankaj would deliver their precious babies, he had long ago given up his obstetrics practice, concentrating instead on helping couples with conception. Therefore, some patients returned to their home countries, while others were referred at three months' gestation to trusted obstetrics practices in Dubai.

Fourth, for those patients who had come long distances to seek the care of Dr. Pankaj, they were able to receive his undivided *clinical atten-*

tion. Getting an initial appointment with Dr. Pankaj typically took one to two months. But once in the clinic, patients did not have to wait for hours to meet with Dr. Pankaj. In the privacy of his spacious, uncluttered office, Dr. Pankaj took the time to communicate clinical details, provide encouraging pep talks, and answer patients' questions. Patients felt that Dr. Pankaj did not rush them through their appointments. His efforts to provide individualized care were aided and abetted by his staff of more than twenty physicians, nurses, embryologists, health educators, and administrators, who also received high praise for their friendliness, responsiveness, and overall warmth. Such personalized attention and care were especially appreciated during the many difficult physical moments women endured as part of the IVF cycle. These included painful injections and subsequent moodiness associated with hormonal stimulation ("You're a bloody pincushion!" "It's like PMS [premenstrual syndrome] for two weeks!"); waiting for ultrasound scans on a full bladder ("It was torture!" "Eventually, you can't wait."); the numerous vaginal penetrations with speculums and ultrasound probes ("It's big—that steel thing that opens you up!" "Oh my God, it's really, really painful!"); and—for those who became pregnant—the many moments of fear when, for example, unexpected cramping or vaginal bleeding suggested an impending miscarriage. At any hour of the day or night, patients could get through to Conceive's emergency service. Thus, Dr. Pankaj's patients told me that they appreciated never being left alone in the midst of a clinical crisis.[7]

Fifth, Dr. Pankaj was seen by his patients as *clinically comforting*. The word "comfort" was one of the terms I heard most frequently at Conceive. Finding comfort in the capable hands of Dr. Pankaj was especially important to patients whose searches for conception had been filled with heartache, broken promises, and sometimes frank malpractice. Dr. Pankaj provided reassurance when it was warranted, and he delivered bad news in a gentle manner that was not perceived as utterly devastating. Patients found peace of mind with Dr. Pankaj, who provided them with hope after despair, courage after defeat. Described as "optimistic," "reassuring," "friendly," and "kind," Dr. Pankaj was known for his wide smile and overall warmth (see figure 4.1). Both men and women—but especially the husbands—also appreciated Dr. Pankaj's sense of humor. Dr. Pankaj loved to joke and engage in witty banter with his patients. This reduced their stress and tension and helped to lift the gloom off the often disheartening clinical process.

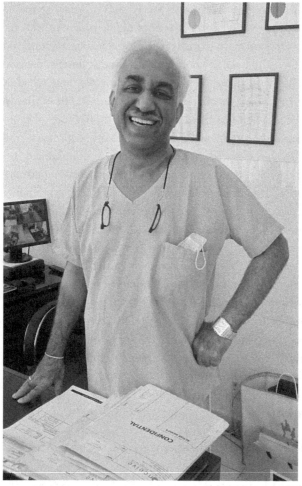

4.1 Conceive's IVF idol, Dr. Pankaj Shrivastav. PHOTOGRAPH BY JUSTINE HOOKS.

Finally, for South Asian couples in my study, Dr. Pankaj was deemed to be *culturally comforting*. Patients from India and Pakistan were often delighted to find an exceptional Indian IVF physician practicing in the Emirates. "I don't know why," one Indian woman put it, "but it *is* important that he understands our language, our comfort levels, our habits, our eating." This was especially important for the many South Asian women who were grappling with PCOS and who therefore required lifestyle changes in order to get their weight and insulin levels under control. Overall, Dr. Pankaj was said to comprehend the tremendous cultural pressures faced by infertile South Asian couples, who were being beseeched by their parents for grandchildren,[8] while receiving heartless comments by others in their social worlds. He understood these couples' urgency to conceive. Furthermore, he was not dismissive of other infertility-related cultural practices. For example, some South Asian couples in my study were taking homeopathic medicines, while others had performed *puja* rituals, appealing to various Hindu gods to increase their chances of conception. In the clinic, they wore threaded bracelets around their wrists and marigold dust on their foreheads, and these signs of Hindu worship were not dismissed by Dr. Pankaj as clinically irrelevant.

Whereas South Asian couples were often comforted by a shared sense of culture, other couples in my study tended to downplay the importance of shared ethnicity or religion in seeking Dr. Pankaj's care. Muslim patients in particular often told me that nothing in Islam prevented them from seeking the care of a Hindu physician. Muslims from Pakistan, for example, cared more about Dr. Pankaj's "South Asian-ness" than about his religion, emphasizing that any differences between Pakistani Muslims and Indian Hindus were due to politics, not the will of the people. Afzaal, a Pakistani Muslim who owned a small business, explained: "It doesn't matter if the doctor is an Indian. It is the *quality* of the doctor only that I care about. I heard about Dr. Pankaj from a French Arabic doctor. She said Dr. Pankaj is doing a *very* good job and is very nice. So it doesn't matter to me. I'm just looking for quality."

Afzaal's feelings about the unimportance of religion were not shared by all of the Muslim couples in my study. Some of them told me that they would have preferred a Muslim IVF physician, who could understand the religious sensitivities surrounding assisted conception. However, Muslims in my study also tended to stress "quality" over religion. Hisham, an infertile Syrian accountant, had much to say on this point:

In Islam, there is no problem if your doctor is Muslim, Christian, Jewish, whatever. It's okay. It's accepted. And you should show respect and appreciation without any concern for religion or nationality. I completely put this point out of my mind when choosing a doctor, and it should be this way for *real* Muslim people. I, myself—I just look for the quality of the person without consideration of nationality. It doesn't matter to me. My wife would prefer her doctor to be an Arab for one reason—the communication will be a bit better. Like, my wife speaks English, but not so proficiently. So in Arabic, she'll be feeling more comfortable. But here in this clinic, there are people speaking Arabic and "Indian" and English, so good communication is available.

The fact the Dr. Pankaj was a male gynecologist was also a matter of concern for some Muslim patients. As I had discovered in my prior research in Lebanon, some particularly pious Muslims, both Sunni and Shia, believe that men and women should be treated by physicians of their own gender, making male gynecologists anathema. This issue frequently surfaced in the Emirates. I heard from several staff members at Conceive that Emirati women often preferred to visit the three female IVF physicians practicing in the country, all of whom were Arab Muslims.[9] Those Emirati women who did seek Dr. Pankaj's care often pulled their black veils over their faces during gynecological exams, and some also asked for their lower bodies to be covered with a sheet, leaving only a small opening available for insertion of the speculum. Indeed, "embarrassment during pelvic examinations" was a major finding in a study conducted with 508 Emirati women in Abu Dhabi.[10] The vast majority (86 percent) of Emirati women surveyed preferred a female gynecologist, and 75 percent also said that religious issues and sociocultural values were significant in their gynecological care. The majority believed that a male physician could not be trusted to offer reproductive counseling, especially about "confidential" gynecological matters.[11] Interestingly, these gender concerns were much less pronounced for other medical specialties such as ophthalmology or cardiology, where Emirati women said that they would be willing to visit a male physician. In my study, a highly educated Emirati woman, Rabab, explained her countrywomen's preferences in this way:

This has to do with religion *and* comfort. Because it's part of our religion that a woman doesn't like to have her body scanned by a man. She has to cover her body before him. But if I'm in a position where I have only one chance and no other choices, and the only thing that can be done is to be seen by a male physician, then I will do it! But let's make sure first that there are no good women physicians out there. I believe in God, and I believe that sometime in the future we will have kids. It's not in our hands, and it's not in the hands of any doctor. It's a test from God about how we will react.

Like the other Emirati women in my study, Rabab had made the decision to travel from Abu Dhabi with her husband to ask Dr. Pankaj for a second opinion, after receiving a discouraging diagnosis of "unexplained infertility" in several other clinics in the country. Another Emirati woman, Latifa, the second wife of a highly ranked Emirati ambassador, was seven months pregnant when I met her at Conceive. She had just undergone an ultrasound scan at a government hospital and was upset to be told that her twins were in "the wrong position." Panicking, Latifa asked her driver to take her immediately to Conceive. There, Dr. Pankaj performed an ultrasound scan, reassuring Latifa that her twins were well placed and that her pregnancy was not in any danger. Feeling much calmer, Latifa told me how she had "followed" Dr. Pankaj to Conceive, when he left his position at the Emirati government hospital in 2004. "He knows what he is doing, and I trust him so much," Latifa explained. "Dr. Pankaj is a very good doctor—so good! There are a lot of [IVF] doctors at other hospitals, but I think every woman I know, everybody found Dr. Pankaj to be very good. I think this is why people—why Emirati people *all want Dr. Pankaj!*"

From Emiratis to Europeans and South Asians to Arabs, praise for Dr. Pankaj was a leitmotif of my study. Most of my interlocutors seemed devoted to Dr. Pankaj, offering unsolicited, laudatory comments during our interviews. In fact, one-fifth of the infertile men and women in my study provided lengthy testimonials about the virtues of Dr. Pankaj and explained why they had traveled great distances to find this patient-centered physician. Patients' desires to tell me their positive feelings about Dr. Pankaj made me realize the importance of patient-centeredness in a physician's delivery of high-quality IVF care. A few selected patient testimonials, delivered by men and women from several different countries, speak to Dr. Pankaj's patient-centered clinical care:

Jamila (from Lebanon): Dr. Pankaj's treatment is *completely* different, completely different from Lebanon!

Imad (Jamila's Lebanese husband): He's not as invasive.

Jamila: And he's very confident, and his team is amazing. It's all been so positive here. What happens if you're panicky, and you call them? They are very positive and helpful. Really, the Indian doctors are the best. They are really good because they "go by the book." They're really excellent.

Imad: It's not because he's Indian! You shouldn't be saying that. It's because he's down to earth. He's not a show-off. He doesn't say he's doing miracles, even though he's doing miracles. This is one of the most difficult things in life—to want to have babies, and you're not having babies.

Jamila: And when you see Dr. Pankaj giving hope, it *really is* incredible after so many years. You don't know how to thank him. When you thank him, he gives you a nice smile, and then just walks away.

Baldvin (from Sweden): That's what I like about Dr. Pankaj. He's fair. I did my first semen test and discovered that I had really poor quality, with crooked tails, and generally very "lazy" sperm, with poor motility. That was in Germany. But Dr. Pankaj said: "That was then, and this is now. There's no reason to speculate why it's like this. Let's just deal with that poor quality." So he's straightforward, professional, and positive. Positive in a way, but also real: "This is your situation. You have maybe a 20 percent chance, but let's take it." It's better to be honest, and he was honest. He was verbal in a way that a lot of doctors are not. They don't have a pedagogical side to talking to people.

Laura (from Canada): My friend found the doctor to be quite abrupt. But to me, he's been nothing but pleasant ever since I first tried IUI [intrauterine insemination]. We talked to him and he said, "Quite frankly, you're getting old." My husband and I were talking on the way home, and we said, "Well, that's quite reasonable." It might have offended someone else, but he said it in a way that made sense to me. Maybe I'm not as sensitive to these kinds of things as my friend. But for us, we both take it in stride. My husband thinks he [Dr. Pankaj] has a good sense of humor. One day I was here with a larger handbag than this one [which was quite large], and he said, "Laura, do you always pack an overnight bag?" I thought this was funny! I've had no bad experiences here. And I think he's been quite genuine. So at the end of the day, for me, he's given me straightforward information. They don't dwell on it when it's not successful. He took the time to answer the phone when I phoned him. And when I got my test results, I was in Canada. And I told him they were giving me certain medicines, and he said: "Don't worry. Use what they gave you there. And when you get back, you can change." If there was a place better for us in Canada, that's what we'd do. But this gentleman [Dr. Pankaj] is very, very successful. You can see that by the many photos on the walls. If you believe in what people are doing for you, you will have success, and that is what we suspect of our particular case.

Svetlana (from Russia): I trust Dr. Pankaj *a lot*—tremendously! Yesterday, I went for a follow-up checkup with [an obstetrician], and he recommended bed rest [to prevent a miscarriage]. But I really trust

Dr. Pankaj, and so I asked Dr. Pankaj, and he said, "I don't really recommend bed rest." So, it's just two different opinions, and they both respect each other. But Dr. Pankaj is *highly* recommended by everyone. Everybody was saying we should come here. And when I came here, I saw the attitude, and spoke to the doctor, and felt really comfortable. Here, it's really hyper-professional, with high technology. Everything is done for the customer.

Kavita (from India): I just do whatever he tells me. He's a blessing for us. I had such a good feeling when I came here for the first time. And now they're threatening to send me off [for obstetric care]. But I refuse to budge! I told Dr. Pankaj, "I don't trust anyone else but you!" For the delivery, they're telling me I have to go elsewhere, but I hope to wangle my way in here for as long as I can! It's such a pity that he doesn't do deliveries. I wish I could do everything in one place. But he has his hands full. I understand this, but I feel it is *such* a good place. I see so many other patients here, and it gives me a good feeling.

Hamid (from Iran): Many people are coming here from all over [the world]. If Dr. Pankaj wanted to have a branch in Iran and make "one package" for Iranians to come over to Dubai, then many people would come here. From *every* part of Iran, they would come! Dr. Pankaj, he never promises anything. He says: "I try my best. Sometimes it happens. Sometimes it doesn't happen." He's not making promises he can't keep. He's very gentlemanly. He never does anything wrong, and he does what he can. He tries his best. We're comfortable with him. Even though there are lots of doctors in our country who have this [IVF] knowledge, he's having more information than in Iran. It's very accidental that I found him, but we're going to keep on coming here.

Sharmeen (from Pakistan): So many people told me about him. They told me to check with him before going back to Pakistan. It's a blessing to find a doctor like him. It's a blessing. In this part of the world, the doctors are *very* commercial, don't you think so? I feel doctors are *very* commercial here, and there are very few good doctors. So it's a blessing if you find a good doctor like Dr. Pankaj.

Manisha (from India): The best part of Dr. Pankaj is that he's very honest, extremely honest, and very, very intelligent and doesn't mislead you. He doesn't misguide you. He tells you the facts. And with somebody like me, who wants to keep this a secret, he's very ethical.

Dr. Pankaj . . . I don't know if he knows this, but he's known as "the magic man of Dubai" in terms of getting people pregnant!

Patient-Centeredness and Psychological Support

At the same time that I was hearing praise about the "magic man of Dubai," a debate was unfolding in the pages of the leading European IVF journal, *Human Reproduction*. In an essay titled "Coming Soon to Your Clinic: Patient-Friendly ART," the prominent Belgian bioethicist Guido Pennings and the physician-activist—and advocate of low-cost IVF— Willem Ombelet argued that too much attention was being focused on IVF clinic success rates.[12] In their view, "patient-friendliness" should also be used to judge IVF clinic quality. Patient-friendly assisted reproduction, they argued, would entail four basic bioethical principles, including equity, cost-effectiveness, minimization of risks, and minimization of emotional and physical burdens. In the next volume of *Human Reproduction*, a team based in the Netherland's Centre for Quality of Care Research agreed in principle with the Belgian authors but criticized the term *patient-friendly* for implying that "being nice" to patients was the same as delivering high-quality care.[13] Instead, they suggested using the term *patient-centered*—or "being respectful of, and responsive to, individual patient preferences, needs, and values, and ensuring that patient values guide all clinical decisions"—to be in line with the definition offered in the seminal report from the US Institute of Medicine (IOM), *Crossing the Quality Chasm: A New Health System for the 21st Century*.[14] According to the IOM, patient-centeredness was one of six key dimensions of quality health care, along with safety, effectiveness, timeliness, efficiency, and equity of access.

As the debate unfolded in Europe, the term "patient-centered" was quickly adopted in IVF circles, and the Dutch and Belgian teams joined forces to launch the first major study of this phenomenon.[15] In a large-scale study involving 925 IVF patients, 227 IVF physicians, and fourteen focus groups collectively containing 103 infertility patients, the European researchers discovered major discrepancies between physicians' and patients' attitudes toward patient-centeredness. Whereas IVF physicians routinely "underestimated" the importance of patient-centeredness in their delivery of infertility care, IVF patients cared greatly about this dimension—so much so that a lack of perceived patient-centeredness was "the most common reason for patients to change clinics," according to the study's authors.[16] One-quarter of the 925 patients surveyed had already switched IVF clinics during their treatment, with most citing nonmedical factors such as "disrespectful staff or contradictory information" as their reason for leaving.[17] Furthermore, the study showed patients' willingness to travel "significant distances for better quality of care," suggesting that patient-centeredness was a key dimension in widespread European repro-travel.[18] In general, European patients had much to say about the importance of patient-centeredness. Their views on the ten key dimensions of patient-centered infertility care are summarized in table 4.1.

Although debates about patient-centeredness were playing out in Europe, the term had yet to enter the local IVF lexicon in the Emirates when I arrived at Conceive in 2007. Instead, Dr. Pankaj liked to think of Conceive as having a "family feeling," which he clearly reinforced in the clinic's motto, "let's make you a family." At Conceive, staff members were encouraged to treat patients in a friendly and familiar manner, making them feel welcomed and comfortable in a home-like setting. Furthermore, Dr. Pankaj liked to view clinic staff as part of "one big family." Both personally and professionally, staff members were expected to trust one another implicitly, to treat each other with kindness and respect, and to form friendship circles both inside and outside of the clinic. For example, on the occasion of Dr. Pankaj's fiftieth birthday, staff members gathered around a large cake on the desk in his office. As soon as the cake was cut into bite-size pieces, Dr. Pankaj moved around the circle, placing a small piece of cake into each staff member's mouth and also feeding me, the newly arrived anthropologist, by hand. Although I had witnessed this gesture of intimacy only between brides and grooms at American weddings, I felt the genuine warmth of this clinical community, into which I was being symbolically initiated.

In this very familial environment, doctors and nurses on staff were expected and encouraged to provide infertile patients with psychological and emotional support, especially when clinical outcomes were disappointing. The need for emotional support was intensified by the fact that many infertile couples were far from home, with no one else to turn to. Some patients had already been deeply disappointed by a lack of compassion among their family members and friends. For example, Olisa, who had come all the way from Sweden to Dubai, described how she had helped an infertile friend through a devastating miscarriage. But when she herself had needed friendly support on the difficult road to IVF, her friends were only minimally helpful. "When you talk to people, you find out that they're not that keen to listen," Olisa told me. "They may ask you

Table 4.1. Ten Dimensions of Patient-Centered Infertility Care

Dimensions	Details
System factors	
Information	Need for concrete information, both general and personal, provided face to face in a timely fashion
Competence of clinic and staff	Desire for clinical expertise, including thorough diagnostic investigation and good medical follow-up without unnecessary care; desire for staff to stick to appointments and be prepared with a complete medical file
Coordination and integration	Appreciation of minimal waiting times for appointments, receiving results, starting cycles, and time spent in waiting rooms; appreciation of smooth organization, including coordination between staff
Accessibility	Importance of telephone accessibility and emergency accessibility to the clinic; desire for appointment flexibility
Continuity and transition	Appreciation of staff continuity, including having a lead physician responsible for each case; desire for follow-up care after medical procedures and assistance with hormone injections; desire for care at the end of treatment, on referral to another clinic, and during early pregnancy
Physical comfort	Preference for accommodations offering privacy, comfort, and a home-like environment that is spacious, peaceful, and well maintained; preference for clinics to be exclusively devoted to infertile (rather than obstetric) patients
Human factors	
Attitude of and relationship with staff	Desire for every staff member to be friendly, respectful, and appropriate in behavior and comportment
Communication	High importance of communication with clinic staff, including taking time and providing opportunities to answer questions; importance of information on what to expect during treatment, including a time schedule; a premium placed on honest and reliable communication, including "bad news conversations"
Patient involvement and privacy	Importance of patient autonomy and informed, shared decision making; high value placed on personalized care, being addressed as a couple, and involving partners; desire for privacy and a limited number of staff members present during consultations; appreciation of openness and recognition of errors
Emotional support	Expectation of emotional support from doctors and nurses during daily care, support to include providing information, paying attention to emotional well-being, and discussing emotional topics; additionally, appreciation of support from specialized staff (such as psychologists) during emotional emergencies and in weeks leading up to pregnancy tests

Adapted from Dancet et al. 2011.

a question, and when you answer, it's too much for them. So I don't need that kind of response."

Furthermore, sharing the details of infertility and IVF with family members was viewed by many couples as a mixed blessing. Mothers were often seen by infertile couples as their best friends and therapeutic allies—always there to offer advice and encouragement; provide tender, loving physical care and nurturance during treatment cycles and ensuing pregnancies; and serve as "the shoulder to cry on" when IVF and ICSI cycles ended in failure. Yet divulging the details of infertility, IVF, and reprotravel to mothers could also induce additional stress. Some mothers were inveterate worriers, while others could not be counted on to keep a couple's infertility problems a secret. Once other family members were informed, invasions of privacy were often the result. "They'll ask you one hundred questions," a young Indian woman, Maya, explained to me. "If you talk on the phone with them, they will keep asking you questions. 'What's going on?' 'When is it going to happen?' 'How is it going to happen?' 'How much are you paying?' They will be *very, very* inquisitive. So we can't brief them on our ICSI. We just told them we're getting treatment in Dubai, but not all of the details."

This desire for medical privacy, including absolute secrecy from prying family members, was one of the main reasons why so many couples in my study, especially those from other parts of the Middle East and South Asia, had traveled to Conceive from their home countries. Of the 125 couples I interviewed, one-fifth—nine Hindu and sixteen Muslim—had not told anyone, including their closest family members, that they were undergoing IVF or ICSI, or the reason for their travel. Terms such as "total secrecy," "absolute confidentiality," "complete privacy," and keeping IVF "hidden" were used over and over again to describe secretive journeys to Dubai. In fact, four of the first ten couples I met at Conceive had not told a single soul what they were doing. Raj, a certified public accountant from India, explained why:

> What I'm telling you is absolutely confidential. I'll tell you frankly, apart from the doctors here and the two of us, you are the only person who knows. If we were doing this treatment back home, we're quite sure that we'd be psychologically more relaxed. But in India, if I'm staying with my mom, I'll be surrounded by my neighbors and my cousins. That's the way it is in our culture. We have big families, not just us. And if you tell one person, they want to announce it to the whole world, and soon everybody knows. So this is *super top secret!*

These desires for secrecy were clearly linked to ongoing issues of stigma. Although infertility is now widely viewed as a treatable medical condition throughout the Middle East,[19] it nonetheless impinges upon both male and female gender identity, as well as the achievement of full adult personhood. Furthermore, in some Muslim societies, IVF is still seen as morally tainted because of suspicions about third-party gamete donation.[20] Thus, "test-tube babies" are implicitly believed to be the product of "illegal" conceptions. Given these damaging views, many Muslim couples in my study considered secrecy to be absolutely mandatory. Jameel, a Sri Lankan man of Malaysian descent, explained why he and his wife, Jinduja, had not told their families the true reason for their "holiday in Dubai": "Not even our mothers know this. We don't want other people to know, so that it will not become a big story. *Insha'Allah* [God willing], when he is born and grows up, we don't want others to say, 'This is an IVF baby!' This is because our parents are not learned. They are old and traditional in their thoughts. Even my mother asked me, 'Are you doing this test-tube baby story?' And I had to say, 'No, no, no—nothing like that!'"

Similarly, Sharifa, a college art professor in Pakistan, laughed when I asked her whether she had told anyone the reason for her travel: "Not at all! Not even our two moms! Because you can say in Pakistan that there's no awareness about test-tube babies. So if someone did IVF or ICSI for their child, they don't feel good! There will be so much gossip. Even at this stage, people still feel it is haram [forbidden]. Even though it's not haram, most of the people there think it's haram. So this is the culture, and if anyone does this [IVF], they don't tell anybody."

Such adamancy about medical privacy was also apparent among the local Emirati population in the clinic. In the backrooms of Conceive, I found Emirati couples who had driven hundreds of miles across the Emirates in their effort to "hide" their infertility from other Emirati couples.[21] Explaining their secret journey to me, Ali, a young Emirati husband who sat by his wife's bedside as she slept, had this to say:

> We like to make this [IVF] secretly. Especially for us "local" guys, the problem is the mentality, our culture. They will think very much less of you if they think you are doing fertility treatment. So if you go, you must keep it secret. No one knows we're here. Even our mothers, brothers, and sisters. No one! It's very difficult, actually, to keep this secret. If we traveled outside [the country], people would ask why we were going outside and staying for a month. It will attract more atten-

tion. So by coming here, we can say, "We are going to the mall," and no one will question that. *Insha'Allah*, she'll become pregnant, and no one will ever know about this. Because they would think it is wrong, and they will call it a "tube baby." They will say things about the baby as if it's not normal. So we came here in secret to protect the child.

Similarly, Mouza, an Emirati woman pregnant with ICSI twins, told me how difficult it was for her, as a "local" woman, to keep her trips to Conceive "top secret":

Nobody knows what I did for my pregnancy! Not even my family, not even my mother. She knows I take medicine, but she doesn't know about the ICSI. She's an old woman. She would tell another old woman. And then talk, talk, talk would happen. I *want* to talk to my mother about this, but I cannot. So this is *completely* secret, between me and my husband. I have to come alone here, because nobody knows. And if people came with me to this clinic called Conceive, they would know what this clinic does. My mother is old, but she is clever. She will ask, "Why did you come here?" So I don't want my mother to think that there is some problem in me or my husband. This is not good for my husband [who is infertile]. This is my life. This is my husband. And I'm keeping my husband's secret. It's not good if some day people know this about my husband. He is the father of my children! This is my future!

In all of these cases, the Conceive staff were infertile couples' only sources of emotional support, a situation that was somewhat untenable. Although a few female staff members prided themselves on their ability to comfort anxious but secretive patients, such psychological support was also a significant burden, given that all of the staff members were busy, and none had been trained as professional counselors. Dr. Pankaj told me that he had initially employed both a clinical psychologist and a "lifestyle consultant," the latter to help the many overweight women to control their diet, exercise, and insulin levels. But few patients ended up keeping their appointments because they were unwilling to pay for these specialized services. Within a year, both counselors were let go.

From the perspective of patient-centeredness, Conceive's lack of on-site counseling was a legitimate concern, expressed to me by a small number of Western patients. For example, Parveen, a Pakistani American woman who suffered from a painful and debilitating case of severe endometriosis, wished that she could speak to a clinical psychologist after her arrival at Conceive. Unburdening herself to me instead, she complained:

> I've been to so many doctors, and this is the third [IVF] center. Honestly, none have a good support system. I don't want to call somebody I don't know. I need someone *in* the clinic to support me, a counselor. In the US, they have Alcoholics Anonymous, so many kinds of support groups. But the US doesn't really have it [counseling] *in* the centers. They've got great doctors, but they're so busy. They're not there to give you emotional support. You really *need* some support, because there's a very high chance you don't succeed. You're not walking out of the clinic with a baby. It's so heartbreaking and devastating. These centers really need a support system. I told Dr. Pankaj this clinic should have a professional therapist, a counselor to deal with this. Here, they don't have this, and he knows that. Dr. Pankaj can give me scientific answers. But it's psychological support I'm looking for.

Evangeline, a British personal trainer who had recently been treated for thyroid cancer in Qatar where she lived, wished that Conceive would offer a more "holistic" approach to treatment. Putting forth her critique both politely and respectfully, Evangeline suggested: "What *I* would like to see—and I mean no disrespect to the doctors—what they need is a more holistic approach. A lifestyle assessment, because there are a lot of other issues, your diet, your nutrients, your stress levels, that can all be taken into account. And psychological things, if you have some sort of latent psychological problems, it could stop you from getting pregnant. But fertility clinics, they just do an initial checkup and treat you from the medical point of view."

As I knew from my previous research in Egypt and Lebanon, psychological therapy of the sort desired by both Parveen and Evangeline has never really taken hold across the Middle East, because of its association with severe mental illness. Furthermore, patient support and advocacy groups, of the kind so common in the West, are also rare in the Middle East, because so few patients are willing to reveal their illness problems to total strangers. As a result, there are no infertility support groups in the Middle East, including in the Emirates. Although Conceive had made its own informal attempts to link willing patients to one another, the clinic had never managed to forge a formal patient alliance. As a result, all "emotion work" was being done by the clinic staff.[22] Still, the staff was sometimes criticized for attending to patients' medical issues at the expense of their psychological needs.

This was true of Dr. Pankaj himself. A few patients complained to me that Dr. Pankaj had become too busy to act as both doctor and patient counselor, especially as Conceive's patient population had grown. For example, Stuart—a very tall, very opinionated British petroleum engineer who was clearly proud of having worked everywhere "from Libya to Syria, all those off-limit places"—delivered a vehement critique of Dr. Pankaj, who he accused of being too busy to deliver personalized care, especially to Western patients:

> His business is booming, and he's totally overbooked, running from lab coat to lab coat, from cubicle to cubicle. He's over-busy, and he's got his balls to the wall. Maybe it's different if you're Indian. A lot of Indians see Dr. Prankage [mispronouncing his name]. Maybe it's a good time of year for them to conceive. Indians very much believe in karma. So it might be our bad timing coming to an Indian doctor. But if someone said, "He gets the job done," I might say that he doesn't explain things to me. It's like, "Go get your carwash!" They lift the hood, spray it, and say nothing. He obviously gets the job done. But there's a certain lack of the personal touch. If I'm a prominent Indian businessman, I'd probably get the personal touch.

Stuart was not the only "white" person to make such disparaging, even racist remarks. A Greek South African woman, Xenia, whose "*huge* big fat Greek family" lived in Capetown, openly confessed her initial uneasiness at being treated by an Indian physician. "Even seeing Dr. Pankaj for the first time," she said, "you notice he is of Indian origin. So you sort of think—somehow you think—is his knowledge not as high?" Similarly, a Russian woman, Svetlana, told me that she and several of her Russian friends living in Dubai had had a major discussion about the baby photos on Conceive's walls. "One of my friends said, 'All the babies look like Dr. Pankaj. Even the European babies look like him.' I told her, 'All babies look like that at first!'" Although Svetlana said that she "didn't mind" coming to the clinic, she felt that other Russians might care a great deal about "the nationality of the doctor," doubting whether an Indian physician could be fully trusted.

In a cosmopolitan clinic such as Conceive, where people of many nationalities come together, it may be shocking to realize that racism still exists, especially among reprotravelers who have presumably chosen to be there. Yet I have encountered racist comments in every study I have ever conducted in the Middle East—usually in the form of paranoid anxieties about "sperm mixing" and resultant "black babies."[23] Sadly, even within Western academic expatriate communities in the Middle East, a "bunker mentality" often exists, with people feeling free to condemn the local Arabs and the imported South Asian workers. Thus, it came as no surprise to me that a few Europeans and Americans in my study used their private, confidential interviews with me as an opportunity to spew racist vitriol. For example, Helen, a stylishly dressed American woman from New York City, had nothing good to say about the two IVF clinics she had visited in Dubai, including Conceive. Assuming that an American anthropologist would share her supercilious views, she grumbled:

> Here, they need to button up! They get angry at the staff in front of people. For example, if someone brings the wrong file, they scream in front of the patients. Also, they come up to you and tell you and the people around you what you're going to have to do. People sitting there hear everything. They should take people aside and do it in a private place. Instead, they come to you: "You have your IUI, and you need a full bladder." They should have a little conference room, just for these kinds of conversations. Privacy is kind of important in this. You feel you're in a "bush hospital," but you grin and bear it and laugh through it.

Helen's depiction of Conceive as a "bush hospital" was utterly inconsistent with everything else I had ever heard or seen at the clinic, with its gleaming corridors; well-trained, multinational staff; and commitment to high-tech reproductive medicine. But it was clear that Helen was not satisfied with the medical care she had received in the Emirates, and she was not alone in her criticism. Although Helen and Stuart were among the very few people in my study (seven, to be exact) to complain about the quality of care that they had received at Conceive, I heard a multitude of complaints about medical care in the Emirates more generally. Despite the the country's growing reputation as a regional medical hub, many men and women I met at Conceive were deeply frustrated with the Emirati medical system, including its gynecology and IVF sectors. Their critiques of poor-quality care that was not patient-centered resonated with the European study cited above in this chapter. From Europe to the Emirates, it appears that poor-quality care is one of the main reasons for twenty-first-century reprotravel.

Emirates Lamentations

In the early days of my study, I met an Emirati gynecologist who happened to be a close friend and colleague of Dr. Pankaj. When I told her that I was studying IVF-related reprotravel into her country, she surprised me by delivering a scathing critique of the poor quality of medical care there. This is how she described the situation in the Emirates:

> Doctors here claim certain degrees and certain training, even if they don't have it [*sic*]. For example, they'll say they have a degree in laparoscopic surgery from Saudi Arabia. But they never did a "degree," even though they tell this to their patients. Or you look at some doctor who has taken a two-day course in colposcopy [a treatment for cervical dysplasia]. He'll be advertising his specialty in cervical cancer screening, but really, he's just making 1,000 dirhams [$367] off each colposcopy. And there are a number of people here doing fertility treatment, but they have no training. Sometimes patients come with fertility protocols that are just a disaster—for example, patients who've been put on Clomid [a common fertility medication] for many years. Furthermore, you look at the people who, unfortunately, are heading certain [medical] associations, and they are not necessarily that fit to decide who has and who hasn't received proper training. We need a [professional] body to see what everyone's degrees really are. There are examples of doctors here who are *not fit*. Whatever they claim, they have managed to get their licenses through *wasta* [personal ties of patronage]. Unfortunately, there are a lot of politics in this country, which is very, very sad. People who talk well will convince somebody that they're good, even though they may be quacks. At the same time, there is a lot of negative competition—not positive competition—between doctors. Instead of everyone having an equal chance—saying "Let's help each other. Let's do our best"—some people say, "Let's take each other's dirhams." [Marcia: "Really?"] Oh my God, medicine here is so commercial! I refer all of my patients for delivery, and they all end up with cesarean, cesarean, cesarean![24] It's a disaster! No one is following this, asking "What is your cesarean rate? What is your morbidity and mortality rate?" Patients have a right to know this information. But here, they don't put any doctor in that position, by asking him, "What's your cesarean rate?" It's easier for him to just get the baby out that way, and there's a lot of cash in it for him. So it's not fair to patients, and I'm really disappointed in the entire medical system.

This stunning indictment of the UAE medical system caught me a bit off guard so early in my study. So I decided to ask the opinion of Dr. Pankaj, a sixteen-year veteran of the expanding Emirati medical sector. Agreeing with his Emirati colleague on a few key points, Dr. Pankaj was succinct in his assessment: "There's zero regulatory environment in this country. So, especially in gynecology, there's a lot of bad medicine. They don't necessarily recruit and keep the best doctors here. There's a lot of pressure to appoint Muslim Arab doctors, so lots of doctors are pouring in from other countries, especially Egypt and more recently Iraq. But many doctors are only here to make a fast buck. They aren't really invested in improving the quality of medicine in this country."

Over the ensuing months, I would hear these kinds of criticisms repeatedly from disgruntled patients. Many had experienced "bad medicine" in the Emirates, and they told me sometimes shocking stories of medical incompetence, complacency, and malpractice. Over time, I came to recognize three categories of complaint—of the medical system overall, of gynecology more specifically, and of particular IVF clinics in the country.

On the most general level, about one-fifth of couples in my study said that they did not trust the Emirates' medical sector. These critics claimed that even the "best" hospitals in the Emirates were filled with "bad" doctors—physicians who were more interested in getting rich than in helping their suffering patients. Patients spoke about the rampant "greed" and "commercialism" among physicians, sometimes calling them "cowboys," "quacks," or "thieves." A Lebanese man, Youssef, felt so strongly about the poor quality of care in the Emirates that he sought me out at the end of his appointment to share his opinion. "I have a general cautiousness about medicine, particularly here," Youssef told me. "There is a Hippocratic oath and everything. But at the end of the day, it is a business. And here, there is no better business bureau! So it's a Darwinian environment." Youssef's belief that the UAE was filled with inferior, mercenary doctors was shared by some Emiratis, who feared that their country was importing the "worst doctors" from other countries. As one Emirati woman, Fatima, put it, "*Alhamdulillah* [praise be to God], my government provides good hospitals, good equipment, and good services. Everything is good, but maybe not the doctors!"

Although Fatima applauded the Emirati government and condemned the foreign doctors, non-Emiratis tended to hold the opposite view; they believed that the Emirati government had created a medical system that lacked incentives for foreign physicians. For example, Krishna, a successful Dubai-based business owner, saw the problem in terms of government labor relations. As a lifelong member of Dubai's "nonresident Indian" (NRI) community, Krishna blamed the policies of the Emirati government—namely, the impossibility of naturalization and citizenship rights for foreign workers—as the key reason why so many doctors lacked a sense of investment in their jobs. In a stinging indictment of the overall service sector in the Emirates, Krishna had this to say about poor-quality medical care:

> I've yet to come across someone in Dubai who comes from a family able to afford medical treatment who would not rather travel to India, the UK, or the US. And this is irrespective of ethnicity, so this would include Arabs who would prefer to go to India over treatment in the UAE. India provides very good care. I've come across many cases, including my grandfather's, where you wouldn't mind paying Indian doctors to come over to Dubai to take care of you, rather than going to local doctors. In fact, this is still a very common practice. For example, there is one visiting Bombay gynecologist—a very famous one over there—who comes over to [a particular] hospital in Dubai, and there's always a long line to see him. He doesn't do deliveries, unfortunately, but he comes over to do checkups, and everyone wants to see him. This is because we don't trust the doctors here, and these sentiments are very common, at least among my generation. If you are a pregnant woman and you deliver here, you will have a C-section. The doctors here apparently are doing C-sections as a money-making scam. They don't even give the mother a chance to give birth! The overall service levels in this country, whether a waiter in a restaurant or a doctor in a hospital, are lagging behind for a developed country. This place lags behind Delhi or Bombay, even though India is *not* the most developed country.
>
> I can describe this because I am an employer. Most employees come over here on three-year contracts, whether they are a general doctor, a surgeon, a waiter, or a cook. Everyone's mind-set is, "I'm here for two or three years. Let's make hay while the sun shines!" They plow their money back into their home countries. And so the fact that the UAE doesn't offer citizenship comes in a roundabout way to be a very negative aspect. Even for us. Even though I've always lived here, as an investor, I'd rather invest in my country [India] than put any funds here. Because, at the end of the day, why park it here when I'm not a UAE national? So we can't blame the educated lot, the doctors and the

teachers, who don't feel an investment in this country. And it affects every aspect of the service economy. Shaikh Makhtoum [the ruler of Dubai] has announced in the papers that there will be a service initiative—to see how to enhance the service levels in the country by 2015. So the ruling family, too, is really concerned that Dubai and the UAE are lagging behind in service. And this is felt the most in medicine, because medicine is something so close to all of us. It really affects the person when it's poor quality. It's life or death. It's very fundamental. But if the medicine is poor quality here, do you blame the employer (the government) or the employee (the foreign doctor)? In my view, it all boils down to a lack of ownership in this country. We're all called second-class citizens, NRIs. And we're made to feel it every day.

In his pointed critique of blocked paths to citizenship and worker alienation, Krishna clearly articulated a major problem in the Emirates—one that the anthropologist Neha Vora has aptly called "impossible citizenship."[25] In her nuanced portrayal of the cosmopolitan Indian families who have lived in Dubai for many generations, Vora shows that even these families—the most "typical residents" and "quintessential citizens" of Dubai—lack the possibility of permanent emigration and Emirati naturalization over time. Thus, many Indians in Dubai—people like Krishna, Dr. Pankaj, and some members of the Conceive medical staff—exist in a state of "permanent temporariness" in an Emirati state that fails to grant them citizenship rights. For young men like Krishna, this "impossible citizenship" is deeply troubling, as evident in his critical commentary. Furthermore, he sees the problem of impossible citizenship as extending well beyond the Indian community in the Emirates. For Krishna, impossible citizenship is what unites all foreigners in the Emirates, from waiters to physicians. Few of them have incentives to offer good service in a country that refuses to embrace them.

It is important to point out that Krishna's rather pessimistic assessment fails to fully account for physicians like Dr. Pankaj—those who are deeply invested in their clinics, their patients, and their long-term medical careers in the Emirates. While I lived in the UAE, I met several foreign-born physicians who were committed to remaining in the country and establishing excellent clinical reputations there. However, these dedicated physicians were an anomaly, according to my interlocutors. In their view, most physicians in the Emirates could not be trusted to deliver appropriate, affordable, reliable, and effective patient-centered care. For example,

Evangeline, who was a cancer survivor, told me that the problem of untrustworthy medical practitioners worried her considerably: "You know, you sit there with a doctor, and at the moment, what he's saying seems like it must be correct. But you hear some scary stories here. From my experience, and from the stories you hear, if something life-threatening did happen to you in the Emirates, you must *always* get a second or a third opinion—that is, if you chose to stay here."

For many couples in my study, these problems of distrust were felt most keenly in the realm of gynecology, the sphere of medicine that includes infertility and its treatment. Women in my study felt that few gynecologists in the Emirates were knowledgeable about infertility. Instead, using "trial-and-error" approaches, both male and female gynecologists tended to prescribe fertility medications such as Clomid, without verifying the source of the problem, including whether the infertility stemmed from a husband's sperm. Female infertility problems such as PCOS were routinely missed or misdiagnosed. More serious cases of premature ovarian failure, ovarian hyperstimulation syndrome, and ectopic pregnancy were often mishandled in ways that were downright dangerous. Furthermore, women with complicated cases of infertility were at a special disadvantage. For example, a thirty-nine-year-old Swedish woman, Rannvig, had come to the Emirates after a decade-long struggle with ovarian cysts, endometriosis, and benign fibroid tumors in her uterus. She had visited several gynecologists in the Emirates who recommended that she be put on Clomid. Not trusting their advice, Rannvig found a "Swedish Polish doctor who was really good" and who told Rannvig, "It's criminal to tell someone thirty-nine years old that you will conceive with [Clomid], especially with your history." Working in Rannvig's best interests, the physician called Conceive directly, telling Dr. Pankaj, "I have a patient who needs your help."

Rannvig was fortunate to encounter a gynecologist of Swedish background who was willing to make a prompt referral. Many other women in my study described how they had wasted valuable weeks, sometimes even months or years, before fleeing from incompetent physicians. For example, Rabab, an Emirati woman from Abu Dhabi, told me how she had endured many "bad experiences" with gynecologists in her home emirate before giving up and driving 120 kilometers to Conceive with her supportive husband, Salman. Angry and exasperated, she exclaimed:

I'm done with medicine here! I'm fed up! They are toying with me as if I'm a mouse, a hamster in a lab. That's why we don't like to try medicine in our own country. They are just trying their experiments with me. Tell me first what my problem is! We go somewhere and do tests, and they say "negative." And then we go somewhere else, and they say "positive." We went to see one doctor who was very firm that I did not have cysts. But then we came to see Dr. Pankaj, and he's the only doctor who said I have polycystic symptoms. My ovaries are symptomatic.

For both Rannvig and Rabab, Conceive was the first IVF clinic that they had visited in the country. But many other couples in my study had started IVF or ICSI elsewhere, sometimes switching to Conceive in the midst of their treatment cycles. Those who had visited other Emirati IVF clinics often had a long list of complaints. Most prominent among them were problems in scheduling timely appointments; lack of clinic hygiene; lack of professionalism on the part of physicians and staff members; a team approach to treatment that precluded being seen consistently by the same doctor; physicians who were inept at the most basic procedures, such as IUI; long waits for appointments; and a lack of medical privacy, including one clinic that announced patients' names and test results over an intercom system! For example, Lamara, a young physician from the country of Georgia, had recently moved to Abu Dhabi after marrying a commercial airline pilot. Visits to two different IVF clinics, one in Abu Dhabi and one in Sharjah, had left her deeply disappointed. Reflecting on her experiences, she told me:

> **Lamara:** We tried to find a place close to home in Abu Dhabi. But unfortunately, we were not happy with their services. Even in Sharjah we tried another clinic, and were *very* unhappy with their services. There was no personal contact as such, and we were very frustrated, *very* frustrated. I had even started [hormonal] regulation at that clinic. But we were so unhappy that we decided to leave in the middle of the down regulation, and we came here. We're very happy here and we started the procedure, which is going to be an ICSI cycle.
> **Marcia:** What problems did you face at the other clinic?
> **Lamara:** Lack of time with the physician. Lack of contact in case of emergency. Or I should say a *total absence* of contact. Lack of a personal touch—let's say, *no personal care*. No patient-doctor contact. Lack of time spent speaking. No psychological support. Because this is very traumatic for a young female, to undergo the procedure, especially for the first time. There was not enough communication, and certainly,

this is very important. So Dr. Pankaj was very kind to accept me in the middle of my [hormonal] regulation, and he's given me what I would call "quality time."

Lamara's disappointment with poor-quality IVF care at other clinics in the country was shared by at least a dozen other couples in my study. Karolin, a teacher from Germany, described how she had found a German-speaking gynecologist practicing IVF in another emirate. But his "bedside manner" was so off-putting that she eventually switched to Conceive:

I don't know. We started with a doctor who, at the end, we decided he probably was doing something he shouldn't have, but we could not know this at the time. He was not able to do this IVF; he was too old for this. I think he just did it to make money. Of course, you have to train to be a doctor, but you should be trained in IVF from the beginning. He probably did some courses and then started to try it out. And from the beginning, he did something which I especially hated. I should say he was really bad about talking on the phone when we had our appointments with him. It doesn't matter if he was speaking German or Arabic or English. But he would talk to his family members, which I don't understand. If it's an emergency, fine, I *can* understand this. But chatting during appointments! The first time, fine. But he did this repeatedly. And for us, we feel it's not very professional to talk about what to have for lunch during our appointments! I could deal with it, but I became very frustrated by this in the end. I didn't want to change doctors because in the long run, that's also not nice. If I had a choice, I would say it's much better to stay with one clinic, to know the doctor, and to have a relationship. But in the end, it was our choice to come here.

Such lamentations about poor-quality medical care and lack of patient-centeredness in the Emirates were a dominant theme of my study. Patients who had experience at clinics other than Conceive were often deeply unhappy with the previous quality of care. Yet to be fair, there were also some Emirates enthusiasts, who believed that they had received excellent care from other physicians, clinics, or hospitals. For example, a few female gynecologists practicing at other medical facilities in the country received high marks for referring their patients to Conceive in a timely and professional manner. For men and women traveling to the Emirates from other countries, many were pleased with the ease of medical access, as well as the significant degree of consumer choice in a medical system that was rapidly expanding. Especially for patients coming from resource-poor countries in Asia and Africa, the quality of care offered in the Emirates was far superior to what they had experienced back home. This favorable contrast was also true of many of the European couples coming to Conceive, who had tried government IVF clinics in their home countries without success. Profound disenchantment with home-country IVF care was expressed by many couples coming to Conceive from around the world. Indeed, patients' stories suggest that poor-quality IVF care and lack of patient-centeredness are global concerns, not problems limited to the Emirates.

Home Country Disenchantments

In a clinic such as Conceive, at the receiving end of global reproflows, couples arrived from many countries after giving up on home-country IVF care. Forty-four of the 125 couples I met in my study had already visited IVF clinics in eighteen home nations: Britain, France, India, Jordan, Lebanon, Pakistan, Philippines, Sri Lanka, Russia, Sweden, Syria, the United States, and six others. Of these traveling couples, twenty had already tried IVF or ICSI back home, sometimes on multiple occasions. In all cases, these IVF or ICSI trials were unsuccessful, leading to feelings of disappointment and demoralization.

During my time at Conceive, I spent many hours listening to stories of medical disenchantment on the part of infertile couples who had once believed that "home" was the best place to undertake IVF or ICSI. Couples explained to me that home represented a comfort zone—a place of deep cultural affinity. Infertile couples were already familiar with their countries' medical systems, had often developed strong connections with particular clinics and physicians, and shared a language and everyday cultural assumptions with home-country medical staff. Furthermore, surrounded by their family and friends, many couples had well-developed social support systems that they could rely on, which were deemed particularly important in cases of medical emergency. The psychosocial and cultural benefits of being at home while pursuing assisted reproduction were felt very strongly by most of the couples in my study. Some believed that the very chance of conception was increased by being "relaxed" in a home-country setting.

In addition, I met about a dozen couples at Conceive who evinced strong beliefs in home-country medical superiority.[26] In my earliest research on IVF in Egypt, I discovered that many Egyptian expatriates working in the Gulf were returning to Cairo for their "test-tube baby-making" out of their firm belief that Egyptian IVF was the best in the region, with Egyptian IVF doctors more experienced than all others. Playing on the words *expatriate* and *patriotism*, I described this phenomenon as *medical ex-patriotism*—intense feelings of patriotic pride in home-country medical services, especially among diasporic communities with feelings of longing and nostalgia for the homeland.[27] People in such diasporic communities often remain proud of home-country medical services, even if they had never lived in the home country or sought medical treatment there. For example, among the large diasporic Lebanese community living in what is known as "Arab Detroit," Michigan, I was often told that IVF back in Beirut was "as good as anywhere in the world."[28] Once I arrived in Beirut to study male infertility, I found scores of proud Lebanese "medical ex-patriots" returning from diasporic communities around the world to undertake their "ICSI holidays" back home in Lebanon.[29]

In the Emirates, I also encountered many of these Lebanese medical ex-patriots. For example, Maha and Ayman had moved from Beirut to Sharjah to work in the emirate's vast "University City" complex.[30] Yet they were convinced that Lebanese universities were far superior, particularly the American University of Beirut, with its "famous" hospital and associated IVF center. Maha stated emphatically that "Lebanese medicine is the best" in the entire Middle Eastern region. "It's their experience, their knowledge," Maha explained, "because of the research studies they do, and their turnover of lots of patients." Ayman then compared Lebanon to the UAE. "Here, you don't trust all doctors," he said, "because most lack experience and knowledge."

I found a similar form of medical ex-patriotism among the diasporic Indian community in the Emirates. Indian couples at Conceive were eager to tell me about their homeland's "advanced" medical system and its "excellent, British-trained doctors." A young Indian teacher, Lakshmi, told me: "In India, they have very good doctors, purely based on their experience. They have vast experience, because of the number of cases and the complications they have to deal with. So their instincts are quite good." Her husband, Harish, who owned a small business in Dubai, said that he trusted Indian medicine much more than medicine in the Emirates, even though neither he nor Lakshmi had ever lived "back home" in India. "The lack of recourse in this country is a problem for us," Harish explained. "You hear these horrible stories. It's hit or miss. Being an expatriate in this part of the world, you just swallow it and suffer. There is no medical malpractice that I can see. And even if there is, it's not easy to get through the system."

Although Harish's feelings of medical ex-patriotism stemmed, in part, from his feelings of expatriate disenchantment in Dubai, Lakshmi believed that Indian doctors were simply superior by virtue of their "vast experience." This is an argument that I heard repeatedly from Indian couples—namely, that India was so large, with so many doctors and patients, that physicians there had superior experience based on the sheer volume of patients treated. This argument about the medical virtue of large numbers was recited repeatedly by Indian patients, especially with regard to IVF. At the time of my study, India's reprotourism sector was beginning to boom, with the country becoming the global go-to site for commercial gestational surrogacy in particular. At Conceive, Indian couples regaled me with the virtues of Indian IVF "writ large"—namely, the country's many clinics and its expansive array of reproductive options, from donor technologies and surrogacy to fetal reduction and sex selection. I also heard about the numerous reproductive tourism websites that were pointing infertile couples to India and about the resulting "international" character of clinics there, which were filled with both Western foreigners and wealthy Indians returning from the diaspora. Lakshmi told me: "What I hear from a lot of my friends—what I understand from them—is that lots of Indians from the [United] States and Europe are coming there for IVF treatment. They have a lot more confidence in the system, just like we have."

Lakshmi and Harish were among the group of enthusiastic Indian medical ex-patriots who wanted to believe that Indian medicine was inherently superior to that found in the Gulf. However, the twelve Indian couples who had actually undergone IVF or ICSI in India had a different story to tell. They painted a picture of medical chaos—throngs of infertile patients, sometimes lined up in rows by the hundreds, waiting to enter overcrowded clinics where no appointment times were given. They told me about teams of IVF physicians who were so rushed and harried that doctor-patient interactions lasted no more than two minutes, even though couples had waited all day to see a doctor. I heard about a lack of medical privacy, where infertile women dressed in hospital gowns waited for gynecological exams in full view of other patients. I also listened to disturbing stories of trial-and-error approaches, including a rather shocking medical disregard for PCOS, which is probably the most common infertility condition among middle-class Indian women. In addition, some couples told me that Indians no longer received preferential treatment in home-country IVF centers, which increasingly catered to foreigners. While Westerners were receiving the best of what India had to offer in IVF and surrogacy, local Indian patients were increasingly being forced out of the local IVF sector via high prices and disrespectful, poor-quality treatment.

The case of a young Indian couple, Shukra and Gopesh, illustrates many of these problems. I met Shukra and Gopesh on the day before they were supposed to move back to Mumbai. Shukra was then nineteen weeks pregnant with IUI twins, one of whom, she was delighted to tell me, was definitely a girl. Now that Shukra's pregnancy was well established at Conceive, she and Gopesh were returning to India, where they had begun their quest for conception, but with somewhat disastrous results. Together, they recounted their experience:

> **Gopesh:** There were hundreds waiting to meet the doctor, and so there was no time. We felt thoroughly rushed. Honestly, these famous ones are getting too busy. They actually don't give appointments anymore. They ask you to come, and then when you reach there, you get a number on a first-come, first-serve basis.
>
> **Shukra:** It could be that the demand is high, but still they should give appointments according to the time that you are there.
>
> **Gopesh:** We went to the clinic at 9:30 in the morning. It was in a big hospital, the biggest hospital, where the doctor was very well known. And when we entered, we were already number seventy-two—at 9:30 in the morning! They gave you numbers, and if you calculated seventy-two in five-minute slots, then it would take 350 minutes to be seen by the doctor.
>
> **Shukra:** We finally got to see the doctor around 1:30 PM, and we only got two to three minutes with him.
>
> **Gopesh:** And we went into the room, and there was somebody else sitting there! So the doctor went in to talk to the other patients, and then came back out to talk to us.
>
> **Shukra:** Before I did my internal exam, patients were asked to line up, six to eight patients in a room, with their clothes off, wearing only a sarong so that the lower part could be covered. I had to stand in line

with many other women! When I saw this, I was very scared, and I ran out the first time. But eventually, I got used to this. I was scanned so many times by Indian female gynecologists. They all said we should go straightaway to ICSI. They just rush to it: "Get something done! IVF! ICSI!" And the female doctor who did my x-ray said that both of my tubes were blocked. She and all the rest said this, including the guy who did the ICSI. When the ICSI didn't work, this Indian doctor told me that I would never get pregnant, because my eggs were all defective. He told me that I would need a donor egg if we did ICSI a second time.

Gopesh: But even that first ICSI was totally unnecessary! We are very happy that things turned out the way they did.

Shukra: You see, we ended up coming here [to Conceive], and after Dr. Pankaj looked at all our reports, he told me that I *would* get pregnant. When he saw my Indian x-ray, he said that my tubes certainly weren't blocked. The x-ray wasn't very clear, but Dr. Pankaj could make out that it was okay. He was surprised by the [poor] quality of the diagnosis in India. He said that IUI would work, and that we didn't need to do a second ICSI. So all of the doctors in India missed everything, including my PCOS, which they never even mentioned.

Gopesh: We had never had any problems with Indian medicine until we started with infertility. People feel that they get the best doctors in India, especially that's the perception over here, among Indians living in the Gulf. But people who say this have *not gone to India*! We've had horrible experiences there, because they're over-busy. They just see you, and the first thing they say, is "ICSI! IVF!"

Shukra and Gopesh were truly lucky to have made their way to Conceive, where PCOS management and a simple IUI had led to a twin conception. But the young couple had paid a heavy price for their Indian misadventure. Between their futile ICSI and their subsequent reprotravel to Dubai, Shukra and Gopesh had spent nearly 30,000 dirhams ($8,200), which was a huge amount for a young middle-class Indian couple. Furthermore, obtaining visitors' visas to Dubai had not been easy for Shukra and Gopesh. Although the Emirates is generally an "easy visa" country—welcoming foreign shoppers at the airport with two-week tourists' visas, or issuing two-month visitors' visas (extendable by a month) for foreign medical travelers who have received a letter of invitation from a doctor—Indians face much stiffer visa restrictions. In the country's attempts to staunch the flow of South Asians into the country, Indian reprotravelers must be "sponsored" by Emirates Air or an Emirates hotel in order to obtain a simple tourist visa. "We didn't know all this before we started," Shukra explained. "But we were helped by this clinic, and we feel so blessed to have found Dr. Pankaj."

Shukra and Gopesh's story was not unique. A dozen other Indian couples in my study had similar tales of disenchantment, with a total of eight failed IVF and ICSI cycles undertaken in five Indian cities. Their descriptions were very similar—crowded, poorly maintained clinics, where patients were rushed through appointments with physicians who had too little time to get to know or really care for them. When I asked Dr. Pankaj why this problematic state of affairs might have arisen in his home country, he told me that many Indian IVF clinics were now "cutting corners." According to him, the global influx of patients into Indian IVF clinics had led to difficult compromises, particularly as physicians attempted to process the high volume of patients.

India was the country about which I heard the most complaints, but it was not alone in being criticized by patients. Nearly twenty other nations were mentioned by once hopeful, but now wary infertile couples coming from other parts of the Middle East, South Asia, and Europe. European couples who were living in countries with subsidized medical care were generally highly critical of the publicly funded IVF services there—with treatment cycles tightly rationed, clinics packed with patients, long and sometimes insurmountable waiting lists, doctors who were often incompetent or complacent, and services overall of low quality. Infertile couples from other parts of the Middle East spoke of bad treatment, misdiagnosis, lack of continuity of care, and lack of monitoring and follow-up in home-country IVF centers. In many cases, home-country IVF services had been less costly than those at Conceive (for example, $2,000 in Lebanon versus $6,000 in the UAE). But couples had become distrustful of "cheap" IVF services back home. For example, Huda, who had visited an IVF clinic in Jordan, had been traumatized by her experience:

> I had been on prednisone, two tablets a day for two years. And then [when I visited] the IVF doctor, [she] told me to stop suddenly. I should have been taken off the medication gradually. So after that, I have had so many problems. I was flushing, like menopause, and I was very afraid that my eggs are finished! But the doctor was very unprofessional in speaking with me. She said, "You are feeling a hot flash, because your biological age is fifty." I was only thirty! So my husband

quarreled with her, and insisted that I make [have] a blood test. That's when we knew that my hormone level was absolutely normal. So the doctor apologized. She told me she was wrong: "I was mistaken." But after that, I still have a big problem, because the heat flushes are not gone, and I can never forget that sentence, "Your biological age is fifty."

Iatrogenesis and Reproductive Damage

As suggested by Huda's experience above, poor-quality IVF care can be physically harmful to women, and even life-threatening. In an opinion piece in *Human Reproduction*, "Is Your IVF Programme Good?," a group of eminent European and American IVF physicians warned that clinics' continuing emphasis on achieving high pregnancy success rates has come at a significant cost to women's health. The authors wrote: "The use of pregnancy rates as the sole or most important criteria for the measure of quality in an IVF centre is misguided. . . . The price takes the form of excluding less than ideal candidates, accepting high order multiple pregnancies, excessive number of cases of ovarian hyperstimulation, and often recommending IVF to patients who would otherwise conceive with simpler approaches."[31] This group of authors made a "plea" for better-quality IVF, including the development of an international standard to evaluate the "goodness" of IVF clinic programs.

As seen in this chapter so far, IVF clinics may not be "good" and, in fact, may be quite "bad," even causing medical harm to patients. The term *iatrogenesis* is often used to designate such medically induced harm. Iatrogenesis is "any adverse condition in a patient occurring as a result of a diagnostic procedure or treatment by a medical team (including physicians, nurses, technicians, laboratories, and anyone involved in patient care)."[32] Iatrogenesis can be broken down into at least ten different categories, including "significant" or "life-threatening" iatrogenic events that result from "medical error" and "bad clinical routines." Iatrogenesis can be "intercepted," "prevented," or "corrected" by a medical team. But without intervention, some forms of iatrogenesis may be deadly. Unfortunately, iatrogenesis occurs far too often in twenty-first-century medical settings, according to some experts; thus, it has become "a major burden of health care systems" that needs to be corrected.[33]

During the many years I have spent studying infertility in the Middle East, I have heard hundreds of stories of iatrogenesis. For example, I have met scores of women whose fallopian tubes have been blocked by unnecessary gynecological surgeries, usually the removal of ovarian cysts that led to scar tissue and adhesions. As a result of unsanitary gynecological and obstetric procedures, other women have developed massive pelvic infections that have rendered them infertile. Many women in my studies have nearly died from ectopic pregnancy emergencies, some of which were the result of assisted reproduction. And as I have shown in this book, some women who have undergone IVF or ICSI have lived through life-threatening ovarian hyperstimulation syndrome, as well as unsettling fetal reductions of high-order multiple pregnancies.

At Conceive, I was not surprised to hear many harrowing tales of iatrogenesis resulting from treatment undertaken in other clinics and countries. I came to think of this genre of lament as *medical horror stories*. Six of these medical horror stories involved ectopic pregnancies; five involved massive pelvic infections; four involved ovarian hyperstimulation syndrome; two involved ovarian cyst removals gone awry; and the rest involved a miscellaneous assortment of missed diagnoses with various unfortunate consequences. In many of these cases, women had sustained permanent *reproductive damage*. Thus, they and their husbands were traveling to Conceive—sometimes actually resettling in the Emirates on a temporary basis—in the hope of achieving some form of *reproductive salvation*.

In the reprotravel stories that follow, we will hear about the untoward consequences of poor-quality reproductive medicine—involving rampant misdiagnosis, botched IVF procedures, care that was not patient-centered, and callous disregard for both women's and men's reproductive health. These cases of medical horror and reproductive damage suggest a discomfiting reality—namely, that reprotravel may be an attempt to escape from medical harm in gynecologists' offices and IVF clinics around the globe.

DISCOMFORTS: REPROTRAVEL STORIES

....

• **Surviving Reproductive Damage**

During my first month at Conceive, I met a pregnant woman, Sheela, whose path to conception had been anything but easy. Eighteen days before her baby's due date, Sheela and her husband, Niels, had stopped by Conceive to pick up a DVD of Sheela's pregnancy ultrasound scans, which Sheela wanted to put in the baby's album. Dr. Pankaj introduced me to the couple, who were eager to share their story with me, appreciating the relevance of their tortuous reproductive journey for my own project.

Both Sheela and Niels worked in the oil industry, and they had met on a business trip. The very blond, blue-eyed Niels came from the Netherlands, where he owned a small business serving the Dutch oil industry. Sheela was from a Mumbai-based Indian Catholic family and had been working in Dubai for twelve years with a Dutch-based oil pipeline manufacturer. Both Niels and Sheela were busy, traveling professionals, and they decided to make their lives together in Dubai. When they wed in 2002, they had no immediate plans to start a family. But a funny thing happened on the way to their wedding:

> **Niels:** We met this person on our wedding day, and she said, "Oh, you're getting married! Are you planning to have kids?" And we said, "No, we want to wait for some time. Get settled. Start our business. Change our home. So we will wait for a year." But that lady told us, "Well, it's not up to you to shape this. I took seven years to conceive." She was just talking to us casually. But even so, it was quite strange.
>
> **Sheela:** She said, "Get a medical checkup!" So we got married in December, and from February, we started trying.

When Sheela did not become pregnant after several months of marriage, she decided to visit a gynecologist in Dubai, who scanned her ovaries, told her that she probably had PCOS, and put her on a six-month course of Clomid. Sheela took the Clomid dutifully, but with each dose she felt acute cramping in her abdomen. One January evening, a year after they had gotten married, Sheela was entertaining visitors while Niels was away on a business trip in Bahrain. Suddenly, Sheila felt excruciating pain—so strong that she fell to her knees and began writhing in pain on her apartment floor. Duly alarmed, Sheila's guests rushed her to the nearest hospital, where an emergency room (ER) doctor performed an abdominal ultrasound scan. Finding nothing, the physician released Sheela with a prescription for a painkiller. However, when Niels returned home from Bahrain the next day, he urged Sheela to make an appointment with a well-known female Indian gynecologist working in Dubai. The Indian physician scanned Sheela's abdomen again—this time finding a huge "chocolate cyst" on her right ovary. Also called an endometrioma and related to endometriosis, this chocolate cyst was filled with unclotted blood and had grown to the size of a tennis ball. Sheela and Niels were astonished by the news:

> **Niels:** What was really amazing to us was that, when we looked on the scan, we could easily see it! It was major—the size of a fist [holding up his fist]. We

ourselves were able to tell what it was straight on the screen! And we had gone to three or four doctors or hospitals by that time, all in the UAE, and they had completely missed it.

Sheela: And it had been there for a long time, not [just] one fine morning!

The gynecologist who finally diagnosed the chocolate cyst told Sheela to head immediately to India for laparoscopic surgery, warning her that physicians in the Emirates had limited experience with removing these kinds of cysts. Although they also discussed going to the Netherlands for the operation, Niels quickly ruled this out:

Niels: In Holland, there is a *huge* wait[ing] list in hospitals. For example, my father had to wait six weeks with a serious heart condition. He was in so much pain, he could hardly walk. It was only because the person on the list before him died that he got his surgery after three weeks! But he was supposed to wait for six weeks. So this is one problem with Holland. And it's *bloody expensive*, and especially for Indians!

Sheela: Because I don't have a Dutch passport.

Marcia: But I thought medicine in Holland is socialized?

Niels: There is a social security system. Basically, there used to be a complete welfare model before. But things have changed. For people with a medium salary, it would be beneficial. But if your salary goes up to a certain level, you have to insure yourself, and it's *only* for employees. Entrepreneurs, people with their own businesses, have to insure themselves.

Marcia: So this is a system mostly for poorer people?

Niels: The objective is to help poorer people, and everybody gets the same medical attention. But the weak point in the system is the long waiting list. And in Holland, first you have to go to your GP [general practitioner]. He will diagnose you. And then he refers you to a specialist. Then you have to take an appointment with the specialist. It would be three to four weeks before you can see the specialist, then he decides. It's a *long* procedure, even when the procedure is allowed. The wait for us would have been months.

Given their sense of urgency, Niels and Sheela headed to Mumbai, where the surgery was performed in early April. When they returned to their own gynecologist in Dubai for a follow-up scan three months later, Sheela and Niels received some more shocking news:

Sheela: The cyst was still there! They did not take it out. The video they gave me [in India] showed a removal, but the video was somebody else's. The doctor in Dubai told us, "This is not you." She could see that in India, they had taken the left cyst out, but not the big chocolate cyst on the right.

Marcia: So they gave you the wrong video *and* performed the wrong surgery?

Niels: Whether this was intentional or not, we don't know. By that point, we had lost confidence in *all* medicine.

Not knowing exactly where to turn, Niels and Sheela did some Internet research, finding another female Indian gynecologist in Dubai who had received a local businesswoman's award. This physician told Sheela that removal of the large cyst was absolutely necessary. But she also warned Sheela, "I've seen your history, and I won't touch you, because you need a specialist. The more they mess with your body, the more scar tissue that will form. Your chances of conceiving at this point are very scarce." The physician recommended an Egyptian surgeon based in Kiel, Germany, who traveled twice a year to the Emirates to handle the most difficult gynecological cases. He ended up performing Sheela's cyst removal, but he was also forced to remove most of Sheela's right ovary. The fallopian tube, which he attempted to preserve, was nonetheless contorted and swollen.

Following the surgery, Sheela's gynecologist was honest with her: "The longer you wait, the more adhesions you'll have. Don't waste your time. You have a high FSH [follicle stimulating hormone; a sign of reproductive aging], and if you wait too much longer, you don't know how many eggs you'll have." She then gave Sheela the name of Dr. Pankaj, recommending that she visit his clinic immediately. "You can keep trying naturally," she said. "But I wouldn't waste time. Go see Dr. Pankaj. He's a fertility specialist, and you should follow his recommendations. If he tells you to try normally, try normally. If he tells you to try IVF, try IVF."

Up until this point, Sheela and Niels had never even considered IVF, but they were beginning to feel "quite desperate," according to Niels. Their first meeting with Dr. Pankaj was a psychological relief. "We were very happy with him," Niels remarked. "He is very well known, and he has a good reputation as well. He was on the spot with everything. From that time on, we trusted him much, much more than other physicians. Whatever decision he made, we were finally getting improvements. Since we met him, he's tackled one problem after another. For us, we have so much faith in Dr. Pankaj."

Given the serious damage to Sheela's reproductive organs, Dr. Pankaj recommended that the couple try IVF. But when two IVF cycles failed for no apparent reason, Dr. Pankaj decided to retest Sheela's insulin level. "It hadn't even crossed his mind, because she had absolutely no symptoms," Niels explained. "So that

[PCOS] was another problem solved." When a third IVF cycle also failed, Dr. Pankaj was truly puzzled, and he recommended that Sheela undergo another diagnostic laparoscopy of her internal reproductive organs. It was only then that Sheela's hydrosalpinx was diagnosed. Over time, her swollen right fallopian tube had filled with fluid that was leaking back into her uterus, preventing any IVF embryos from implanting. Dr. Pankaj recommended surgery to remove the tube altogether. The next day, Sheela and Niels were on the plane to Mumbai to undertake the surgery with one of Dr. Pankaj's most trusted Indian colleagues.

More concerned about Sheela's health than about having a baby, Niels took Sheela on a late spring vacation to Canada, where they decided to put IVF out of their minds until the following fall. But a funny thing happened on the way back from Canada. Sheela missed her period, and a drugstore pregnancy test confirmed the news of an utterly "spontaneous" holiday pregnancy!

From that point on, Dr. Pankaj undertook all of Sheela's pregnancy monitoring, since she refused to be seen by any other doctor. When I asked Sheela if she planned to deliver the baby in Dubai or back home in India, she was emphatic on this point: "No, it's out of the question to go back to India! Maybe it was just bad luck our first time there. But I would think twice about going back again. The *only* reason I went the second time is because we were following Dr. Pankaj's advice. Otherwise, I wouldn't have ever considered going back there for medical care." Niels chimed in:

Niels: You may be interested in this for your research. We've had both good and bad experiences with medicine in this region. Our problem was finally solved here when we found Dr. Pankaj, but some of our worst examples are here in the Emirates as well. And in Bombay, we've also had some of our worst experiences, and some good medicine as well. So we've had both experiences in both places.

Sheela: To give you an example, after the first surgery in India, when I came back to pick up Zolodex [a medication] from a pharmacy in Dubai, I asked the pharmacist what the medicine was for, and he said, "What do you have? Cancer or something?" I was just curious, but he said, "It's used for cancer patients." **Niels:** She was completely shell-shocked! It was crazy for the guy to make this statement! There is no continuity of care here.

Sheela: And here is another interesting thing for your study. Dr. Pankaj diagnosed me with placenta previa. My placenta is a bit low, a bit on the edge [near the birth canal]. There is only one hospital [in Dubai] that can save your baby if it's between twenty-four and thirty-two weeks premature, because they specialize in these kinds of things.

Niels: That is the best part, that they specialize in these kinds of things. But here comes the worst part again. They did the intake interview with her. She got registered with the hospital, because you have to be registered there first. If you aren't registered, then you can't get in on an emergency basis. So we go there, thinking it is better to register, because they give priority to you then. During the intake interview, she tells them about her history of IVFs and her severe endometriosis. I don't know if she was a doctor, but the person doing the intake interview asked, "What is endometriosis?"

Sheela: She was scanning me, and I said to myself, "Man, this is the last time I'm going here!"

Niels: It's like they're thirty years back in time here. They were so old-fashioned that it was shocking. They diagnosed her with placenta previa, and they wanted to put her in the hospital for the last two months of her pregnancy.

Sheela: They admitted me, and I said, "If they don't let me out, I will commit suicide!" There were no private rooms, and it was more the thought of staying two months there.

Niels: They had the best intentions, but they were very old-fashioned. I checked with Dr. Pankaj, and he said, "They are way back in time. Go home, and nothing will happen."

Sheela: I was only in the hospital for two to three days, but even then, every time a different doctor would come by, each one would have a different recommendation. One would say that I had to stay in the hospital after twenty-four weeks. Another at thirty-seven weeks. One said, "Take this." Another one said, "Take that." Now we just follow whatever Dr. Pankaj says!

Niels: Let me tell you a third incident. At some point in time, we were doing IVF, and she had a kidney stone. At the same time, she was getting heavy injections, and she got an attack of vomiting. We thought it might be ovarian hyperstimulation, so we rushed to a hospital. We were in the ER, and she was crying in pain on the table. They had taken a urine test, and they said, "You're pregnant." I told them that we were doing IVF, that she was on gonal F, and that she was definitely not pregnant. And he said, "No, you're pregnant." I had to fight with the guy! We had a big fight! So we just left, and we went to the next hospital. At least they had a good ER there, and I was able to get through to Dr. Pankaj on his mobile [cell phone].

Sheela: So maybe we just have bad luck or something. But I've already had my share! Without Niels, I wouldn't have been able to go through all of this—three laparoscopies in two years, and all of these incompetent doctors.

Niels: It was mostly about figuring out the exact problems. In that way, Dr. Pankaj was very good. When he diagnosed something, he was on point.

Even when she had this kidney stone and I was fighting with the doctor in the hospital, I phoned Dr. Pankaj, and he agreed with me. He said, "No, she has a kidney stone."

Sheela: For me, he's like a god!

Niels: He also has a good personality, and professionally he's on the spot. It's been nearly two years that we're with him. And the only time he was wrong was when he didn't diagnose the insulin problem right away, and he was disappointed that he missed it. He apologized to us for that. So, to be honest, here in the UAE, the subject of medicine can be quite good, *if* you have bumped into the right person at the right time.

Sheela: We feel very blessed with Dr. Pankaj. We can't complain.

Niels: And with regard to traveling, here's something else that's interesting. At least we're lucky to have good jobs and good incomes. When we were in India, we saw a woman being sent *out* of the hospital with severe endometriosis because she didn't have the money to pay. In Europe, it may take you a helluva lot of time to get an appointment, but they will not leave you stranded.

Sheela: But in India, there are *so many* people.

Niels: And what we found quite sick in India, if you're from the UAE, an NRI, you pay *much more* for treatment. And it is blunt—in your face! They ask: "Where are you from?" If you say the UAE or the Gulf, then you're an NRI, and you will pay 25 percent more. But if we used the address of her mother [in Mumbai], our hospital bill was 20 percent less. Cost is the least of our concerns, because fortunately, we have enough money. But for a lot of people, many can't afford this, especially infertility treatment. In this country [the UAE], maybe 50 percent of the people coming for IVF are from India. And they have a lot of family pressure to have children. They have to take out a loan to do this infertility treatment, just to keep the family happy. In this region of the world, it's much more conservative. It's like twenty years ago in Europe. "Is something wrong?" "Why don't you have a kid?" In Europe all the couples are open about this now. But in this region, if you have Indian relatives, they are asking you all the time!

Fortunately for Sheela and Niels, they could now tell their Indian relatives that they were expecting a baby any day. Furthermore, there would have to be no lies to cover up an IVF for, in the end, IVF was not responsible for the couple's pregnancy. Yet in many ways, Sheela and Niels considered their IVF physician, Dr. Pankaj, responsible for their joyous conception. As they told me time and time again, he was the only one who had eliminated all of the reproductive obstacles in their way. In the end, Niels and Sheela felt very lucky to have found the right clinic and the right doctor who could guide them. "I mean, if European people knew about this place, they would flock to it!" Niels opined.

As they left the clinic that day, with Niel's arm wrapped protectively around his very pregnant wife Sheela, they were looking forward to the birth of a little daughter—conceived in Canada and born in Dubai to a Dutch dad and Indian mom, whose struggles to have her would make her all the more precious.

• A Young Wife's Ruptured Uterus

In the substantial corpus of medical horror stories that I collected at Conceive, Sheela and Niels stood out among the lucky ones. Sheela's poor-quality medical care had been quite traumatic, but it had not rendered her unfit to carry a child. Daniyah, however, was not so lucky. When I met her and her devoted husband Abner, I learned that the couple had made a difficult decision to move forward with IVF, despite the fragility of Daniyah's ruptured womb.

Like Sheela, Daniyah and Abner were Christian Indians who had made their home in the Emirates. Hailing from the southern state of Kerala, Abner and Daniyah were proud of their communist government's achievements, including Kerala's 100 percent literacy rate and its equal sex ratio due to the carefully enforced legal ban on sex selection. Considering themselves to be "progressive," college-educated, middle-class Indians, Abner was pursuing a banking career in Dubai while Daniyah had a good job in logistics. Abner was the eldest son, and at thirty-six he was under considerable pressure to provide his parents with grandchildren. However, Abner was devoted to his now infertile wife Daniyah, who had experienced untold reproductive horrors throughout their eight-year marriage.

As a newlywed in Dubai, Daniyah easily became pregnant. But not trusting the hospitals in the Emirates, she flew back to India to deliver the baby in a well-known hospital in Gujarat. Although the infant boy seemed healthy, he was slightly premature, and after two months, he succumbed to a lung infection. Grief-stricken, Daniyah returned to her mother's home in Kerala. Her mother noticed Daniyah's ongoing postpartum bleeding and took her to a local hospital, where physicians performed a dilatation and curettage to remove the many pieces of placenta that remained in her uterus. Daniyah's botched delivery had also caused a severe postpartum infection, which required her to take prescription antibiotics for nine months.

When Daniyah returned to Dubai, she and Abner decided to wait for a year to give Daniyah's infected womb a chance to heal. Daniyah had no trouble becoming pregnant again, but due to pelvic scarring her second pregnancy was an ectopic emergency. Her treatment included surgically removing her left fallopian tube. The next year, she experienced a second ectopic pregnancy, this time in the right tube—which was tied off to prevent another tubal pregnancy.

With two functioning ovaries but no functioning tubes, Daniyah had no choice but to try IVF. Abner was supportive, surveying the regional landscape of IVF in India and the Emirates. Choosing the best of both worlds, Daniyah and Abner decided to try IVF with an Indian gynecologist based in Dubai, who referred all of his IVF patients back to the hospital he owned in Kerala. Abner explained this unusual, two-country arrangement to me: "He [the gynecologist] works here, but he owns a hospital in Kerala. He's usually in Dubai. But every fortnight, he travels to Kerala. Someone referred us to him. They call him the 'traveling IVF doctor.' He does all of his [IVF] operations in Kerala only, because he owns a big private hospital there, and it's full of Indian patients from Kerala, the Gulf, and many other places." Accepting this arrangement, Daniyah underwent hormonal stimulation in Dubai. Then she and Abner flew with three other Dubai-based Indian couples to Kerala. "We got to know them all," Daniyah explained. "We used to meet them at the clinic, and we kind of became friends. In fact, we still see them. We all live here, but we were together in Kerala for about twenty days. We each stayed in a room at the hospital. There were already ten girls who had just gone [through IVF]. Among them, only one was positive [pregnant following IVF]. But then, out of the four couples from Dubai, two couples got pregnant, including us. So we went for a scan, and everything was okay. So we returned back here after that."

On the first day back in Dubai, Daniyah's condition deteriorated. Abner recalled the traumatic events:

It was the next day, and I was about to leave for work. She was feeling dizzy. I thought maybe it was [low blood] sugar or something. I tried to call up the [IVF] doctor, but he wasn't there. He was in Kerala, actually. But a female gynecologist who works with him in his Dubai office said, "Give her a bottle of sugar water, a sugary drink." I was about to tell this to Daniyah when, all of a sudden, she collapsed [unconscious] in the room. She was on the ground. We have a clinic in the same building where we stay, so I called the doctor. They came up right away and started an IV. We called an ambulance right away to take her to the hospital. When we got there, they said that there must be some bleeding inside. There was no bleeding externally, so she must be bleeding inside. And then we found out that it was another ectopic pregnancy, but this time a cornual pregnancy in the cornum [where the fallopian tube connects to the uterus]. And her uterus had ruptured also. Even though her tube was surgically blocked, the pregnancy was right in the cornum, so her uterus ruptured, and they had to repair it. It was an emergency, and she had to spend two weeks in the hospital after they repaired her uterus. They said they repaired her uterus. But they told us that it might rupture again if she ever gets pregnant.

For the three years following this life-threatening event, Daniyah and Abner remained traumatized, fearing that a pregnancy might lead to Daniyah's death. Ever supportive, Abner convinced Daniyah, who was only twenty-eight and very much wanted to become a mother, to consider using a gestational surrogate back home in India. Abner had done his homework, reading as much as he could on the Internet and in the Indian popular media. On Daniyah's behalf, Abner contacted one of the most famous Indian surrogacy centers in Gujarat. There, they told him that a surrogate could be ready for them within a matter of months.

Yet Daniyah was not convinced, because she realized that using a surrogate would involve an elaborate subterfuge. During the past seven years of their marriage, Daniyah's mother was the only one who knew about all of her reproductive setbacks, including her "hidden" IVF procedure in Kerala. Abner explained their desire for secrecy in this way:

We *should* have shared it with them, because they don't know what we're doing. It's better to share with the parents. After she got pregnant [from IVF], we were back with my parents in Kerala for ten days. They knew we were doing some treatments, but what treatments, they were not aware. You can say that IVF is stigmatized. In that part of Kerala, doing IVF is "something." People tend to talk about it. But later on, we did tell my parents. Daniyah was a bit reluctant. She was more skeptical initially. But I wanted to inform them. She was skeptical about telling them because you can say that, even though India is a big country, there is still a conservative mind-set. Even in educated places, such things are not that common. When people say "test-tube baby"—the word "test-tube" itself, even *I* found it very odd. "Test-tube baby"—I know that it's not made in a test tube. But from the beginning, it's been called that, and that's part of the problem, I think. People don't understand. So not telling people about this is the only way to protect the child.

Suspecting that surrogacy would be even more controversial and potentially stigmatizing, Daniyah and Abner decided to seek a second opinion on Daniyah's case, especially to determine whether she could carry a pregnancy to term in her fragile uterus. The traveling Indian IVF physician urged them to "come back for a second look" regarding this possibility. By this point, however, the couple felt a "mental block" toward him, and they rejected his offer out of hand.

Meanwhile, friends in Dubai urged Daniyah and Abner to visit Conceive, telling them that many Indian couples had been successful with Dr. Pankaj. At their first meeting, Dr. Pankaj reviewed Daniyah's medical records, concluding that most of her medical care had been poorly handled. Still he was hopeful, believeing that Daniyah could carry an IVF pregnancy to term. He told her that she would have to remain on strict bed rest, submit to careful pregnancy monitoring, and undergo an elective C-section. Although hers would be considered a very high-risk pregnancy, she still had the chance to become an IVF mother. After surviving eleven significant reproductive events—including four pregnancies (three ectopic, one preterm delivery), one neonatal death, two laparoscopic tubal surgeries, two IVF cycles, one uterine rupture, and one uterine repair—Daniyah and Abner were convinced to give IVF a go, hoping that twelve might be their lucky number.

The day I met the couple in the clinic, Abner was sitting at Daniyah's bed-side, comforting her after her egg retrieval operation. Dr. Pankaj popped his head behind the curtain to tell Daniyah and Abner that twelve "beautiful eggs" had been successfully collected from Daniyah's still healthy ovaries. Already the number twelve was feeling very auspicious. As the three of us readied ourselves to leave the clinic, Abner shared these parting thoughts:

> Sometimes we feel that all of this could have been avoided. We always thought it would be better to go back to India, because we didn't know about the quality of medicine here in the UAE. We didn't think it was a problem to go back to India, where everything is also cheaper. But now we think that we wouldn't have gone through any of these serious issues if we'd only stayed here, especially initially. But it's too late now. God willing, it will happen this time. Just one child would be more than enough for me and Daniyah.

• A Young Husband's Hidden Sperm

Reproductive damage is not restricted to women. Men too may suffer from poor-quality reproductive care and may be forced to seek solutions through repro-travel. Such was the case of Nourreddine, a young Moroccan man who was born and raised in Britain. Expected to be independent by the age of eighteen, Nourreddine had opened a small cell phone shop in London that was so successful he could afford to marry within his first year of business. He chose Fadwa as his bride. Also a Moroccan immigrant to Britain, Fadwa was seventeen at the time. Pale-skinned with an East London cockney accent, Fadwa seemed more British than North African. But her long djellaba and modest headscarf signaled that she, like Nourreddine, was a pious Muslim.

As teenage newlyweds, Nourreddine and Fadwa were very much in love and hoped to become young parents. "I've always said to myself that I wanted to have my children by the time I was thirty," Nourreddine explained to me. "I want to be running with my children in the park, being close to their age. Having a child at an old, old age doesn't appeal to me. I'd rather be done when I'm young. I did want a child at an even younger age, but God didn't want it. I would have had a four-and-a-half-year-old child by now if things had gone my way." But Nourreddine continued: "I never really took it seriously, because you come across a lot of people who are trying, trying, trying. I can certainly say that we did try! But, obviously, nothing happened. Really, over the years, nothing happened. Nothing happened at all."

Two years of marriage without any form of contraception led the couple to visit the local National Health Service (NHS) clinic. "I did all the blood tests, and I had ultrasounds, and a [diagnostic] laparoscopy," Fadwa explained. "And they said at the end of the day that everything is fine, everything is fine." When Fadwa's tests all came back normal, Nourreddine was asked to undergo semen analysis, which he repeated several times. The South African Muslim physician working in the NHS clinic delivered the bad news to Nourreddine in this way: "Look. You have no sperm. You've only got, basically, a couple of options. Either use donor sperm, or try to do ICSI. But the probability of ICSI succeeding is not very high. We would have to do an operation on you—to take out some tissue from your testicles and see if we can find any sperm."

As pious Sunni Muslims, Nourreddine and Fadwa were horrified by the first option of sperm donation. "Because of our religion, for us, it wasn't an option at all," Nourreddine told me. "But over there, they do it! The guy who recommended donor sperm to us, he is a Muslim! And he kept saying, 'Why not? You should do it! You should do it!' He was trying to convince us to do it, even though he's Muslim. I don't think he was a very religious person himself. So we spoke to my parents about this, and my father spoke to some imams in London. And, oh no! They did *not* recommend that we do that."

Having rejected sperm donation altogether, Nourreddine was willing to accept the second recommendation of testicular biopsy. This would determine whether Nourreddine was suffering from a simple blockage in sperm transport or a more serious form of nonobstructive azoospermia, in which sperm were simply not produced in his testicles. "This is not a part of the body that you like to be operated on—not for a man!" Nourreddine exclaimed. "And I would not like to do this again. But really, I had no choice. In other cases with no sperm, he was telling [those men] to go to Spain, because there they have fertility units where his clients from the NHS can get donor sperm. But for me, this was basically out of the question. So instead, they took three samples of specimens from my testicles. And they found nothing, nothing, nothing." When I asked Nourreddine how he felt about this bad news, both he and Fadwa were philosophical:

> **Nourreddine:** I don't know. I didn't find it too serious. I didn't really look at it as being serious. It was just a normal problem.
>
> **Fadwa:** I see it as an illness, not something we asked for, not something within our control. It's just like a cancer patient. They don't ask for their disease. No one asks for their illnesses. You just have to deal with it. Cancer patients do their chemotherapy, and we had to find our treatment.
>
> **Nourreddine:** But for me, it's a bit more difficult. I don't have a problem admitting my condition. But for men, I think there's pride involved, a lot of pride involved.
>
> **Fadwa:** If anything happens in conception, they always say, "Oh, what's wrong with that lady?" They always think it's the lady first. No one thinks that men can also have reproductive problems.

Facing the problem of azoospermia together, Nourreddine and Fadwa turned to their religion and community for support. They asked a local Moroccan imam to read the Qur'an over them to ward off any "black magic," which could have resulted from envy over their happy marriage. Nourreddine also ingested several herbal remedies, including ground nutmeg and whole milk, which he was told would "strengthen" him as much as eating ground sheep's testicles. The couple also consulted with their Moroccan neighbors, who had been childless for sixteen years. The older couple told them their story of failed IVF in the NHS, which resulted in the wife's ten-day hospitalization for hyperstimulation, followed by five unsuccessful attempts at ICSI back home in Morocco, and, finally, the birth of an ICSI daughter on the sixth attempt. Encouraged by this news, Nourreddine and Fadwa thought about traveling home to Fez for a cycle of ICSI. But first they made their annual trip to Dubai to visit their closest friends, who had moved there from London five years before. It was in Dubai that Fadwa and her friend hatched a plan:

> To be quite honest, I was with my friend in Dubai, staying with her and just talking. We brought out the yellow pages, and she opened it up to see if we could find a clinic. It opened right to the page of Conceive! So what she did is to phone it up, and she phoned up a couple of hospitals as well. But *everyone* referred us to this clinic. Everyone she asked from Dubai to Sharjah. So my friend said we should just give it a try. We only had four days left before we were supposed to go back to the UK. But Dr. Pankaj said we should just come in and see his clinic and have a checkup. And as soon as he saw me, he said,

"It's possible that you've got polycystic ovaries." Because I have really large spots [pimples] on my chin. He said, "You should have a scan, and I'll show you." And so I did a scan, and I saw loads of these cysts. Dr. Pankaj sent me to have blood tests, to be sure. My insulin levels were really high, because PCOS causes insulin to be high. My insulin was 209 when it should have been 75. See, it was sky high! And he prescribed medication to reduce it, to bring my insulin levels down. He said that I must try to control it before I start any IVF treatment. But no one in the NHS had ever picked up this problem on me at all, after two to three years of going there. Dr. Pankaj picked it up right away just by looking at me. He knows what he's talking about. Sometimes you don't have confidence with what someone says. To be quite honest, I did every diagnosis in the NHS, and I was told I was fine: "Everything is fine. Absolutely nothing wrong." This NHS doctor would say, "I'm not going to talk about you. Let's deal with your husband."

Nourreddine had his own story to tell about Dr. Pankaj's comparatively excellent diagnostic acumen:

When we got here, we saw this Dr. Pankaj, who consulted our files. Once he saw these results, he said, "Look, we're going to do your sperm test again." I done [sic] it here, and then we waited. And within half an hour, he came back to me and said, "We found sperm. We found maybe 5 percent sperm." We didn't believe him! We thought it was somebody else's. So many years in England, we were told, "Absolutely nothing. Not at all!" Here they showed me under the microscope. Just for me—I got "special treatment." They said, "We spun it. We spun it in the machine." I'm sure they did this in the UK, or at least I reckon they did. But maybe they didn't. So Dr. Pankaj suggested to freeze it, and I didn't want to because I didn't know this clinic. And you never know what goes on inside clinics these days! Leaving your sperm, and it's live sperm! But I have a bit of confidence because (a) you see the pictures [of babies] here on the walls, and (b) he knew our South African doctor back in London. So we froze it, and we came back three days later to give some more sperm. We left two samples. You see, the more you have, the better, because some of the sperm can die. I was—I was honestly thinking that I'd have to do another [testicular] biopsy. So as soon as they found sperm [in the normal ejaculate], I couldn't believe it! Because when I walked in here, the first thing I said is, "I've got no sperm." I brought my test results from England, and all the reports said zero, zero, zero. But Dr. Pankaj said, "Throw it in the [trash] bin!" He didn't want to look at the reports. He said: "I found sperm. I don't need to see that."

As it turned out, Nourreddine had a classic case of cryptospermia, or "hidden sperm" in his ejaculate. The Palestinian Muslim laboratory director at Conceive had taken special care to centrifuge Nourreddine's semen sample, creating a "pellet sample" in which even the smallest number of spermatozoa could be detected. Although Nourreddine was seriously infertile—with fewer than 1,000 sperm found, when a fertile man would have at least fifteen million sperm per milliliter under the microscope—nonetheless he produced enough viable spermatozoa to be a candidate for ICSI. With routine IVF laboratory techniques, this was easy to determine. Thus, what Nourreddine came to realize in the Emirates is that the NHS had utterly failed him—convincing a twenty-two-year-old Muslim man who was opposed to sperm donation that he would never father a biological child.

In a happy state of shock over the recovery of his hidden sperm, Nourreddine was eager to get on with the ICSI procedure. The only problem now was finding the financing. A price tag of 20,000 dirhams ($5,445) was much more money than the young couple could easily afford, especially given that they were used to free health care under the NHS. Nourreddine explained their financial dilemma in this way:

> In England the blood work and all the consultations are free. But here you spend literally five minutes with Dr. Pankaj, and it's 500 dirhams [$136]. Yesterday, I paid again 300 dirhams [$82], and [Fadwa's] medicine is like about 600–700 dirhams [$163–$191] as well. The flights are £600 [$947] for both of us together. So, in dirhams, that's about 6,000–7,000 dirhams [$1,633–$1,906]. Luckily, our friends are here, so we are staying with them. But we had to rent a car for 3,000 dirhams [$817] a month. Because now we have to stay for a month. With the 20,000 dirhams [$5,445] for the actual treatment, plus the medicines that we have yet to buy, Dr. Pankaj said that we should be prepared to spend £3,000 [$4,735] for the whole treatment. And maybe with the scans, it will crop up to 21,000 dirhams [$5,717], on top of which we already spent well over 30,000 dirhams just to get here [$8,167]! So I've spoken to Dr. Pankaj to give me some kind of discount, because we're trying to save our pennies. We're living in the UK, which is not the cheapest country. He is going to speak to the owner, some Arab guy [about offering a charitable discount], because it will be at least 20,000 dirhams [$5,445] to do this ICSI.

Despite the high cost of the ICSI and the associated reprotravel, Dr. Pankaj was very honest with Nourreddine and Fadwa that their chances of success on the first ICSI cycle were no higher than 38 percent. As believing Muslims, the couple took this in stride. "I believe that God will give me a child if he wants to,"

Nourreddine opined. "If I do have a child, it comes with its own *rizk* [financial sustenance]. I already say that it's like I'm buying a child, though I try not to think like this! With all this expense, you might buy one and get one free! They say you have a higher chance of twins with ICSI."

Telling me that they would feel lucky to have even one ICSI child, Fadwa then asked if I would be telling their story in some future publication. I told the couple that I planned to write a book and would change their names to protect their confidentiality. This led to a brief, but interesting, conversation about secrecy and disclosure:

> **Nourreddine:** I have always thought of this as something confidential—not necessarily private, just confidential. I don't want anyone to say, "Oh, you have a child from IVF?" I won't say, "Oh, I have a child from IVF." It's just not a nice thing. It's abnormal.
>
> **Fadwa:** I don't know . . .
>
> **Nourreddine:** So will you tell your friends about IVF?
>
> **Fadwa:** I would tell my family, because it's not abnormal. Lots of people do it now.
>
> **Nourreddine:** So if someone *asks* you, you can't be dishonest?
>
> **Fadwa:** It would be silly for someone to make comments about IVF. That would be very uneducated.
>
> **Nourreddine:** Well, I'll tell you what I'm going to do. I told Dr. Pankaj that when I get back to the UK, I'm going to tell that doctor who is referring lots of his customers to Spain that lots of his customers should be coming straight here! I'm sure that there are lots of clients like me with the same problem, and they're telling them in the NHS to use donor sperm! It's the worst thing that they could do—to tell people like me that they can never have kids.

Fortunately for Nourreddine and Fadwa, Conceive was their *nasib* (destiny), as they told me. Nourreddine's once hidden sperm were effective in producing several viable ICSI embryos, three of which were transferred into Fadwa's waiting womb. On the day of the pregnancy test, I was at the clinic eagerly awaiting the news, along with the couple and several Conceive staff members. Fadwa was seated on a red couch in the clinic administrator's office, while Nourreddine stood beside her. When the Palestinian lab director came in to deliver the news, the happy smile on her face presaged the results of a clearly positive pregnancy test. Everyone cheered and hugged each other, with several other staff members coming by to congratulate the young couple.

Nourreddine and Fadwa remained in Dubai for the next six weeks, determined as they were that Dr. Pankaj himself would undertake the initial pregnancy ultrasound. The ultrasound showed that two of the couple's three embryos had not implanted in Fadwa's womb. However, Fadwa was definitely pregnant with a single fetus—the product of her eggs and Nourreddine's hidden sperm, which, though lost in the British NHS labyrinth, had been found in a patient-centered clinic in the Emirates.

• **Transnational Malpractice**

Foreigners such as Nourreddine and Fadwa, Daniyah and Abner, and Sheela and Niels were not the only ones to seek reproductive salvation at Conceive after years spent in a wide world of poor-quality medical care. Some Emirati couples, too, had suffered terribly. Such was the case of Maitha and Ateef, an attractive Emirati career couple whom I met in Conceive's recovery room. Sitting up in bed and dressed in a hospital gown, Maitha had long, straight, jet-black hair and intricate floral henna decorations winding up both her arms and legs. When I admired Maitha's henna design, she sighed, "It's ruined now," pointing to the IV still stuck in her arm following her egg retrieval operation.

Both Maitha and Ateef spoke excellent English, but it was Maitha who wanted to tell me her difficult reproductive history. Ateef was clearly concerned about the couple's privacy. He was circumspect in the interview, even adopting a kind of Emirati "cool pose" by slouching back in his long white *dishdasha* robe as he sat at Maitha's bedside. Nonetheless, Ateef did answer all of my questions politely, and he listened attentively as Maitha described her harrowing tale of transnational medical malpractice.

Now thirty-two, Maitha was one of the new generation of educated Emirati women, who had a busy career as the marketing manager of her father's real estate firm. Both she and Ateef had obtained bachelor's and master's degrees in the United Kingdom, so they were comfortable with Britain and its medical system. When Maitha failed to become pregnant after two years of marriage, she decided to seek the care of the only British IVF physician operating in the Emirates, one who commuted regularly between Dubai and his busy London-based IVF practice. When the physician saw Maitha for the first time, he diagnosed her with PCOS and a "T-shaped" uterus,[34] which he said would prevent her from undergoing IVF in a normal fashion. Instead, he prescribed several rounds of IUI, which resulted in an ectopic pregnancy and the blockage of Maitha's right fallopian tube.

Still convinced that Maitha could not become pregnant through IVF because of her uterine malformation, the doctor prescribed a procedure called gamete intrafallopian transfer (GIFT). GIFT differs from IVF in that eggs are extracted from a woman's hormonally stimulated ovaries and then placed directly into her fallopian tube, along with her partner's sperm. The rationale for GIFT is that it more closely resembles the "natural" process of conception. However, because it does not involve laboratory-based methods of vitro fertilization, GIFT is not as successful as IVF, nor is it used with regularity in most reputable IVF clinics. Not knowing this—and inherently trusting the British physician's superior judgment—Maitha and Ateef agreed to the GIFT. Maitha began her hormonal stimulation in Dubai and then flew with Ateef and her mother to London to undergo the egg retrieval and GIFT in the physician's London clinic.

Unfortunately, GIFT was no gift for Maitha. A "miscommunication" occurred between the physicians in Dubai and London that led to a critical overdose of Maitha's ovulation induction medication. Before leaving for London, Maitha was told by her doctors in Dubai that she might be at risk for ovarian hyperstimulation. But it was too late to cancel her GIFT, so Maitha boarded the plane for London. Once she reached the United Kingdom, a medical emergency began to unfold, as Maitha recounted in painful detail:

> I got severe hyperstimulation while in London. They had made a mistake on my ovulation induction, with too many injections. They basically gave me an overdose. The [British] doctor told me so. He literally told me that it was a mistake—a communication problem between the doctors. I don't know where the mistake occurred, in Dubai or London, but the last time they scanned me in Dubai, it looked like I might be at risk for hyperstimulation, and I don't know if this [risk] was communicated to them at the clinic in London. But when the hyperstimulation started to happen, I literally became bloated. I came back to Dubai very sick, and they had to put me in the American hospital for around one month. And while in hyperstimulation, I got pregnant with another ectopic. [The British physician] had transferred over twelve eggs into my tube, which I now understand is an "extreme thing." I thought he was a professor who knew what he was doing! I was only thirty years old, and I suffered through a tubal pregnancy and hyperstimulation at the same time. After that, we took a long break. But I still had some frozen embryos in London, which they had fertilized after my GIFT treatment. So a year ago, we went back to London for the embryo transfer. They put two embryos back in at the five-day blastocyst stage.[35] We came back here, and the result was that

I got pregnant—my pregnancy hormones were very good. But then it turned out to be a blighted ovum.[36] So that was it—*khalas* [finished].

Maitha was fortunate that this transnational medical mishap had not cost her the use of her remaining fallopian tube or the forced removal of her ovaries. But the financial cost of two international trips, the medically mismanaged GIFT, and all of the attendant complications had been significant for Maitha and Ateef, who decided to appeal their case to the UAE Ministry of Health. As they pointed out, Maitha's reproductive complications had begun at an Emirati government hospital. Taking pity on the young local couple, the Abu Dhabi–based ministry eventually paid for all of their medical expenses, including their international reprotravel, thereby effectively footing the bill for a transnational case of medical malpractice.

Not knowing where to turn next, Maitha considered heading to another IVF clinic in London that belonged to an Egyptian physician who had been featured in a BBC documentary on assisted reproduction. Maitha and Ateef also thought about traveling to Amman, Jordan, home to one of the Middle East's most famous IVF clinics and a hub for regional reprotravel. However, Maitha had already "had her share" of Arab male gynecologists, including the mostly Egyptian and Syrian doctors who worked in the Dubai and London IVF clinics that she had visited. Therefore, Maitha and Ateef considered traveling to Belgium, where ICSI had been invented.

Yet the thought of more European reprotravel did not appeal to the Emirati couple, who were now in their early thirties. After serious deliberation, Maitha decided that she was simply more comfortable in her home country, where she could continue her work and be surrounded by her loving family. Maitha also wanted to be seen by a female physician from this point on, so she visited one of the major Dubai hospitals that employed several well-known female gynecologists. The Australian doctor who reviewed Maitha's complicated case urged her to abandon any future IVF plans. Her message to Maitha was both frightening and familiar. Maitha recalled the painful conversation:

Some doctors are very technical and emphasize the worst-case scenario, especially regarding hyperstimulation: "You can get blood clots! There are so many risks! And even if you get pregnant, fluid could build up in your tube and be toxic to the pregnancy." I guess she was trying to be frank and straightforward, just in case it happened. But I was freaked out. This was unintentional on her part—she was just trying to be honest, but it never works to give so much detail. Just tell me that it happens, but don't tell me any more. I'm used to this now, because I've seen doctors from lots of nationalities! But the way they communicate with you is the most important thing that I concentrate on.

"Too much information," and none of it hopeful, turned Maitha away from the Australian physician. Back to square one, Maitha heard from acquaintances that a male Indian IVF physician named Dr. Pankaj was supposed to be an excellent clinical communicator. Maitha looked him up and made an initial appointment for herself and Ateef. When Dr. Pankaj reviewed Maitha's medical records, he saw no particular obstacles to IVF, insisting that she could become pregnant even with a congenitally misshapen uterus. However, he needed to manage Maitha's significant case of PCOS, even cancelling Maitha's first IVF cycle when her PCOS-affected ovaries failed to respond well enough to hormonal stimulation.

From that point on, Maitha was determined to become an IVF mother at Conceive. "I always say that I am going to get pregnant, and we just have to try," Maitha explained. "This is my second cycle of IVF, but I've done lots of IUIs, lots of timed cycles, lots of injections. I even learned how to give myself injections! I don't even know anymore all the things that I've done, but now I do whatever Dr. Pankaj tells me!"

When I asked Maitha how many IVF children she would eventually like to have, she took a moment to reflect on motherhood, the importance of work, and changing aspirations for Emirati women. "Actually, I like to work, and I have a career," Maitha explained. "So it is changing here. Especially in my generation and among my friends, people are settling for two [children].[37] Women are more active with their work. And because of Emiratization,[38] there is recently a lot of pressure to hire Emiratis in the private sector. There are even special programs to encourage young [Emirati] graduates to get into the private sector. I work in the private sector and so does Ateef, so two or three kids is all that we can handle. I definitely want only two or three children."

Lest Maitha's definitive desire somehow tempt fate, the truculent Ateef ended the interview on a cautionary note: "But let us just have one for now!"

- **Reproductive Resettlement and Anchor Babies**

Walking down the hallway of Conceive in February 2007, I saw a couple who looked strangely familiar to me. This feeling of déjà vu overwhelmed the young couple as well, so we approached each other in greeting. There in the hallway, we realized that we had met four years before, during my earlier study of ICSI in Lebanon. In this "tale of two studies," the husband, Abdullah, was an eager participant,[39] differing significantly from Maitha's cautious husband, Ateef. Abdullah was a loquacious Lebanese man who had spent two years in an MBA program in St. Louis and who loved American culture. He and his infertile wife, Muna, wanted to tell me their complex story of reprotravel, which involved the trials and tribulations of a "commuting marriage" between two Arab cities; many failed IVF cycles back in Lebanon, which led to profound disenchantment with the Lebanese medical system; religious concerns over being treated by a non-Muslim physician in the Emirates; and the couple's eventual struggles to secure an IVF "anchor baby" in Canada,[40] thereby ensuring the child's safe future outside of the turbulent Middle Eastern region. This final concern was prescient, for Muna's family hailed from Syria—which, four years later, would become embroiled in a bloody civil war.

Muna's reproductive troubles had begun in Syria. As a teenager in Damascus, she suffered from menstrual irregularities that landed her in the office of a male gynecologist. The physician diagnosed ovarian cysts and insisted that Muna needed surgery. Whether the ovarian cyst removal was warranted remains unclear. But as a result, Muna was left with two blocked fallopian tubes, which were discovered eight years later when she married Abdullah.

Muna met Abdullah while she was completing pharmacy school in Beirut, and Abdullah had returned from his MBA program in St. Louis. Abdullah quickly fell in love with Muna, whose strawberry blonde hair, blue eyes, and alabaster skin reminded him of the American women he had met in the United States. Following the couple's wedding, Muna quickly found a position in a hospital pharmacy in Beirut. But well-paid jobs for Abdullah were few and far between in Lebanon's impoverished post-war economy. Thus, Abdullah headed off alone to the Emirates. There he worked as a certified financial analyst, helping Emiratis manage their considerable assets.

But Abdullah's life in the Emirates was not easy. At least once a month, he flew back to Beirut to spend time with Muna and to help her overcome her tubal infertility problem. Together, they visited a Beirut-based IVF physician, who was reputed to be "number one in Lebanon." Their first IVF cycle was successful, resulting in a joyful twin pregnancy. But then disaster struck, as Abdullah and Muna recounted:

Abdullah: The first time, we got pregnant with two. Everything was going well, but all of the sudden, at the fifth month, something happened. There was bacteria, something in her water [amniotic fluid].

Muna: Suddenly, I got contractions. They thought it might be strep B [group B streptococcus], but they were not sure.[41] They gave me too many antibiotics, but my white blood cell count was still not going down. They also gave me medicines to stop the contractions. So I spent one week in the hospital, but I woke up one morning and found too much blood. I was in the middle of delivering one boy and one girl. *Alhamdulillah* [praise be to God], I delivered Mohamed and Fatima in May 2002, my first pregnancy.

Abdullah: The doctor in that hospital did not try seriously enough to save them. Part of the problem is that we could not afford the right hospital. Our financial situation did not help us to get access to the American hospital—the only one that can handle high-risk pregnancies. She needed to spend one to two weeks in the American hospital. But we didn't have enough funds for the American hospital. So she had to go to the only hospital where our insurance would take her. Because she is a pharmacist in Lebanon, she had insurance from the Lebanese pharmacists' association. It is supposed to be number one in Lebanon! The insurance covers two weeks if the delivery is premature, and a lot of other things. But it will *not* cover the American hospital! And there are other restrictions, like you *cannot* be pregnant for one year before taking the insurance. We had to take this insurance to fit into our budget, but that's why we couldn't go to the American hospital. So instead, she had to go to a hospital that was not equipped enough to handle high-risk pregnancies. That's what we learned from them.

Following this most devastating pregnancy loss, Muna and Abdullah tried IVF again, this time in a different hospital-based Beirut IVF clinic. That is where I met them in 2003 in the midst of their second IVF cycle. But after two IVF cycles at the hospital were unsuccessful, the couple returned to their original Lebanese IVF doctor. Two more IVF cycles in his clinic failed to produce a viable pregnancy, and Abdullah's dissatisfaction with Lebanese IVF medicine was mounting:

Commercialism in Lebanese medicine is a real problem. One of our IVF doctors was a real gentleman, and he tried his best. But otherwise I have a problem with these people. There are still honest doctors in Lebanon, but this is not true of everyone. For example, we saw a doctor who was honest with us. He told us, "Don't do *anything* until her insulin level [from PCOS] comes down." He had a clinic across from the American hospital, and he was a gentleman. But when we asked one of the IVF doctors about her insulin problem, he said: "No problem. This does not affect [IVF]." Actually, we were looking for the right doctor and not really finding one, which made us upset. So we left him, because honesty and trust are most important. Don't lie to us! Tell me exactly what's going on! To give you another example, my wife was supposed to be told about her eggs [following the surgical egg retrieval]. But the doctor didn't come by, and he was late by at least two to three hours. When I asked, "Where is the doctor? My wife is waiting in the recovery room," they told us, "He's tied up. He has a health emergency, and he has to go to the hospital." They gave us an excuse. The nurse said, "He has an emergency. He has to see another patient." But then when the doctor came by many hours later, he said, "Sorry, I was at the hospital, and I was not feeling good, so I went home to rest." It freaked me out! I didn't argue with him. But these were not the right people to deal with. They were not being honest with us. We needed to get away from these people, because we were wasting our time and money. Especially, we heard back in Lebanon that they were supporting and helping certain people, certain [political] groups. They were taking $3,000 from us, and taking it to help "certain groups," if you know what I mean. They help [infertile couples from those groups] without even charging them! So it's their right, But then help me with the right to treatment! I'm paying money—not asking for free treatments.

And there's something else about the doctor that made me think he's commercial. I tried to entertain him. I invited him out for dinner, because I appreciate that he's helping us.[42] But when I was with him in the car, he was talking with one of the other physicians on his mobile phone. "How many did you do today?" He's not asking, "How is she doing? Is she feeling good?" Things are being done to generate money, not "How are these people? How are *my* people?" He is not in touch with these people as his patients. So when we decided to quit, he tried to e-mail me many times. But I did not respond. I just ignored him. Just respect the fact that I've been traveling to your clinic—taking my vacation time, having a difficult time, just to come and help my wife and save this marriage—and all you're interested in is money!

Abdullah's indictment of Lebanese medicine as highly "commercial" was one that I had heard many times in my earlier study in Lebanon. But his statement about "saving this marriage" was intriguing to me, as relatively few Lebanese men considered a wife's infertility to be grounds for divorce.[43] When Muna stepped briefly outside of the room, I asked Abdullah if his marriage was in trouble because of Muna's infertility. He responded adamantly:

No, no, no! I'm an independent person. Everything is my own decision. It could have been me, not her [as the infertile spouse]. I don't believe in this thing called divorce. It is God's word; it's something to be fixed, and she can't be punished for something that is not in her hands. I can't destroy someone else's life because God created her like that. But you feel that you're *exhausted*. Her parents, my parents, they're not showing it, but they're making us feel under pressure. They're telling us, "Don't worry. It's gonna be okay." But we *know* that from the inside, they're hurt, and they're panicking *more* than us. But they're not showing it at all.

In Arabic culture, in Middle Eastern culture, they tell you, "Go marry! Go get yourself another wife." But I will not, because I believe maybe God sent me to help my wife, to be there for her. And maybe because we have been patient with each other, our life is always happy. We accept each other. She accepts me when I've been having financial problems. And I accept her with this problem. It's all about sharing and accepting each other. No one is perfect; everyone has something wrong. I felt unhappy, but I was trying not to show it; I was trying to help her. Especially in the Middle East, the mentality is that if your wife doesn't have babies, you must have a second wife. A lot of families indirectly or directly push their sons [to remarry]. But I try to reassure her that if she hasn't any babies, our marriage is all about her and not about babies only. I think that if the [infertility] problem was [from] me, I would need the same help. I wouldn't need someone to destroy me! Plus she's educated, a pharmacist, and very clever. So I don't want to put her down.

Abdullah clearly loved Muna, did not blame her for their childlessness, and was willing to finance multiple expensive IVF cycles on her behalf. But he admitted that his patience with IVF was wearing thin: "At the end, I started getting sick and tired of this thing. Perhaps I didn't mention this to her, but I was thinking, 'My God! How long do I have to put up with this?' All the trips and going and coming. All of my bonuses being spent on this. All of my perks being spent on treatment. All my perks just going down the tube. I'm not improving in life. I'm running, and the dollars are running ahead of me!" Furthermore, Abdullah was entirely "fed up" with Lebanon and wanted Muna to join him in the Emirates. However, Muna appreciated the finer aspects of Lebanese medicine, because she worked in the country's pharmacy system. Thus, Muna was "attached" to Lebanon, and felt deeply conflicted about moving to the Emirates, as she explained:

I don't have confidence in just *any* doctor. For example, for my teeth, I prefer to be in Lebanon. I think there's more education, and they give more care in Lebanon. There are some doctors [in Lebanon] who are very good. You hear a lot more in your own country, because you know more people who can tell you a lot. I didn't hear about good doctors in the Emirates. I was not so confident. But it was very difficult for my husband and me to be separated during this time. You need your husband beside you. So, after all this time, I decided to give the Emirates a try.

After Abdullah settled Muna in his apartment in the Emirates, he decided to obtain "multiple opinions" from a variety of doctors. "I learned from my mistakes back in Lebanon," Abdullah told me. "So this time, I decided to put three doctors in front of my wife. I wanted to hear many opinions. And for the first time, our finances were okay, so we were able to afford three doctors—to review her records, to do her scans, to check everything. I can see then if a doctor is okay after listening to how they would handle her case."

The first physician to review the couple's records was the same Australian female gynecologist who had put off Maitha with her candor, as described above. However, Muna and Abdullah appreciated this physician's detailed communication style. "I really liked her," Muna said. "She sits with you for a half hour, forty-five minutes. She sits with you and explains *everything*. And you can ask her questions." Abdullah added his two cents' worth: "She was good. You can sit down with her, and she explains step by step, 'the German way,' in detail. She explains to you the problem, the odds, everything. She gives you her time. So this one I liked, because she knows what's going on. We bought a Christmas gift for this doctor, because we liked her so much. And she was very surprised and happy, because she didn't expect that! But after Christmas, she came back and told us that she was leaving to go back to Australia. I was very upset about that."

Feeling that they were back to square one, Abdullah started doing his homework, and learned that a "famous" Indian IVF physician had just opened a clinic called Conceive. Abdullah convinced Muna to come with him to see Dr. Pankaj, even though she was uncertain. Abdullah was frank about Muna's misgivings:

My wife still had the feeling, "How am I going to start treatment with a non-Muslim?" First of all, he's a man, but she prefers a lady. Second, he's non-Muslim. She mentioned it one time, and I changed the way she was thinking, and then she didn't mention it anymore. It was a kind of anxiety; she was not feeling comfortable because he is not Muslim. But that's stupid, I believe, and wrong. I do believe that people, whatever their religion, if they behave to you properly, and you behave properly, then people will behave right with you. But my wife is scared. If the hospital is Christian, she's afraid that they will not treat her the right way. But that's wrong. We are not all the same. In a Christian or Jewish hospital, in a medical center, people are supposed to treat you right, no matter what religion you are.

According to Abdullah, Muna's "traditional" Syrian family only served to fuel her fears. "I'm lucky because my wife is not around her family here," he said. "Her family [members] are religious, and they practice the religion, and they are sharing her decision about the need for a Muslim doctor. So I'm lucky that they are not involved."

Once Muna started coming to Conceive to consult with Dr. Pankaj, she felt good about her decision to "give up on Lebanon." She explained: "I am a Sunni

Muslim and so is my husband. But in this country, it's regular to see Indians because they live in this country, and almost all of the doctors are Indian. The most important thing is to search for a good doctor. Indian doctors *are* good. They respect you; they treat you better sometimes than Arabs." Abdullah himself had nothing but praise for Dr. Pankaj:

My wife had this religious problem—"Oh, he's not Muslim, Dr. Pankaj." But I told her, "You never look at this person's religion. You look at the *result*, not whether he's Christian or Hindu or Muslim." I told her, "Don't worry. He's okay." Then she started treatment and she was *amazed* at the way Dr. Pankaj was treating her. Everything he does, he mentions God's name. When inside the operating room, the Qur'an was being read [on tape] and he's not even Muslim! She said, "I can't believe this doctor is not Muslim. Look at how much he respects his people!" [Dr. Pankaj] was very smart, intelligent, polite, respectful. He's not just treating the causes; he's also psychologically treating us, because he's being *positive*, and making us feel that the baby is next door, not far away. But we have to do what we have to do. If something is wrong [an infertility problem], we have to know it. So this is a point. I did feel that he is also updated on medical research. One time, he checked something on a website; he always has his [medical] sources. So this is very, very good.

Dr. Pankaj was the first IVF physician in seven years to confront Muna's PCOS, which was probably implicated in her multiple IVF failures. Before Dr. Pankaj would initiate an IVF cycle, he insisted that Muna lose considerable weight, while he attempted to bring down her very high insulin levels through medication. Abdullah appreciated Dr. Pankaj's sensitivity on the subject of weight control:

When we met Dr. Pankaj, he said right away two things: First, lose your weight. So she lost around twelve kilograms. She went on a diet, which helped, and she did exercise, and I tried to help her by not eating out. We are "restaurant people"; we like eating out at restaurants. And second, he told us he has to bring down her insulin level. He treated this problem *before* she started treatment, and after three months she was ready to go! What's special about Dr. Pankaj is that he's always a positive person. He's very calm, and he thinks positively, which makes you feel very relaxed. He says: "It's not a big problem. It's not a big deal." And if there *is* a problem, he always has a solution. For example, he told my wife to reduce to 84 [kilograms; 185 pounds], but she only got down to 86 [190 pounds]. I was upset, but he said, "No! This is very good! She did a great job!" He didn't shame her, so that if the [IVF] operation failed, he could say that this happened because she should have been 84 [kilograms]. He didn't try to find a glitch and blame it on us.

On their first cycle of IVF at Conceive—their sixth cycle overall—Muna became pregnant, eventually giving birth to a healthy baby daughter named Sarah. I was delighted to meet Sarah at Conceive—a cherubic one-year-old, dressed fashionably in a red jumper, white turtleneck, white tights, and little gold earrings. While I gushed over Sarah, Muna told me that her daughter was already a "frequent flyer." "She's only one year old," Muna explained, "but how many times she has traveled already! Maybe ten to fifteen times—to Canada, and back to Beirut, then Dubai. We've already been to Canada two to three times this year."

When I asked about Canada, Muna and Abdullah told me another part of their reprotravel story, which had involved their desire to deliver their "anchor baby" in Canada.[44] In the years since I had met them in Beirut, Muna and Abdullah had become citizens of Canada, a country that still welcomes educated Arab professionals. But for their daughter to obtain full Canadian citizenship rights—including a birth certificate, passport, and visa—she needed to be born in Canada. This desire to deliver their first IVF child in Canada involved a painstaking decision for Muna and Abdullah, one in which Dr. Pankaj's input proved essential. The couple told me their "anchor baby" story in this way:

Muna: If I didn't deliver in Canada, then it would be very difficult for our daughter to get a visa. One of our friends with Canadian citizenship delivered here in the Emirates, and for one-and-a-half years, she couldn't take her daughter with her to Canada, because she had no visa for her daughter. So we were very concerned to go to Canada and deliver there. But it was our first baby, and I was worried that I might miscarry again on the plane. What if there is bleeding, or something happens? Many times, we reserved tickets, then canceled. We reserved, then canceled. Because everyone told us, "Don't go! This is your first child after waiting seven years!" They were creating fear. But, you know, from early on, from seven weeks of pregnancy, all I could think about was whether to go or not.

Abdullah: My wife met with an Indian obstetrician in Dubai, and she was very negative. She said, "Do not move one step! Do not think of traveling! Are you crazy?" It was a very difficult decision to make. You've been waiting six years, and people are not helping you, and a few people are *not* accepting the idea at all. All we heard was, "Not a good idea!" "You've waited six years!" So we consulted some doctor friends, and they also said, "Are you crazy? Are you willing to lose what you've waited for for six to seven years?" And this really freaked me out! I also believe that some doctors only want to do the delivery themselves. They look for money more than they look for what you want.

Muna: And that Indian lady doctor, I didn't like her. When I asked her about traveling, she told me, "I say no!"

Abdullah: So this is when we decided that we should only rely on Dr. Pankaj. If Dr. Pankaj says "no," then we will not travel. But if Dr. Pankaj says everything is okay—that now she can travel without any problems—then we will go. When Muna told Dr. Pankaj about that lady doctor, he said, "No, don't listen to her! You're all set for traveling." So I told Muna, "Let's go to the travel agency!"

Muna: It was only two days before we traveled. *Insha'Allah, khalas!* Let's go get the ticket!

Abdullah: I said that we should go business class on British Airways. In business class, she could sit a little bit more comfortably, with her legs out like this [he stretched his legs out to show me]. She can sleep, have a bed, to take this fear away. So it was a smooth flight. We went to London first, and she relaxed there a couple of hours.

Muna: It was a long trip—seven hours to London on British Air, one hour of waiting, then seven hours to Toronto. So maybe fifteen hours, and I was already thirty-five weeks [pregnant]!

Abdullah: One hour before we landed in Toronto, she started feeling some pain in her legs. So I very much tried to manage the pain in her legs, tried to help her, tried to talk to her to make her forget. And when we made it to Canada, the weather was beautiful! It was the 24th of December in Toronto, and there was no snow! We did not see any snow.

Muna: I thought I would deliver directly once we arrived in Canada. But we got there, and I waited four more weeks. *Exactly* four weeks later, at thirty-nine weeks, I delivered Sarah.

Marcia: Where did you deliver her?

Muna: In Mt. Sinai Hospital in Toronto. I didn't have a history there. We told them we were coming from overseas. So the resident called a doctor, and he was very good. Actually, they don't usually accept patients at the end of pregnancy. But he was very kind, and he accepted us. I told him that this is an IVF baby, and I had a history of strep B. So maybe this is why he accepted me.

Abdullah: Actually, before we got there, I had done my homework about this hospital. Mt. Sinai delivers more than 7,300 babies in one year! They have a high record, with very, very good ways of treatment. I knew that it was a hospital for Jewish people, but I didn't care. As long as we received the right treatment, in a clean place, we just needed someone to help us. So we decided to go to Mt. Sinai on our second day in Canada. We didn't have a doctor or anything. And usually, no one will take you so far along in a pregnancy. But one of the professors, he came to me, and he spoke to me in a very friendly way. He tried to speak some Arabic with me. I could kind of tell that he was a Jew, because of the way he talked Arabic with an Israeli accent. But he was very, very friendly. So I said to Muna, "People behave to you the way you behave to them." He was very gentlemanly, and he did not want to bother us. He sent us to see a Palestinian Israeli lady doctor, to find out how we felt about having him as our doctor. So the lady spoke Arabic with us, and we told her that we liked him [the Israeli physician], and that we wanted him to be our doctor. We told her that we didn't mind [that he was Israeli], if he was willing to accept us. He was Israeli-Canadian Jewish, and he ended up being our doctor and our friend. After I sat down and spoke with him, I came to know that he had served in the Israeli military in Gaza and all that. But he gave us every option. He helped us to the maximum! He knew that we were coming from the Middle East, and that we don't have anybody in Toronto. He was a true gentleman. For example, something else I liked about this doctor, if the vagina needed to be checked, he'd ask one of the ladies to do that. He didn't want to put her [Muna] in a position to say no. So my wife very much liked him. The *politeness*! And maybe he also understood our religious background. And during Muna's labor, there was a midwife in the room, but he was watching us on the monitor, so as not to bother her. He came in at the end, and I helped pull Sarah out. That was a tough job! And to see Muna in pain for such a long time. In Lebanon, usually, the doctor just goes inside [without the husband], and he is in charge of everything.

Clearly, Muna and Abdullah's "interfaith" delivery had been a positive experience for them in many different ways. But Abdullah was also delighted that Muna's maternity care had been entirely free in Canada's subsidized health care system. "Because I have a Canadian passport, I didn't pay anything! Nothing!" Abdullah exclaimed. "I would have ended up paying $7,000–$10,000 if we had delivered in the US. But we're Canadian, and Canada is much better because of its free health care. So I figured that we could afford the business class flight, because we would have a free delivery. It was roughly $8,000 for each."

I then asked Abdullah why they were still in the Emirates, when they could be receiving "free" IVF in Canada. Abdullah explained that subsidized IVF cycles were strictly rationed in the Canadian health care system. Thus, they would probably be forced to pay for private IVF, which was more expensive in Toronto than in

Dubai. Furthermore, Dr. Pankaj had earned the couple's undying devotion and trust, and they hoped to conceive their second child in his clinic.

At the end of our interview, Abdullah told me of his many hopes and dreams. Once they conceived their second IVF child, Abdullah planned to move his family permanently to Toronto, where he could establish his own investment firm, Muna could get her Canadian pharmacist's license, Sarah could start public nursery school, and their family could be "free," living in a safe, secure, and stable country. Having grown up in war-torn Lebanon, Abdullah wanted to spare his half-Syrian half-Lebanese children from a similar fate, as he explained to me with great feeling and intensity:

> It's not only about the citizenship matter. I want my daughter to be raised in Canadian society. I don't want her to go to Lebanese schools. I don't want her to experience the same mentality that I was raised in. Lebanese people are addicted to political issues! Even in school, they ask, "Are you Christian or Muslim?" So I don't like for my kids to be raised in Lebanon. I want my daughter to have the right English accent, and to be raised with the right people, *healthy* people. So I want her to be raised there in Canada. In this area, no! There are too many religious headaches. Too many conflicts in the Middle East. I don't want to stay here and raise my kids in this place. My wife—the good thing about her is that she's a happy person. She doesn't misjudge people. If someone is late, she says, "Oh, maybe he has some emergency. Let's give him a chance." She helps me very much to relax and not be in tension. She's being friendly and nice with people. But she is too trusting. In Lebanon right now, everyone asks you, "Sunni? Shia?" Everywhere you go, it's politics, politics, politics! I'm *tired* of this politics! I don't want to talk this politics and religion all the time. Lebanon has not been free from conflict for the last thirty years. We'll spend all our lives waiting until it will be okay. So I'm lucky I left, and we're not going back. We left because it is not a good place to raise our children.

Little did Abdullah realize that much of the Middle East would soon erupt into violence. Four years after our meeting at Conceive, Muna's home country of Syria was plunged into horrifying violence, dragging Lebanon into its military and refugee crisis. As of this writing, Syria remains in the throes of war, with Lebanon deeply implicated in the neighboring tragedy.

Muna and Abdullah's seventh IVF cycle did not succeed at Conceive, and I lost track of the couple once they left the clinic. I could only hope that they had made their way safely to Canada. In Toronto, their precious IVF daughter Sarah—who was conceived with the help of a patient-centered, Indian Hindu IVF physician in the Emirates by a loving Syrian Muslim mother and a prescient Lebanese Muslim father, and who was delivered by a sensitive, caring, Israeli-Jewish obstetrician in friendly and welcoming Canada—could live a happy childhood. Settled in Canada, Sarah could be free from the violence and strife surrounding so many other less fortunate Syrian and Lebanese children, whose parents had been unable to "anchor" them in safe havens far away.

CONCLUSION

Cosmopolitan Conceptions

It was very hard to conceive, very hard. But I'm very optimistic.
I see bright light at the end of the tunnel.
—Rahnia

Postscript

"At the end of the day"—an expression that I heard often in Dubai—I
would like to return to the story of Rahnia, whose reproductive journey
was chronicled in the prologue. As readers may recall, Rahnia was an
Eritrean-Ethiopian Muslim woman, who was grateful to the United Kingdom for taking her in as a teenage refugee. Rahnia and her Sudanese refugee husband, Ahmed, became British citizens. Yet Rahnia and Ahmed's
path to reproduction in Britain was anything but straightforward. Eight
cycles of in vitro fertilization (IVF) there led to the birth of only one child,
a daughter named Wisal. Feeling "desperate" to provide Wisal with a sibling, Rahnia began a global search to find a trustworthy IVF clinic. Her
journey led her to Dubai, which she perceived to be the Middle East's
most cosmopolitan city. There, Rahnia was lucky to find Conceive. Yet it
was in Conceive that Rahnia almost died, due to a dangerous reproductive tract infection that was lingering in her swollen fallopian tube. Once
the infectious agent was released into her bloodstream via IVF, Rahnia
developed a life-threatening infection, which Dr. Pankaj managed to cure
with intravenous antibiotics. The toxicity of the pelvic infection caused
Rahnia's eighth IVF attempt to fail. That is where her story ended in the
autumn of 2007.

However, Rahnia was a woman of steely determination. She followed
Dr. Pankaj's advice to return to the British National Health Service.

There, she had her infected fallopian tube removed through a government-subsidized laparoscopic surgery. This surgery left her ovary intact. Thus, she was able to return to Conceive in 2009 to undergo her ninth attempt at assisted conception. Happily, Rahnia became pregnant with an intra-cytoplasmic sperm injection (ICSI) daughter, who was delivered in the United Kingdom in 2010. Still wanting to bear a son for her husband Ahmed, Rahnia returned to Conceive in 2011, delivering a male ICSI child nine months later. Buoyed by this experience of two rapid ICSI successes, Rahnia traveled to Conceive again in 2012, becoming pregnant with another male child. However, after returning to London, Rahnia went into premature labor at twenty weeks of gestation, delivering an extremely premature infant, who did not survive his untimely delivery.

At the age of forty-four, Rahnia decided to return to Conceive one last time. Having undertaken twelve attempts at assisted conception—eight in London and four in Dubai—Rahnia hoped that her last IVF sojourn would allow her to beat the odds, to "make the impossible possible," as she was fond of saying. At Conceive, Rahnia produced enough eggs to create two viable embryos, which were transferred into her womb in early 2014. Following the embryo transfer, Rahnia returned to London and was not heard from again. The assumption of the Conceive staff was that Rahnia's thirteenth ICSI cycle had been unlucky, and that she had therefore been unable to replace her lost ICSI son. Yet, when compared to many others, Rahnia could be considered quite lucky. Through assisted reproduction, she had been able to become a mother of three children, two daughters and one son, thereby triumphing over her infertility and her social and embodied suffering.

Reproductive Aspirations

Over the years, I have thought a great deal about the infertile women I have encountered who, like Rahnia, have traveled great distances—often at considerable cost to their reproductive bodies and their pocketbooks—in order to conceive a longed-for child. Rahnia's reprotravel epitomizes a journey of aspiration, one woman's attempt to find the "bright light at the end of the tunnel." Indeed, it is these aspirations for parenthood, these feelings of child desire—or the yearning to become parents of children who are wanted, needed, and cherished—that undergird the global movements of all reprotravelers. Such parenthood aspirations and child desires are found among both men and women, in a world where nearly

95 percent of all adults still express the desire to have children at some point in their reproductive lives.

In cases of infertility, where reproduction becomes thwarted, these parenthood aspirations and child desires are even more keenly felt, often becoming paramount, even engulfing. "It is hard to explain," said a thirty-seven-year-old Indian artist, Indira, whom I met at Conceive. "But this is my project. When you want something so bad, you really want it." A thirty-one-year-old infertile man, Rein, who is now the proud father of an ICSI daughter after making his way to Conceive from the Netherlands, explained the aspirations for parenthood and child desire in a similar way: "People who are going into fertility treatment and traveling thousands of miles *really, really* want to have kids. And if they manage to conceive and get a kid, I'm pretty sure that they will be good parents. Optimum parents, in fact! And we have a vision of how to bring our children up and to make them balanced people. We would have been very much sad if we couldn't have babies. We both have always envisioned our future with children. We're very family oriented."

Such widely held desires for parenthood and children belie the view—widely held in the West—that "childfree living" has become a new normative aspiration. For example, *Time* magazine recently ran a cover story on "The Childfree Life: When Having It All Means Not Having Children."[1] The glossy cover photo showed a white couple, lying intertwined in their matching bathing suits on a bed of white sand. Evoking images of an elite, paradisical idyll (with the implied message of "Don't spend your money on children . . . spend it on vacation!"), the article conveyed the fact that childlessness by choice is now a viable option in the Western world. Indeed, for a growing number of Western couples, childlessness may be a preferred life choice. Nonetheless, a powerful rejoinder in the *Atlantic*—"When Being Childless Isn't a Choice," written by a British journalist of West African heritage—reminded readers that most couples around the world desire children.[2] Childlessness is usually not a "choice," but rather a painfully visible reminder of a hidden infertility problem. Rahnia called this the "invisible disability"—something that "cannot be discussed openly" and that makes an infertile individual "isolated in your own world."

For the estimated 48–186 million infertile people worldwide, IVF and other assisted reproductive technologies (ARTs) have offered the possibility for technological salvation. IVF is, after all, the quintessential "hope technology," to use Sarah Franklin's well-turned phrase.[3] Franklin reminds us that the "pursuit of IVF offers a newly valid social role as a would-be

parent, an active consumer and a 'trier' as opposed to a 'do nothing'. . . .
Above all, the pursuit of ARTs offers a path forward that is sustained by
hope, and offers proof of a commitment to a normative aspiration, even
if it never delivers on its promise."[4] As she points out in her most recent
book, *Biological Relatives: IVF, Stem Cells, and the Future of Kinship*, IVF has
also served as a kind of "platform technology," being the biological fore-
bear of many IVF-related innovations.[5] These include preimplantation
genetic diagnosis (PGD),[6] which—as we have seen—can be used for sex
selection as well as for genetic screening of embryos; mammalian cloning
(as in the sheep, Dolly),[7] with the phantasmagorical future potential of
autonomous, asexual human reproduction; and human embryonic stem
cells,[8] which can be created from excess IVF embryos and which hold the
promise of future therapeutic modalities for debilitating conditions such
as Parkinson's disease and spinal cord injury.

IVF's potential often seems limitless, as new variants of the technology continue to unfold. Take, for example, egg freezing, the "newest" new
reproductive technology. Called "oocyte cryopreservation" in medical
parlance, egg freezing involves half of an IVF cycle (the retrieval of eggs
from hormonally stimulated ovaries) and holds the promise of "revers-
ing the biological clock."[9] Recently made available in the United States,
the United Kingdom, Israel, and several other Western countries, egg
freezing is currently being used by two groups of women, known as "social" egg freezers, who are the older, single, professional women who are
concerned about aging out of their fertility, and "medical" egg freezers,
who are generally younger women seeking to preserve their fertility in
the face of life-threatening diseases such as cancer.[10] Whether IVF-related
egg freezing will become the next "reproductive revolution" remains uncertain, but egg banks are now being rapidly developed across Europe and
America in order to accommodate millions of future frozen oocytes.[11]

Other revolutionary technologies are also coming down the pike. In
an article in the *Atlantic* titled "Making Babies: Five Predictions about
the Future of Reproduction,"[12] reproductive scientists speculated about
five possible reproductive scenarios: first, the development of new
forms of reproductive donation, including uterine transplantation and
techniques that combine the genetic material of three people to make a
baby free of certain mitochondrial defects;[13] second, ways to "personal-
ize" each woman's biological clock through predictive information that
will help women to understand their own fertility profiles better; third,
new fertility-tracking apps to precisely time procreation (that is, to cal-

culate the best time for sex); fourth, the creation of artificial gametes—synthetic eggs and sperm—through the manipulation of a person's stem cells; and finally, more precise forms of embryo screening and genotyping to create the genetically "best" IVF baby.

Despite the ethical questions posed by some of these techniques, a number of them are already being used. For example, in the United States, more than seventeen babies have been born from cytoplasmic transfer, in which cytoplasm from the eggs of healthy fertile women is transferred into infertile women's eggs. The babies born from this procedure share the DNA of three people—father, infertile mother, and fertile cytoplasm donor.[14] In February 2015, a similar "three-person IVF" technique was endorsed by the government of the United Kingdom. Members of the British parliament overwhelmingly passed a mitochondrial donation law, designed to help women suffering from serious mitochondrial genetic diseases that can be passed on to children with devastating effects.[15] Indeed, the new law makes Britain the first country in the world to permit IVF babies to be conceived using the genetic material of three people (or, as the *Guardian* put it, "two mommies, one daddy").[16]

Furthermore, in the past few years, uterine transplantation has been tried in several Western and Middle Eastern countries (for example, Saudi Arabia, Sweden, and Turkey). A twenty-two-year-old Turkish woman who was born without a uterus became pregnant in 2013 with an IVF embryo that was transferred into her transplanted womb. The IVF pregnancy ended in fetal demise at eight weeks of gestation,[17] but the young woman, named Derya Sert, told reporters that she would try again: "If I had a magic wand, I would want to be pregnant now. I just want to hold my baby in my arms, to be a mother."[18] A year later, in September 2014, the first living "womb-transplant baby"—a premature boy, delivered at thirty-two weeks gestation and weighing 1.8 kilograms (3.9 pounds)—was born in Sweden under the careful watch of his mother's uterine transplant and gynecological surgery team.[19] Meanwhile in Japan, the country with the largest number of IVF clinics in the world (around 600), IVF physicians have successfully reimplanted ovarian tissue into the bodies of women facing premature menopause.[20] At least one healthy baby has been born this way, suggesting that ovarian transplantation may be the next new hope for women with the poorest ovarian function and the worst reproductive potential.

This stream of IVF innovations bespeaks new hopes and dreams—what Henrietta Moore has aptly described as the "ethical imagination," or "new forms of the imagination and of knowledge, new ways of connecting to each other and their object worlds, new forms of desire and satisfaction."[21] In her recent book, *Still Life: Hopes, Desires and Satisfactions*, Moore attempts to elucidate the "arts of the possible," the "acts of hoping" that make new possibilities come into clear vision.[22] Moore argues that hope is an "animating force" in all social life, reorienting new generations toward possible futures in imagined spaces beyond the borders of quotidian experience.

New technologies of reproduction are part of this ethical imagination—an aspirational approach to life among the reproductive scientists who invent these futuristic conceptive techniques and the infertile men and women who clamor to use them. This is why Rahnia and millions like her travel around the globe in pursuit of the latest forms of assisted conception. There is also a clear commercial impetus: companies such as Planet Hospital and Global IVF are cashing in on these hopes and dreams by assisting infertile couples (as well as single people and gay couples) to find the right "reproductive destination," where they can achieve their parenthood aspirations and child desires. This is why countries such as India, Thailand, Singapore, and the UAE are investing in their countries' medical infrastructures to boost so-called reproductive tourism.[23] And this is why clinics such as Conceive—located in the center of new global reproscapes—receive reproflows from many different directions. In short, a new global reproductive assemblage is being formed in response to individuals' and couples' parenthood aspirations and to the steady stream of technological innovations in the world of assisted reproduction. These reproductive aspirations and technological innovations are at the very core of twenty-first-century reprotravel, the growing magnitude of which cannot be underestimated.

Cosmopolitan Dubai

If aspirations are an inextricable element of globalization, as Moore and several other globalization theorists have argued,[24] then Dubai represents an example par excellence of global aspirations on multiple levels. An early cosmopolitan trading hub for seafaring merchants, coastal pearl divers, and Bedouin nomads, Dubai has transformed itself into one of the world's emergent global cities—a cosmopolitan techno-hub unparalleled in any other part of the Muslim Middle East. Having survived the

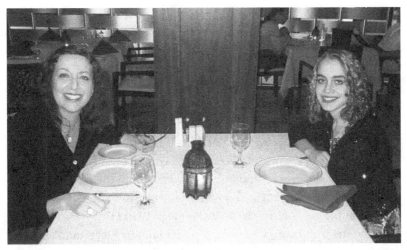

C.1 The author (left) and her daughter, Justine Hooks, at a Lebanese restaurant in the Emirates Towers, Dubai.

economic downturn of 2008–9 with the help of Abu Dhabi, and having been spared from the regional violence at the turn of the millennium, Dubai is currently booming, with tourists pouring in from every corner of the planet. In Dubai, one senses a cosmopolitan "intermingling" that is quite palpable and exciting, even to an anthropologist who has studied and lived in the Middle Eastern region for many years.

When I last visited Dubai, in the spring of 2013, I could not help but notice the ever-increasing diversity of the city. New influxes of people from East and Central Asia, East and West Africa, and Latin America and the Caribbean were evident throughout the cityscape. In addition, Arabs from many countries were frequenting the malls and restaurants. I saw numerous young Arab Gulf couples holding hands while they shopped, a sign of "couplehood" that I never observed on my first visit to the gender-segregated Gulf in 1983. These glittering cosmopolitan malls, with their strolling throngs and restaurants serving an enormous variety of international cuisines, fascinated my teenage daughter, Justine, who accompanied me to Dubai and who took many of the photos found in the pages of this book (figure C.1). As part of our trip, Justine interviewed a dear friend, an American University of Sharjah faculty member, for a school project on comparative cultures. The Canadian-born professor told Justine that one of the best aspects of living in the UAE is its diversity and multiculturalism—the ability to live, work, and "play" with people from many different nations and cultures. This sentiment was certainly echoed by my interlocutors at Conceive, who considered Dubai's cultural cosmopolitanism to be one of its most attractive features.

Without a doubt, Dubai is the Middle East's most multicultural city and its most technologically sophisticated. As holder of more than a hundred Guinness records, Dubai brims with architectural marvels, including the world's largest human-made archipelago, World Islands, and the world's tallest building, Burj Khalifa, which is shaped like a glittering stalagmite and is the world's tallest building (figure C.2). Dubai's status as an emergent global techno-hub is also obvious in the city's hosting of numerous technology-themed conferences and exhibitions. These include the Dubai Bio Expo-2015; the Biotechnology World Congress, designed to promote "the translational nature of modern biotechnological research"; the Forensic Science and Law Middle East Congress, featuring innovations in modern forensic science to improve criminal justice; the Dubai Airshow, one of the world's largest aerospace events and the major marketplace for commercial and military aircraft sales in the region; and the Dubai International Film Festival, a global media extravaganza, featuring many films that would be censored in most other Middle Eastern countries. Furthermore, in December 2013, Dubai was named the site of the World Expo 2020, thereby becoming the first Middle Eastern city to host the world's most important global technology and culture exhibition.[25] To accommodate the World Expo, as well as many other international events, Dubai has announced the construction of what will be the world's largest airport.[26] Named after Dubai's ruling family, the Al Makhtoum International Airport will be able to handle 160 million passengers and twelve million tons of cargo each year, quadrupling the capacity of the already impressive Dubai International Airport. To accommodate the new travelers, Dubai has also announced construction of the world's biggest, climate-controlled, hotel-mall complex—with one hundred hotels, 20,000 hotel rooms, four miles of streets and promenades, eight million square feet of stores and retail outlets, a theater district, the world's largest theme park, and—of particular relevance to medical travelers—a "wellness center" that will offer various surgical options, including cosmetic procedures.[27]

The wellness center in the newly planned hotel-mall complex reflects Dubai's aspirations to become the medical tourism hub of the Middle East. Already hosting the region's only medi-city (Dubai Healthcare City, discussed in chapter 1), Dubai has made the top-ten list of global medical

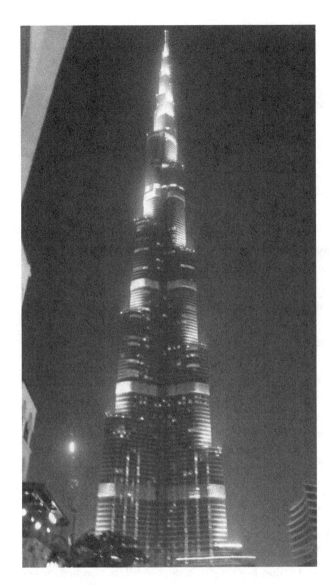

c.2 The Burj Khalifa at night.
PHOTOGRAPH BY JUSTINE HOOKS.

tourism destinations and aims to capture much of the regional Middle Eastern medical market as well. This is especially important for patients coming from other parts of the Arab Gulf, who often feel forced to travel to places like Thailand, the United States, and the United Kingdom for specialized medical services.[28] For Gulf Arabs, Dubai is closer to home on both geographic and cultural levels, and going to Dubai instead of farther afield thus spares sick travelers the feelings of disconnection and foreignness that they experience when they travel abroad.[29]

Conceive has clearly benefitted from Dubai's growing reputation as a global medical tourism hub. Conceive represents an example par excellence of a medically cosmopolitan clinic—a place where patients from many different countries can find high-quality care and enjoy a sense of clinical comfort across national, ethnic, religious, linguistic, and cultural lines. Coupled with its technological sophistication and high IVF success rates, Conceive has managed to attract reprotravelers from around the world, even without marketing itself as a "destination" clinic. For example, Conceive has never offered "fertility tourism packages" for clients coming from overseas. The clinic has also never cut deals with particular hotels in Dubai, nor does it offer spa services or trips to Jumeirah Beach as enticements for reprotravelers. Instead, Conceive flourishes by virtue of its consistently high-quality, patient-centered care, which has led to a growing global network of referrals. Like Dubai itself, Conceive is a place of cosmopolitan conceptions—a clinic where self-consciously crafted medical cosmopolitanism has worked to create a vibrant, international clientele.

On my last research trip to Dubai in 2013, I found Conceive to be pulsing with new energy. The clinic had undergone substantial remodeling to accommodate even more patients, including those coming from new countries such as Kenya, Mauritius, and Senegal. Furthermore, when I asked Dr. Pankaj about how the 2008–9 financial crisis and the 2011 Arab uprisings had affected Conceive's business, he was characteristically sanguine:

> I thought we *would* be affected because fertility is at the luxury end of the medical market. When finances are tight, people can say, "Let's wait." But, on the contrary, in times like that, people seem to relook at their priorities. Is a holiday more important, or is this more important? We found that since 2008, it is only uphill—a pleasant surprise! The UAE is still in trouble, but they're being careful. The Europeans are all coming back now, but at lower salaries. And the Arab Spring did affect business, but in a surprising way. We did have a few patients who would have normally gone to their home countries—mostly Egypt or Syria—for treatment, but who opted to have their treatment in Dubai instead. So our business has doubled. We're doing 65–70 cycles a month, which is more than 800 cycles a year.

Cautions and Concerns

Although Dubai itself is flourishing, the Middle Eastern region as a whole is more unstable than it has been in many decades, and Dubai has become the unwitting beneficiary of the surrounding regional violence. Millions of Arab men, women, and children are now caught up in the region's violent upheavals. IVF clinics have been forced to shut down in countries such as Iraq and Syria, and many Middle Eastern expatriates are afraid to travel home, including to undertake their IVF cycles on annual holidays. As of this writing, there is no end in sight to the ongoing Israeli-Palestinian conflict. Warring factions in Libya are fighting in Tripoli and Benghazi. Egypt is still shaking from the violence of its revolution. And at least two Arab Gulf countries, Bahrain and Yemen, are attempting to deal with ongoing sectarian violence and Islamic militancy. Indeed, in Yemen, a group of Shia Houthi rebels has recently taken over the government,[30] while Bahrain—with its Sunni-minority government and Shia-majority population—has joined its Sunni-dominant neighbors, Saudi Arabia and the UAE, in the US-led coalition of sixty countries battling ISIS, a Sunni insurgent group that has taken over large swaths of Iraq and Syria. These regional coalitions and sectarian-infused tensions sometimes defy easy interpretation. But what is clear is that the Middle East is facing unprecedented levels of violence in the beginning of the twenty-first century.

Although spared so far from violence on its own soil, the UAE may eventually become caught up in the regional turmoil. In his book, *After the Sheikhs: The Coming Collapse of the Gulf Monarchies*, the political scientist Christopher Davidson predicts the eventual downfall of the Arab Gulf monarchies, including the confederated monarchies of the Emirates.[31] According to Davidson, regional violence is inherently destabilizing for the Gulf monarchies. But the monarchies themselves are also politically unstable, for they are incapable of brooking dissent within their own countries or enacting meaningful political reforms. Davidson's critique is seconded by the Middle East feminist scholar miriam cooke. In her book, *Tribal Modern: Branding New Nations in the Arab Gulf*, she argues that the Arab Gulf monarchies, which are tribally organized, have attempted to impress the world with a modernist veneer.[32] But beneath the surface, tribalism in the Gulf is inimical to modernity; it is elitist, exclusive, racist, intolerant, and backward, and thus ripe for overthrow.

The Emirati scholar Noor Al-Qasimi describes her own nation as "indebted and disinherited."[33] The UAE, she argues, has allied itself with the "pan-Gulfian neo-liberal block that exercises control over the future through capitalist accumulation" (for example, in the growth of tourism, shopping malls, and the information technology sector). Yet, according to Al-Qasimi, the UAE is actually threatened by multiple instabilities. These include climate change and erosion of its landmass; depletion of its oil reserves; a demographic imbalance whereby Emiratis themselves face a "state of extinction" amid an ever-growing foreign labor force; uprisings of disenfranchised groups, including foreign workers who lack citizenship rights; ethno-sectarian revolt from within; the rise of the Muslim Brotherhood and other Islamic insurgent groups; and the threat that monarchical rulers will be unable to maintain their sovereignty over time, which is what Davidson, mentioned above, has also predicted.

Political transformation in the Gulf—either through violent, internal revolutions or broad-scale regional war—remains a threat to the status quo. Whether such events will occur in the UAE is, of course, uncertain. But what is clear is that Dubai is located in the thick of things—built on an unstable political foundation, in the midst of one of the world's most volatile regions. As critical Gulf studies scholars have already argued, many contradictions and tensions are simmering just beneath the surface.[34] Thus, Dubai's foundation may eventually crumble under the weight of increasing turmoil and political repression.

Among my own interlocutors, none of whom were scholars, I found a different set of critiques, which were directed at the Emirates' medical sector. Although these critics took great pains to tell me that Conceive existed in a state of exception—as an isolated island of medical competence in a sea of medical negligence—they often viewed the Emirates' medical system as a whole as inherently untrustworthy. Disenchantment with Emirati medicine, including on the part of Emiratis themselves, was not what I anticipated to find in a neoliberal medical tourism hub. But according to my interlocutors, health care in the Emirates was uneven and often poorly delivered by a corps of foreign physicians with questionable medical acumen and little long-term investment in their jobs. Dubai has made significant financial investments in its health care infrastructure—particularly in its government hospitals, which command 54 percent of the total health care budget.[35] But Dubai has not made similar investments in its health care personnel. This is especially true in the private medical sector, which accounts for two-thirds of all health care expenditures, but where quality control and regulatory oversight appear difficult to achieve.[36] There, poor-quality medical care may be the norm. But according to patient testimonies, bad medicine is practiced in government-run facilities as well. An implicit acknowledgment of these inadequacies may be found in the fact that Dubai spends 14 percent of its total health care budget to send its Emirati citizens abroad for specialized medical services.[37]

Such "medical outsourcing" is apparent in the IVF sector.[38] For many years, infertile Emiratis were flown by their government to other countries, in particular to the United Kingdom. However, IVF outsourcing has diminished over time as the local IVF industry in the Emirates has expanded to more than a dozen clinics. At the same time, legislators in the Emirates have transformed what was once the Middle East's most permissive IVF regime into the region's most restrictive. Legal devolution in the Emirates has led to enforcement of the world's toughest IVF law—more prohibitive than legislation in any other Middle Eastern Muslim country and more stringent than Italy's Vatican-inspired IVF law, which is often held up as the "poster child" of legal retrogression.[39] The Emirates' 2010 ART law has forced some IVF patients to become reproductive outlaws. Others are manipulating the new legal requirements in questionable ways, for example, by using permitted PGD technologies to enable son preference through sex selection. The first court cases related to reproductive illegality are beginning to unfold in the Emirates,[40] suggesting that the country's strict new law is engendering a new brand of reproductive criminality.

In this regard, it will be interesting to see whether the UAE eventually follows the path of Turkey, which is the only country in the world to have made cross-border reprotravel illegal.[41] As reported by the medical sociologist Zeynep Gürtin, the 2010 Turkish law prohibits citizens from using donor gametes or surrogates, either domestically or abroad.[42] The Turkish law is probably unenforceable and is thus largely symbolic. Nonetheless, it legally instantiates the Sunni Muslim religious ban on gamete donation and surrogacy by preventing Turks from traveling to countries where these reproductive practices are available. Other Muslim countries, including the UAE, may eventually follow suit, even though outlawing reprotravel may only serve to push this practice further underground.

Partly because of patients' fears that they may be breaking the law—or at least doing something in a moral "gray zone"—many are already undertaking reprotravel under strict conditions of secrecy. At Conceive, some infertile couples had left their home countries to protect their privacy, and the majority believed that they could not find safe, legal, trustworthy, and affordable IVF services back home. These infertile couples' feelings of being "pushed out" of their home countries for a variety of frustrating, sometimes infuriating, reasons constituted their overarching and abiding complaint. Their choice to use IVF to produce a child was voluntary, but their travel abroad was not. Thus, few if any reprotravelers in my study could conceive of themselves as reproductive tourists. Instead, their IVF sojourns in Dubai symbolized the reproductive rejections that they had faced in countries that were either unable or unwilling to meet their reproductive needs. Unsurprisingly, many reprotravelers to Conceive felt that their nations had betrayed and abandoned them.[43]

Reproductive Justice

Clearly, compassion for the infertile and respect for their reproductive rights through the provision of safe, affordable IVF is far from being fully realized. In fact, a group of prominent IVF scholar-activists has joined forces to publish a scathing critique titled "Assisted Reproductive Technologies in Developing Countries: Are We Caring Yet?"[44] As they point out, relatively little progress has been made on a global level in ensuring access to IVF for the world's infertile. The vast majority of IVF cycles are delivered in the private medical sector, meaning that costs may be prohibitive for most citizens, and certainly for the infertile poor.

Thus, on a most basic level, ensuring reproductive justice for the world's infertile people means providing affordable IVF as a basic right and expectation of citizenship. To do so, nation-states (including the United States[45]) must resolve a number of important issues, including, first, whether the infertile have a disease needing treatment or whether having a baby is a "luxury" and thus of little or no concern to the state; second, whether health services are a right or entitlement of citizens and, if so, whether IVF services should be considered as a part of basic health care; third, whether IVF and all its variants should be fully legalized or whether some aspects are to be constrained by the law; and finally, whether IVF services are an entitlement of citizens only or whether noncitizens (migrants, refugees, guest workers, expatriates, and the like) can claim the same services.[46]

The idea of "biological citizenship"—in which sufferers of disease make demands on the state by virtue of their biological afflictions and their sense of entitlement to health[47]—is generally missing from the world of assisted reproduction. Exceptions are found in Israel and parts of Europe, where generous health care subsidies cover IVF treatment cycles. However, few reprotravelers feel empowered by their nation-states to demand IVF as a basic health care right. Even Emiratis, despite being granted many privileges by their government, do not have automatic access to state-sponsored IVF services. Instead, like the foreign residents in their country, most Emiratis seek IVF services in the private sector, with varying results and experiences. Thus, some Emiratis also become reprotravelers, seeking IVF services outside of their emirates or nation-state as a whole.

Furthermore, some reprotravelers seeking IVF in the Emirates exist betwixt and between home and host countries. Like Rahnia, many reprotravelers are Arab, African, or South Asian migrants, expatriates, or refugees who have left their home countries for political and economic reasons. As we have seen, many of the infertile patients at Conceive were political exiles from war-torn Middle Eastern and African nations. Others were economic migrants from resource-poor countries, especially in South and Southeast Asia. During my time in the Emirates, I came to think of these kinds of reprotravelers as *reproductive exiles* or *reproductive refugees*— terms that were never used by reprotravelers themselves, but that nonetheless seemed to capture their sense of being "pushed" or "forced out" of a home country.[48] For those seeking permanent residence in the Emirates, the country was not a safe haven. The UAE does not grant citizenship rights to foreigners, leaving large numbers of political exiles and economic refugees in limbo.

In short, reprotravel often connotes the failures of states to grant safe, legal, affordable, and effective IVF as a right of citizenship. Much like "abortion tourism," reprotravel often bespeaks the desperate border crossings of women like Rahnia, who feel expelled by their home countries in their darkest moments of reproductive need.[49] Reprotravel is about politics— about what states are willing to do for their citizens to ensure their reproductive rights. Although not all reprotravel is about fleeing the state—for example, some infertile couples travel by choice, and most of them also enjoy the right of return[50]—reprotravel often evokes bitter experiences of rejection and escape, of being evicted from pathological health care systems, of circumventing restrictive IVF laws, and of seeking safety and refuge through reproductive services delivered abroad.

Compassion for the infertile, respect for reproductive autonomy, and access to IVF as an entitlement of citizenship would thus appear to be important reproductive rights goals. If infertility is accepted as a source of profound human suffering, and reprotravel for IVF is acknowledged as logistically challenging, time-consuming, impoverishing, frightening, and even life-threatening, then ensuring access to IVF must be viewed as an important humanitarian and reproductive justice issue.

Activist Futures

What can be done to achieve this kind of reproductive justice? I want to end by suggesting three major avenues for reproductive health activism, all of which would help to prevent the need for costly reprotravel among the world's infertile citizens.

The first avenue for activism involves *infertility prevention*, or averting the preventable forms of infertility before they take hold in men's and women's reproductive bodies. Infertility prevention entails many different strategies and the work of both reproductive health specialists and public health educators. Infertility prevention involves the early detection and treatment of reproductive tract infections, including sexually transmitted diseases such as gonorrhea and chlamydia, which can wreak havoc on the male and female reproductive organs; and of postpartum, postabortion, and iatrogenic infections, which are a major cause of both primary and secondary infertility in women. In addition, the world's women need better education about fertility over the life course, so that they are aware of the ways in which fertility postponement may lead to infertility outcomes. Furthermore, in some parts of the world, including the Arab Gulf and South Asia, an infertility "epidemic" is raging and is linked to the triad of overweight/obesity, insulin resistance/diabetes, and PCOS/infertility. The solution for this growing problem remains obscure, as noted in a 2014 *New York Times* article titled "PCOS: An Infertility Issue That Is Little Understood."[51] In my experience, very few women, including highly educated ones, have ever heard of PCOS. Health education about PCOS is desperately needed to explain the genetic and lifestyle factors that are linked to this globally pervasive cause of infertility.

The same goes for men's health. Of the world's billion smokers, 81 percent are men. Yet very few men, including highly educated ones, seem to have any idea that smoking is toxic for sperm. Antismoking campaigns need to address the reproductive health outcomes of tobacco consumption for men, not just for pregnant women. Furthermore, men who work in agriculture, heavy industry, and the military should be aware of the ways in which various environmental risk factors—including toxic metals and weaponry, certain pesticides, and endocrine disruptors found in plastics—can deleteriously affect male fertility.[52]

Increasing global awareness of these kinds of risk factors is an important avenue for prevention. However, not all infertility can be prevented, especially the millions of cases of male infertility that are due to genetic factors. Thus, a second important activist avenue involves *support of the infertile*. In my view, much more global effort must be directed at destigmatizing infertility and supporting the men and women who find themselves infertile in societies where parenthood is socially mandatory. Infertility support groups need to be developed and sustained in the global South, perhaps with input from nongovernmental organizations dedicated to reproductive health and reproductive rights. Furthermore, efforts should be directed at creating new routes to social parenthood, particularly through the encouragement of adoption and fostering. Although legal adoption of the kind found in the West is not allowed throughout most of the Muslim world, fostering has a solid foundation in the social institution of *kafala*, or guardianship/sponsorship. Avenues to foster parenthood need to be encouraged among infertile Muslim couples, including across the Middle East, where the practice remains relatively uncommon.[53]

Moreover, in parts of the world where marriage and parenting have provided exclusive routes to adulthood, entirely new social paths need to be forged. These new ways of being need to include categories such as "single by choice," "happy couples," "dual-income, no kids" (DINKS), and "child-free living." In my many years of working in the Middle East, I have discovered support for these ideas among some infertile couples who are often happy in their childless marriages and wish that others would simply leave them alone. Similarly, Amrita Nandy has studied women in India who have chosen not to become mothers, often with the support of their husbands.[54] Over time, I hope that these kinds of childless options—coupled with increasing educational and career opportunities of all kinds—will become more viable as alternatives for men, women, and couples. Only then will the stigma of infertility and the social agony of childlessness lessen.

Finally, the third avenue—which is my biggest hope and my personal activist commitment[55]—is the *low-cost IVF (LCIVF) movement*, which has emerged in the past five years. The mission of LCIVF is to make safe, affordable, effective IVF accessible to everyone who needs it, but primarily to people in the global South. Making LCIVF a global reality remains a formidable challenge, but recent efforts and technological innovations to make a simple, transportable IVF laboratory system are certainly a step in the right direction. (Although technologically more difficult, a low-cost ICSI system also needs to be developed, to address the millions of cases of male infertility.) So far, LCIVF has gained support from the World Health Organization and the European Society for Human Reproduction and Embryology. My hope is that other global health agencies and philanthropic organizations will eventually take up this charge, including infertility and the LCIVF movement in the global reproductive rights and reproductive justice agendas.

Through activism directed at preventing infertility, supporting infertile couples, and encouraging the LCIVF movement, we can begin to mitigate the suffering of infertility, facilitate the parenthood aspirations of women like Rahnia, and reduce the need for costly reprotravel to places like Dubai. But until then, infertile people will keep on traveling in their desperate but aspirational attempts to conceive the IVF babies of their dreams.

ACKNOWLEDGMENTS

While conducting a study of male infertility in Beirut, Lebanon, in 2003, I kept hearing about the UAE, particularly Dubai. Many of the Lebanese men I interviewed aspired to migrate to the Emirates for work—"the best place to live in the Arab world"—and they intrigued me with their favorable depictions of this global mecca. It was in Beirut that the seeds of this present book were planted. I want to thank Dr. Michael Hassan Fakih and Hamzah Tahan in particular for encouraging me to head to the Emirates as a researcher. It was Dr. Fakih who introduced me to the assisted reproduction community in the UAE, even though his own IVF clinics—based in Abu Dhabi and Dubai—would not open until months after my study had been completed. I am deeply grateful to Dr. Fakih and to his Emirati partner, Dr. Amal Shunnar, for their support and for their introduction to Conceive, the IVF clinic where I ultimately carried out my research.

At Conceive, Dr. Pankaj Shrivastav did everything in his power to facilitate my study and to make me feel at home in his global clinic. I cannot thank "Dr. Pankaj" enough for agreeing to host me as a researcher and to recruit "reprotravelers" into my ethnographic project. In addition, many of the staff members of Conceive welcomed me warmly into their offices, their labs, and their homes, which enriched my life in the UAE and the pages of this volume.

However, it is the patients who traveled to Conceive who are at the heart of this book. Nearly 220 men and women—from 50 different nations—agreed to tell me their reprotravel stories, filled with hardship and heartbreak but also with hope and aspiration. These reprotravel stories, shared with me in clinic back rooms and at hospital bedsides, reveal the still arduous nature of infertility and its treatment in the twenty-first century. My most heartfelt thanks go to these reproductive sojourners. I hope that they may all come to meet the test-tube babies of their dreams.

This study of reprotravel to and within the UAE could not have been carried out without the institutional support of the American University of Sharjah (AUS), where I lived with my family throughout my stay in the Emirates. I thank my colleague at the University of Michigan, Professor Mark Tessler, for introducing me to AUS and to Professor Nada Mourtada-Sabbah, who arranged my institutional affiliation and a lovely office in AUS's Department of International Studies, which she chaired at the time. Paula Doyle, AUS's director of human resources, deserves special thanks for securing our residence visas, a lovely AUS townhouse for my family and me, a student counseling position for my husband, places for our two children in the Sharjah English School, and my appointment as AUS's first visiting research scholar. At AUS, we formed a lasting friendship with Professor Cindi Gunn, Professor John Raven, and their two children, who introduced us to the world of Arabian horses and many other local delights.

My study was generously funded by the US Department of Education's Fulbright-Hays Faculty Abroad Research Program, as well as the Cultural Anthropology Program of the National Science Foundation (NSF). Both the NSF and Fulbright-Hays have funded my multiple, extended research trips to the Middle East, including time spent living with my family in Egypt, Lebanon, and the UAE. I am deeply grateful to these two granting agencies, and to their program officers, for being enthusiastic supporters of my Middle Eastern medical anthropology scholarship.

This study was carried out while I was a professor at the University of Michigan (2001–8). I owe many thanks to that great "Research I" public university—especially for impressing on me the need to keep working in the Middle East, even in the tumultuous aftermath of September 11, 2011, the wars in Iraq and Afghanistan, and the 2006 "summer war" in Lebanon. Since moving to Yale University in 2008, I have been well supported in my return visits to both Lebanon and the Emirates in 2009, 2010, and 2013. During those years, I was also able to co-organize a Yale-supported conference—called Global Health and the UAE: Middle East–Asia Connections—at the United Arab Emirates University (UAEU), where I first presented my research on reproductive travel to a local audience. I thank Michael Dalby and Molly Moran for being wonderful conference co-organizers and the administration of UAEU for hosting such a unique global gathering.

At Yale, my interdisciplinary life is supported by the Department of Anthropology, the Council on Middle East Studies of The Whitney and Betty MacMillan Center for International and Area Studies, the Women's

Gender and Sexuality Studies Program, and the Global Health Initiative in the Yale School of Public Health. I am particularly grateful to my colleagues Julia Adams, Elizabeth Bradley, Richard Bribiescas, Linda Lorimer, Frances Rosenbluth, Ian Shapiro, and Laura Wexler for the many ways in which they have supported me and my research since I came to Yale. In 2012 my colleague in medical history, John Warner, brought together all of Yale's faculty in the medical social sciences and humanities. We call ourselves MASH (for medical anthropology, sociology, and history), and we have become a wonderful Friday afternoon reading group. I thank my MASH colleagues, Rene Almeling, Gretchen Berland, Richard Bribiescas, Danya Keene, Catherine Panter-Brick, Joanna Radin, Naomi Rogers, and Frank Snowden—as well as my visiting MASH colleagues Astrid Blystad of the University of Bergen, Norway, and Fiona Parrott of the University of Amsterdam—who read the prologue and introduction to this book, offering invaluable and incisive commentary. I am also fortunate to collaborate closely with Dr. Pasquale Patrizio, the director of the Yale Fertility Center, who has welcomed me as a researcher and who has been a great intellectual collaborator and coauthor on the bioethics of reprotravel. We are both part of a new group called Friends of Low-Cost IVF: Empowering Women Globally, which, if successful, may obviate the need for reprotravel by locating affordable IVF services in resource-poor settings.

Several chapters of this book were formulated and partially written at the University of Cambridge, where I was honored to be the inaugural Diane Middlebrook and Carl Djerassi Visiting Professor in the Centre for Gender Studies, in the Department of Geography. I want to thank Professor Carl Djerassi, who recently passed away at the age of 91, and Professor Jude Browne, the Frankopan Director of the Cambridge Centre for Gender Studies, for making possible one of the most fruitful and enjoyable periods of my academic career. Lesley Dixon facilitated my visit at the Centre for Gender Studies, and the fellows of Downing College—including Master Barry Everitt, Dick Taplin, and the late Richard Stibbs—provided great conviviality. Most fortunately, the dazzling Zeynep Gürtin became a close friend and colleague of mine during that period. We brought together, for the first time, an international and interdisciplinary group of scholars working on the topic of cross-border reproductive care. At that workshop, I presented my first paper on the return reproductive tourism of diasporic Arabs to the Middle East. Papers from that workshop have since been published as a special issue of *Reproductive BioMedicine Online* on cross-border reproductive care in November 2011, for which Zeynep and I served as guest editors. While I was based in England, Zeynep accompanied me to conferences in both Turkey and Singapore. At the National University of Singapore, supported by the Social Science Research Council, I was able to present my first paper on "Reproductive Exile: South Asian Stories," parts of which appear in chapters 2 and 3 of this book. In addition, Zeynep has been an amazing colleague, who gave me the first invaluable feedback on my prologue and introduction. (Zeynep's positive feedback truly bolstered me during a summer in which I was immobile and confined to my home following foot surgery. However, that foot surgery, performed by the talented female orthopedic surgeon Dr. Sanda Tomak, allowed me to walk without pain. And, during my "confinement," a book was born!)

I have been fortunate to present my ideas on the topic of reprotravel to multiple academic audiences, who have given me very useful feedback. These include audiences at Brown University, Claremont Graduate University, Columbia University, the Graduate Center of the City University of New York, Florida State University, King's College London, McGill University, New York University, the Norwegian University of Science and Technology, Princeton University, the Rockefeller Foundation's Bellagio Center, Swarthmore College, the University of Arizona, the University of Bergen, the University of California at Berkeley, the University of Lisbon, the University of Lyon, and the University of Michigan. In 2012 I was the keynote speaker for a conference on medical tourism sponsored by the Center for Medical Tourism Research in San Antonio, Texas, a research unit ably headed by Dr. David Vequist. In 2014 I was asked to speak about the medical travel of Gulf Arab patients to the United States at both Cincinnati Children's Hospital Medical Center and the Children's Hospital of Philadelphia.

My life is greatly enriched by academic colleagues and students. Mira Vale, a brilliant Yale undergraduate and my advisee, helped me immeasurably by reading, summarizing, and organizing everything I had ever written about reprotravel, thereby facilitating this book's architecture (and, in the end, its index). Her partner, Nick Allen, also a Yale undergraduate, used his geographical skills to craft the maps accompanying chapter 1. Jennifer DeChello, the faculty services assistant in the Yale Department of Anthropology, provided wonderful assistance with multiple literature reviews, thereby enhancing my scholarship and the bibliography of this book. Although he has departed for a wonderful position at the University of Chicago, my former Yale medical anthropology colleague, Sean

Brotherton, helped me track down the origin of the phrase *cosmopolitan medicine*, an early term in our field that was introduced by one of my mentors, Frederick L. Dunn. Fred passed away in May 2014, before this book was published. But his conception of "cosmopolitan medicine" shines through the pages of this volume, which I dedicate to his memory as a great mentor and pioneering physician-anthropologist.

My life as a medical anthropologist would never be the same without a global assemblage of anthropologists who are also my close friends and who work on similar topics in the Middle East and South Asia. They include Aditya Bharadwaj (United Kingdom and India), Daphna Birenbaum-Carmeli (Israel), Morgan Clarke (United Kingdom and Lebanon), Zeynep Gürtin (United Kingdom and Turkey), Susan Martha Kahn (United States and Israel), and Soraya Tremayne (United Kingdom and Iran). The amazing cadre of IVF scholars in the United Kingdom who are my friends and intellectual compatriots include Lorraine Culley, Jeannette Edwards, Sarah Franklin, Kate Hampshire, Nicky Hudson, Robert Simpson, Marilyn Strathern, and Charis Thompson. In Scandinavia my cohort of fellow IVF scholars and friends includes Charlotte Krolokke, Merete Lie, and Marit Melhuus. I am also fortunate to know some of the most important bioethicists and legal scholars working on cross-border reproductive care and IVF in resource-poor settings, including Willem Ombelet, Guido Pennings, Francoise Shenfield, and Richard Storrow. Richard Storrow deserves special recognition for helping me to think through the concept of legal devolution and for his close reading of chapter 3, on assisted reproduction and the law. I am also grateful to Sharmila Rudrappa for sharing her work and insights on surrogacy tourism to India.

In the Middle East, my work and life are enriched by a number of colleagues, including Mohammad Jalal Abbasi-Shavazi (Iran and Australia); Hatem Nabih (Egypt and United Kingdom); Nefissa Naguib (Egypt and Norway); Gamal Serour (Egypt); Sallama Shaker (Egypt and United States); and several Moroccan collaborators, including Hakima Fassi-Fihri and El Mokhtar Ghambou (International University of Rabat); Hsain Ilahiane (University of Kentucky); and Fatima Sadiqi and Moha Ennaji (University of Fez).

I am also fortunate to have three beloved mentors from my graduate school days, Joan Ablon, Nelson Graburn, and Ira Lapidus—all of whom are still going strong. Nelson Graburn was one of the pioneering anthropologists of tourism. Joan Ablon was one of the most influential medical anthropologists of stigma and suffering. And I would not be the kind of

Middle Eastern scholar that I am had I not found a supportive role model in Ira Lapidus.

Working with Duke University Press has been a truly pleasurable experience. Ken Wissoker is an extremely brilliant, responsive, and supportive editor, and I am lucky to have worked with him on two books so far. Thanks also go to Elizabeth Ault for her excellent editorial assistance. Two anonymous reviewers provided incredible insights in their close readings of the manuscript, for which I am very grateful. I also thank the Duke University Press editorial advisory board for providing important suggestions on the book's introduction and tables. Once the book moved into production, Danielle Szulczewski carefully shepherded it through to the end.

Finally, my family deserves the utmost gratitude. My husband, Kirk Hooks, and our children, Carl and Justine Hooks, have embarked with me on every one of my Middle Eastern sojourns since 1996, including half a school year spent living in the UAE in 2007. Kirk, Carl, and Justine are a great group of fellow travelers, and I cannot imagine having made these journeys without their good natures and their spirits of adventure. Most of the photographs in this book were taken by Justine, then a teenager, on our return trip to the Emirates in 2013. Kirk read every chapter "hot off the press," providing insightful editorial comments, line editing, and his invaluable skills as my human dictionary. My parents, Shirley and Stanley Inhorn, have always kept the home fires burning during our absences, for which I am deeply grateful. In a book describing the work of caring physicians, it is especially important to note that my two brothers, Lowell and Roger Inhorn, are both compassionate cancer doctors, who not only care for their patients but also have cheered me on from afar. Another devoted physician, Kristina ("Kris") Austin Nicholls, has been my BFF since fifth grade and is now one of the most esteemed and popular cataract surgeons in the Kaiser Permanente medical system. I dedicate this book to them.

GLOSSARY OF MEDICAL TERMS

Advanced maternal age (AMA): Traditionally defined as when a woman is older than thirty-five at the time of delivery. In women older than thirty-five there are increased genetic risks in pregnancy, due to the aging process of the human egg and resultant chromosomal abnormalities. Fertility rates decline and miscarriage rates increase with AMA.

Assisted reproduction: Also known as *assisted conception,* a number of advanced medical techniques to aid fertilization, thereby achieving pregnancy in couples with *infertility* (see below). *In vitro fertilization* (see below) is the best-known of the assisted reproduction techniques.

Assisted reproductive technology (ART): All fertility treatments in which both eggs and sperm are handled. In general, ART procedures involve surgically removing eggs from a woman's ovaries, combining them with sperm in the laboratory, and returning them to the woman's body or donating them to another woman. *In vitro fertilization* (see below) is the best-known ART.

Azoospermia: See *male infertility,* below.

Blastocyst transfer: A recent advance in infertility treatment, which involves growing human embryos in the laboratory to a later "blastocyst" stage before transferring them into the uterus following a cycle of *in vitro fertilization* (see below). With a blastocyst transfer, fewer embryos are transferred, but pregnancy rates are just as high. The technique thus virtually eliminates the risk of a *high-order multiple pregnancy* (see below).

Blighted ovum: Also known as an *anembryonic pregnancy,* this occurs when a fertilized egg is implanted in the uterus but does not develop into an embryo. The condition causes nearly half of all miscarriages in the first trimester of pregnancy and thus is a leading cause of early miscarriage.

Chocolate cyst: Also called an *endometrioma* or an *endometrial cyst,* an ovarian cyst that contains fluid and sometimes semisolid material, including old, dark blood that grossly resembles chocolate. These cysts are related to severe *endometriosis* (see below).

Cloning: Autonomous, asexual reproduction, involving the creation of a genetically identical copy of a human. Human cloning is ethically controversial and widely banned; it has yet to be successfully achieved in humans, despite its success in other mammals.

Congenital bilateral absence of the vas deferens: An inherited condition in males where the tubes that carry sperm out of the testes (the *vas deferens*, see below) fail to develop properly. Although the testes usually develop and function normally, sperm cannot become part of the semen because the vas deferens is missing. As a result, men with this condition are unable to father children unless they use an *assisted reproductive technology* (see above). This condition is one of the signs of cystic fibrosis, an inherited disease of the mucus glands; when absence of the vas deferens occurs alone, it is considered a mild, genital form of cystic fibrosis.

Cornual pregnancy: Also known as an *interstitial pregnancy*, a rare type of *ectopic pregnancy* (see below) that occurs when the fertilized egg is implanted in the part of the fallopian tube that is buried deep in the wall of the uterus. Pregnancies of this kind are particularly dangerous because they can progress and tend to rupture later, having the potential to damage both the wall of the uterus and the fallopian tube.

Cryopreservation: The freezing of tissue or cells in order to preserve them for future use. Sperm samples and excess embryos are routinely frozen for future cycles using *assisted reproductive technology* (see above). Eggs and ovarian tissue can also be cryopreserved.

Cryptospermia: Also known as *cryptozoospermia*, a form of male infertility in which very low numbers of sperm are "hidden" in the semen. The semen sample must be centrifuged into a "pellet" sample and examined very carefully by laboratory technicians experienced with *in vitro fertilization* (see below). If semen analysis is performed in a laboratory where the technicians are inexperienced, then misleading zero sperm counts will be reported, which could lead to an unnecessary *testicular biopsy* (see below) due to an incorrect diagnosis of *azoospermia* (see *male infertility*, below).

Cytoplasmic transfer: An experimental fertility technique that involves injecting a small amount of cytoplasm from eggs of fertile women into eggs of other women whose fertility is compromised (usually by age). The modified egg is then fertilized with sperm and implanted in the uterus of the woman who is attempting to become pregnant. Children born from this procedure have been reported to possess cytoplasmic organelles called mitochondria from both their biological mother and the ooplasmic donor, a condition referred to as mitochondrial heteroplasmy.

Diagnostic laparoscopy: A surgical procedure that allows a health care provider to view a woman's reproductive organs. Several gynecological problems can be diagnosed (and treated) this way.

Donor insemination (DI): The process by which sperm from a male donor is placed into the reproductive tract of a female for the purpose of impregnation without sexual intercourse. DI is used in cases where the male partner produces no sperm or the woman has no male partner (for example, she is unmarried or a lesbian). In the Middle East, DI is practiced only in cases of *male infertility* (see below) and only in two countries, Iran and Lebanon.

Donor technologies: All forms of third-party reproductive assistance, including *sperm donation* (see below), *egg donation* (see below), *embryo donation* (see below), and gestational surrogacy (see *surrogacy,* below). In the Middle East, donor technologies are used in only two countries, Iran and Lebanon.

Ectopic pregnancy: A complication of pregnancy in which the embryo is implanted outside the uterine cavity. Most ectopic pregnancies occur in the fallopian tube (these are known as tubal pregnancies), but implantation can also occur in the cervix, ovaries, and abdomen. With rare exceptions (abdominal pregnancies), ectopic pregnancies are not viable. An ectopic pregnancy is a potential medical emergency and, if not recognized and treated properly, can lead to death of the woman and demise of the fetus.

Egg donation: Also known as *oocyte donation,* the process by which a woman known as an *egg donor* provides one or more (usually 10–15) *donor eggs* (also known as donor ova or oocytes) for purposes of assisted reproduction or biomedical research.

Embryo: A fertilized egg that has begun cell division, first called a pre-embryo (or pre-implantation embryo) and then called an embryo at the completion of the pre-embryonic stage, which is considered to end at about day fourteen of gestation. In general, the term *embryo* is used to describe the early stages of fetal growth, from conception to the eighth week of pregnancy.

Embryo disposition: Decisions about the future use of excess embryos produced through cycles of *assisted reproductive technology* (see above). The choices include *cryopreservation* (see above), disposal, donation to other couples, or donation for medical research.

Embryo donation: A process in which excess embryos produced in one couple's cycle of *assisted reproductive technology* (see above) are donated to other couples for their use. In the Middle East, embryo donation is currently practiced in only one country, Iran.

Endometriosis: A gynecological condition in which the tissue that behaves like the cells lining the uterus (endometrium) grows in other areas of the body, causing pain, irregular bleeding, and possible infertility.

Epididymis: A narrow, tightly coiled tube connecting the efferent ducts from the rear of each testicle to the *vas deferens* (see below); spermatozoa formed in the testis undergo maturation in the epididymis before exiting the body through ejaculation.

Fibroid tumor: Also known as *leiomyoma*, a noncancerous growth of the uterus, which often appears during the reproductive years, including during pregnancy. Uterine fibroid tumors, or fibroids, develop from the smooth muscular tissue of the uterus and may grow slowly or rapidly, ranging in size from small "seedlings" to large, bulky masses. Fibroids may go through growth spurts and may also shrink on their own. In extreme cases, they may obstruct or expand the uterus, causing problems with conception or loss of a pregnancy.

Follicle stimulating hormone (FSH): A hormone synthesized and secreted by gonadotrophs of the anterior pituitary gland in the brain. FSH regulates the development, growth, pubertal maturation, and reproductive processes of the body. In women, FSH helps to control the production of eggs by the ovaries; thus an FSH test can help to determine a woman's egg supply (or the ovarian reserve) and whether a woman has gone through menopause. The more elevated the level of FSH, the lower the level of the woman's ovarian function.

Gamete: A mature sexual reproductive cell, either a sperm or an egg, that unites with another cell to form a new organism.

Gamete donation: See *egg donation* (above) and *sperm donation* (below).

Gamete intrafallopian transfer (GIFT): An *assisted reproductive technology* (see above) that involves removing a woman's eggs from her hormonally stimulated ovaries and immediately placing them with her partner's sperm into the fallopian tube. With GIFT, fertilization takes place inside the fallopian tube rather than in an *in vitro fertilization* (IVF; see above) laboratory, and the rationale for GIFT is that it more closely resembles natural conception than IVF does. However, GIFT requires at least one healthy fallopian tube in order to be performed, and it is considerably less successful than IVF.

High-order multiple pregnancy (HOMP): A pregnancy with triplets, quadruplets, or more fetuses, often the result of a cycle of *assisted reproductive technology* (see above) or treatment with fertility drugs.

Hydrosalpinx: A fallopian tube that is blocked, usually as a result of infection, and filled with clear fluid. The blocked tube may become substantially distended, giving the tube a characteristic sausage-like shape on an x-ray. Fluid from the tube may leak back into the uterus, causing problems with embryo implantation.

Hyperstimulation: See *ovarian hyperstimulation syndrome*, below.

Hysteroscopy: The inspection of the uterine cavity by a lighted scope with access through the cervix. Hysteroscopy allows for the diagnosis of intrauterine pathology and serves as a method for surgical intervention inside the uterus.

Iatrogenesis: Inadvertent adverse effects or complications caused by or resulting from medical treatment or advice; physician-induced harm.

In vitro fertilization (IVF): A process by which egg cells are fertilized by sperm outside the body, or in vitro. The process involves hormonally controlling the ovulatory process, removing oocytes (eggs) from the woman's ovaries, and letting sperm fertilize them in a fluid medium in a laboratory. The resulting embryo is then transferred to the patient's uterus, with the intent to establish a successful pregnancy. IVF is the best-known *assisted reproductive technology* (see above). It was introduced in 1978, the year of the first successful birth of a "test-tube baby," Louise Brown. Robert G. Edwards, the reproductive physiology professor at the University of Cambridge who developed the treatment, was awarded the Nobel Prize in Physiology or Medicine in 2010.

Infertility: The failure of a couple to conceive after trying to do so for at least one full year (the World Health Organization considers the diagnosis of infertility to occur after two years of trying to conceive). In *primary infertility*, pregnancy has never occurred. In *secondary infertility*, one or both members of the couple have previously conceived but are unable to conceive again after a full year of trying. See also *male infertility*, below.

Intracytoplasmic sperm injection (ICSI): A variant of *in vitro fertilization* (IVF; see above) that was introduced in Belgium in 1991, in which a single sperm is injected directly into an egg to "aid" fertilization. The procedure was designed to overcome problems of *male infertility* (see below), although it is now beginning to supplant IVF because of improved fertilization rates. ICSI is carried out in IVF laboratories under a high-powered microscope using multiple micromanipulation devices. Although ICSI is considered a safe and effective way to overcome male infertility, it may carry an increased risk for the transmission of selected genetic abnormalities to offspring, either through the procedure itself or through the increased inherent risk of such abnormalities in males who require the procedure to conceive.

Intrauterine insemination (IUI): The process by which sperm is placed into the reproductive tract of a female for the purpose of impregnation by means other than sexual intercourse. In humans, it is an *assisted reproductive technology* (see above), using either sperm from the woman's male partner or sperm from a sperm donor in cases where the male partner produces no sperm or the woman has no male partner (for example, she is single or a lesbian). Generally in IUI, "washed sperm"—sperm that have been removed from most other components of the seminal fluids—are injected directly into a woman's uterus.

Laparoscopy: See *diagnostic laparoscopy* above.

Male infertility: Defects of spermatozoa, consisting of the following five main types (see also *cryptospermia* and *infertility*, above):

1. *Asthenozoospermia:* The condition in which a male has poor sperm motility (that is, movement); normally, at least 50 percent of sperm should be motile;

2. *Azoospermia:* The condition in which a male has complete absence of sperm in the ejaculate, which can be of two types. The first is *nonobstructive azoospermia*, in which the absence of sperm in the ejaculate is because sperm production is severely disturbed or absent; the testes are abnormal, atrophic, or poorly developed, and levels of *follicle stimulating hormone* (see above) tend to be elevated. Causes of nonobstructive azoospermia include congenital and genetic issues, undescended testicles, mumps orchitis, surgery, and radiation treatment for cancer. Men with unexplained nonobstructive azoospermia need to undergo a chromosomal and genetic evaluation and ultimately may need a *testicular biopsy* (see below) to clarify the diagnosis. The second type is *obstructive azoospermia*, in which the passage of sperm out of the testes, where they are produced, is somehow blocked, leading to azoospermia. Obstructive azoospermia can be caused by *congenital absence of the vas deferens* (see above) or a vasectomy; furthermore, sexually transmitted infections such as chlamydia and gonorrhea may cause inflammation of the *epididymis* (see above), thereby obstructing the tubules that conduct mature sperm out of the testes into the vas deferens;

3. *Oligoasthenozoospermia:* The condition in which a male with a low sperm count will also have poor sperm motility;

4. *Oligozoospermia:* The condition in which a male has semen with a low concentration of sperm (low sperm count). For many decades, sperm concentrations of less than twenty million sperm per milliliter were considered low or oligozoospermic. Recently, however, the World Health Organization reassessed sperm criteria and established a lower reference point, less than fifteen million sperm per milliliter, which is consistent with the fifth percentile for fertile men; and

5. *Teratozoospermia:* The condition in which a male has abnormally shaped sperm, which can negatively affect fertility by preventing sperm from adhering to the ovum. These abnormalities include heads that are large, small, tapered, or misshapen and tails that are abnormally shaped.

Motility: Movement. Motility of the sperm is required for successful fertilization.

Multifetal pregnancy: A pregnancy with two or more fetuses. The incidence of such pregnancies has increased dramatically over the past two decades, mainly because of the widespread use of ovulation induction agents and *assisted reproductive technology* (see above). Pregnancies with multiple fetuses have long been associated with an increased risk of maternal complications as well as a high prevalence of prenatal and neonatal morbidity and mortality.

Multifetal pregnancy reduction (MFPR): Also known as *fetal reduction*, a procedure of selective therapeutic abortion that, in recent years, has become both clinically and ethically accepted as a therapeutic option in pregnancies with three, four, or more fetuses and in any *multifetal pregnancy* (see above) in which one or more of the fetuses has congenital abnormalities. In cases of pregnancies with two or three fetuses, however, this option remains controversial. Although several techniques of *MFPR* have been reported, the most popular is the injection of potassium chloride into the fetal heart through the mother's abdomen at 10–12 weeks of gestation.

Oocyte: Also known as *ovum* or *egg*, the female gamete in many sexually reproducing organisms, including humans.

Oocyte donation: See *egg donation* above.

Ovarian hyperstimulation syndrome (OHSS): A complication from some forms of fertility medication. The syndrome has three categories: (1) *mild*, in which symptoms include abdominal bloating and a feeling of fullness, nausea, diarrhea, and slight weight gain; (2) *moderate*, in which symptoms include excessive weight gain (a gain of more than two pounds per day), increased abdominal girth, vomiting, diarrhea, darker and less plentiful urine, excessive thirst, and dryness of skin and/or hair; and (3) *severe*, in which symptoms are fullness or bloating above the waist, shortness of breath, pleural effusion, significantly darker urine or no urination, calf and chest pains, marked abdominal bloating or distention, and lower abdominal pains. Although most cases of the syndrome are mild, severe OHSS is life-threatening.

Percutaneous epididymal sperm aspiration (PESA): One of the surgical techniques used to harvest sperm in patients with obstructive *azoospermia* (see *male infertility*, above), especially following a vasectomy. In PESA a small needle is inserted through the skin of the scrotum to collect sperm from the *epididymis* (see above), where sperm are usually stored after production in the testes. PESA is now also widely used to extract sperm for *intracytoplasmic sperm injection* (see above).

Placenta previa: A complication of pregnancy in which the placenta grows in the lowest part of the uterus, covering all or part of the opening to the cervix. If the cervix is partly or complete covered, a vaginal delivery can cause severe bleeding, which can be deadly to both the mother and the baby. Thus, nearly all women with placenta previa need a C-section.

Polycystic ovary syndrome (PCOS): One of the most common female endocrine disorders. It is of uncertain cause but largely classified as a genetic disease. PCOS produces symptoms in approximately 5–10 percent of women of reproductive age (12–45 years old) and is thought to be one of the leading causes of female infertility. The principal features are anovulation, resulting in irregular menstruation, amenorrhea, ovulation-related infertility, and multiple cysts on the ovaries; excessive amounts or effects of androgenic (masculinizing) hormones, resulting in acne and excess facial hair; and insulin resistance, often associated with obesity, type 2 diabetes, and high cholesterol levels. The symptoms and severity of PCOS vary greatly among affected women.

Preimplantation genetic diagnosis (PGD): A technique used to identify genetic defects in embryos created through *in vitro fertilization* (see above) before their transfer into the uterus. When one or both genetic parents has a known genetic abnormality, the testing is performed on one of the cells of the embryo to determine if it also carries a genetic abnormality. Controversial uses of PGD include sex selection and the creation of "savior siblings" for children with life-threatening illnesses.

Premature menopause: Also known as *premature ovarian failure*, the loss of function of the ovaries before age forty.

Premature rupture of membranes (PROM): The rupture of the membrane of the amniotic sac more than one hour before the onset of labor. Preterm premature rupture of membranes means that the rupture has occurred before thirty-seven weeks of gestation. Risk factors for PROM include a bacterial infection caused by group B streptococcus. In some cases of PROM, the rupture can spontaneously heal, but in most cases, labor begins within forty-eight hours.

Septicemia: A serious, life-threatening infection that rapidly worsens. It can arise from infections throughout the body, including those in the lungs, abdomen, urinary, or reproductive tract.

Sexually transmitted infection (STI): An illness that has a significant probability of transmission between humans by means of sexual behavior, including vaginal intercourse, oral sex, and anal sex. A person may be infected, and may potentially infect others, without showing signs of disease.

Sperm donation: The provision (donation) by a man known as a *sperm donor* of his sperm (*donor sperm*), with the intention that it be used to impregnate a woman who is usually not the man's sexual partner to produce a child.

Spermatogenesis: The process by which *spermatozoa* (see below) are produced. In mammals, it occurs in the male testes in a stepwise fashion and for humans takes approximately sixty-four days. Spermatogenesis is highly dependent on optimal conditions for the process to occur correctly and is essential for sexual reproduction.

Spermatozoa: The mature male gametes in many sexually reproducing organisms, including humans.

Surrogacy: An arrangement in which a woman carries and delivers a child for another woman or a couple. She may also be the child's genetic mother by contributing her own egg (*traditional surrogacy*), or she may carry the pregnancy to delivery after having another couple's embryo is transferred to her uterus (*gestational surrogacy*).

Testicular biopsy: One of the surgical techniques used for harvesting sperm in patients with *azoospermia* (see *male infertility*, above). After local or general anesthesia is administered, a testicular biopsy removes a small sample of tissue from one or both testicles and examines it under a microscope to evaluate the presence of sperm and a man's ability to father a child.

Testicular sperm aspiration (TESA): One of the surgical techniques used for harvesting sperm from patients with *azoospermia* (see *male infertility*, above). After a local anesthetic is administered, a small needle and a special syringe are used to extract sperm directly from the testicles to be used for diagnosis and/or sperm freezing.

Testicular sperm extraction (TESE): One of the surgical techniques used for harvesting sperm from patients with *azoospermia* (see *male infertility*, above). Sperm are extracted from testicular tissue obtained through a small incision in the scrotum and in the testicles (see *testicular biopsy*, above).

Third-party reproductive assistance: Also known as *donation*, see *donor technologies*, above.

Varicocele: An abnormal enlargement of the vein in the scrotum that drains the testicles. A varicocele occurs when the valves in the veins along the spermatic cord do not work properly. This is essentially the same process as in varicose veins, which are common in the legs; the backflow of blood and increased pressure may lead to damage to the testicular tissue, causing male infertility.

Varicocelectomy: The surgical correction of a *varicocele* (see above), which is present in approximately 40 percent of men with infertility. Although varicocelectomy is the most common male infertility surgery, including in the Middle East, its effectiveness has been intensely debated, and it is no longer recommended by many infertility specialists or the World Health Organization.

Vas deferens: Part of the male anatomy involved in transport of sperm from the *epididymis* (see above) in anticipation of ejaculation.

NOTES

Prologue: Rahnia's Reproductive Journey

1. The nation called the United Arab Emirates (UAE) is made up of seven emirates, or principalities, each governed by a heredity ruler, or emir. The seven confederated emirates are Abu Dhabi (in which the nation's capital is located), Ajman, Dubai, Fujairah, Ras al-Khaimah, Sharjah, and Umm al-Quwain. Sharjah and Dubai are neighboring emirates. Sharjah offers lower-cost housing than Dubai and thus is often considered a suburb of the much glitzier Dubai.

2. From 1961 until 1991, Eritrea fought a long war with Ethiopia, eventually gaining its independence. This was followed by the Eritrean–Ethiopian War, which lasted from May 1998 to June 2000. Taken together, these wars in the Horn of Africa constitute one of the world's longest running conflicts, between two of the world's poorest countries. Millions of dollars were spent on the Eritrean-Ethiopian War, tens of thousands of casualties occurred, and thousands of people fled as refugees. Fought over disputed territory, the war resulted in minor border changes, but Ethiopia still occupies land claimed by Eritrea.

3. Excess embryos produced in a couple's IVF cycle can be cryopreserved, or frozen, for later use. A so-called frozen cycle is much less complicated than a "fresh cycle" of IVF. A frozen cycle requires only the transferring of an embryo to a woman's uterus. It bypasses the preliminary steps of an IVF cycle, which are hormonal stimulation, egg collection, sperm collection, fertilization of the egg by the sperm in a laboratory, and the production of the embryos.

4. A clinical pregnancy is a pregnancy in which an ultrasound scan has shown at least one fetal heartbeat. However, as in Rahnia's case, not all clinical pregnancies lead to live births.

5. Because it is disallowed in Sunni Islam, egg donation from one woman to another is not practiced by most Sunni Muslims, who make up 80–90 percent of the world's Muslims.

6. Most Shia Muslim religious authorities have allowed egg donation for their followers since the new millennium; thus, egg donation is now practiced in the two Shia-dominant countries of Iran and Lebanon. However, a Sunni Islamic ban on egg donation stretches from Morocco to Malaysia.

7. Legal adoption, as practiced in the West—in which a child receives the adoptive parents' surname, inherits their assets, and receives loving treatment like their genetic offspring—is not allowed in Islam and is explicitly forbidden in the Islamic scriptures, including the Qur'an. However, Islam views the permanent guardianship and financial support of orphans as a good deed to be practiced by Muslims.

Introduction. IVF Sojourns

1. Pennings 2002, 337.
2. *Newsweek*, July 23, 2012, 5.
3. Franklin 2012.
4. Knoppers and LeBris 1991; Pennings 2002, 2004, 2005, 2006.
5. Lee 2005.
6. Briggs 2006a, 2006b; Tesoriero 2008.
7. Hudson et al. 2011.
8. Ikemoto 2009; Martin 2009, Pfeffer 2011.
9. Storrow 2005–6, 326–27.
10. Culley et al. 2011; Whittaker 2009; Whittaker and Speier 2010; Pennings et al. 2009; Shenfield et al. 2010.
11. For example, in December 2010, the University of Cambridge hosted the world's first scholarly symposium on reproductive travel. Ten of the seventeen scholars presenting their work at the meeting were either anthropologists or sociologists—most of whom were from the United States or Europe. Thus, their ethnographic studies of reproductive travel focused on Europe and America, but also India, Thailand, and the Middle East (Gürtin 2011; Inhorn 2011a; Pande 2011; Whittaker 2011). When papers from this inaugural symposium were published in a November 2011 special issue of *Reproductive BioMedicine Online*, the editors chose to call the issue "Cross-Border Reproductive Care," since that was the term that had gained the most traction within the medical and legal communities.
12. Blyth, Thorn, and Wischmann 2011; Blyth and Auffrey 2008; Blyth and Farrand 2005.
13. Gürtin and Inhorn 2011; Inhorn and Gürtin 2011.
14. Speier 2011a; Bergmann 2011b; Whittaker 2011.
15. In my previous work I used the term *reproductive exile*, arguing that it may come closest to capturing patients' subjective experiences of being "forced" to travel across borders for IVF and related forms of assisted conception (Inhorn and Patrizio 2009). The term *exile* has two meanings: a forced removal from one's native country and a voluntary absence. In most cases,

reprotravelers describe feeling forced out of their home country's IVF services for a variety of specific reasons. Their choice to use IVF to overcome infertility is voluntary, but their travel abroad is not. However, the term exile connotes political or religiously based asylum seeking. Such exile may be indefinite, foreclosing any right of return. Thus, it may not be the most precise term for describing the "forced" nature of reprotravel, especially since most travelers return to their home countries following IVF cycles. This point has been made within the larger terminological debates about cross-border reproductive care. One of the anonymous reviewers of this manuscript also argued strongly for a term other than exile.

16. Inhorn 2003.
17. Shenfield et al. 2010.
18. Nygren et al. 2010.
19. Inhorn 2012.
20. De Sutter 2011; Pennings et al. 2009.
21. Bergmann 2011b; Matorras 2005. These remarks about Spanish women's superior "altruism" have been made by Spanish IVF practitioners at international meetings that I have attended.
22. Pennings 2010.
23. Smith et al. 2009.
24. In his trenchant critique of the Indian transplant industry, the medical anthropologist Lawrence Cohen has coined three important concepts— "bioavailability," "operability," and "supplementarity." Bioavailability, Cohen explains, signifies the "selective disaggregation of persons' cells or tissues for reincorporation into another body" (2005, 83) as in gamete donation or kidney transplantation. Bioavailability is "selective," in that some persons, particularly in resource-poor settings, are more "bioavailable" than others. "Operability" refers to the "degree to which one's belonging to and legitimate demands of the state are mediated through invasive medical commitment" (86). In India poor men and women have already been made "operable" by the state, through state-sponsored support of other kinds of invasive bodily practices. These include, for example, tubal ligations and vasectomies, which the poor have come to accept as "family planning operations." Finally, in more recent work, Cohen has advanced the concept of "supplementarity," or the "ability of an individual or population to secure longevity through the mobilization or acquisition of the organic form of others" (2011, 31). Some individuals are able to "supplement" their own well-being through, for example, the purchase of a kidney, while others—whose very lives are deemed "supplementary" by the state—relinquish their "supplementary" organs simply because they are poor and in desperate need of the cash they can get for an organ.
25. Chopra 2012, Dolnick 2007, Rudrappa 2012; Stephenson 2009.
26. Rudrappa 2010.
27. Pande 2009, 2010a, 2010b, 2011; Rudrappa 2010, 2012.

28. Sengupta 2011.

29. Whittaker 2008, 2011, 2015a.

30. Sengupta 2011.

31. Storrow 2005–6, 300.

32. Burkett 2007; Connell 2006; Crooks et al. 2011; Horowitz and Rosensweig 2007; Johnston et al. 2011; Turner 2007, 2010.

33. Bharadwaj and Glasner 2008; Song 2010.

34. Clarke et al. 2010.

35. Horowitz and Rosensweig 2007; Sobo, Herlihy, and Bicker 2011.

36. Burkett 2007.

37. Horowitz and Rosensweig 2007; Solomon 2011.

38. Petryna 2009.

39. These figures on the scope of the medical tourism industry can be found in Burkett 2007; Connell 2006; Sengupta 2011; Whittaker 2010.

40. Connell 2006; Horowitz and Rosensweig 2007.

41. For overviews of India's medical tourism sector, see Crooks et al. 2011; Sengupta 2011; and Solomon 2011.

42. Sengupta 2011, 315.

43. Sengupta 2011, 316.

44. The medical anthropologist Nancy Scheper-Hughes situates the origins of transplant tourism firmly in the Arab Gulf region: "Organized 'transplant tourism' began in the Middle East in the 1970s, when Arab patients from the Gulf States began to travel abroad for transplant surgeries they could not get at home. They went to India to buy kidneys in the Bombay Organs Bazaar until they came home infected with hepatitis and later with HIV. Then they went to private hospitals in the Philippines staffed by American-trained surgeons and with 'guaranteed' fresh and healthy screened kidneys from paid donors. Those requiring hearts, livers and other less divisible organs, went to China, where organs were in plentiful supply on the dates that multiple executions were held. In China and the Philippines Saudis and Kuwaitis met with Japanese and a smaller number of transplant tourists from Canada, Europe and the United States" (2011, 64–65). She goes on to describe the macabre details of Arab transplant tourism in Saddam Hussein's Iraq, where, prior to the first Gulf War, wealthy Gulf Arabs could find a "fresh" kidney taken from a poor Palestinian refugee or from a member of a vulnerable Iraqi ethnic minority. She asserts that "many people from the Middle East (both Saudis and Israelis) travel illegally on tourist visas with the full understanding that they are engaged in clandestine and illegal transplants that are against the law in the countries where these operations take place from Azerbaijan to Turkey" (quoted in Roberts and Scheper-Hughes 2011a, 3). However, it is important to point out that this work is not based on ethnographic research carried out in the Arab world. Furthermore, the depiction of Gulf Arabs—using their wealth and illegal means to extract kidneys from the world's most

vulnerable members—is in keeping with the new Orientalism found not only in the media, but also among conservative scholars and policy makers. Such stereotypes of Arab barbarity are addressed in my recent book, *The New Arab Man* (Inhorn 2012).

45. Since Kangas's early research, other medical anthropologists have taken up the topic of medical tourism, focusing on transplants (L. Cohen 1999, 2002, 2005, 2011; Scheper-Hughes 2000, 2002a, 2002b, 2004, 2005, 2011); plastic surgery, including gender reassignment (Ackerman 2010; Aizura 2010; Edmonds 2011; Mazzaschi 2011); therapeutic stem cells (Bharadwaj and Glasner 2008; Song 2010); and health spas (Bastos 2011; Naraindas 2011; Quintela 2011; Speier 2011b). Between 2010 and 2011, special issues on medical tourism appeared in five journals: "Healing Holidays? Itinerant Patients, Therapeutic Locales and the Quest for Health," in *Anthropology and Medicine* (Naraindas and Bastos 2011); "Medical Migrations," in *Body and Society* (Roberts and Scheper-Hughes 2011b); "Why Is Medical Travel of Concern to Global Social Policy?," in *Global Social Policy* (Leng and Whittaker 2010); "Patients without Borders: Understanding Medical Travel," in *Medical Anthropology* (Whittaker, Manderson, and Cartwright 2010); and "Comparative Perspectives Symposium: Gender and Medical Tourism," in *Signs*. There are articles on reproductive tourism in four of these issues (Bergmann 2011a; Crozier 2010; Inhorn 2011b; Qadeer 2010; Whittaker and Speier 2010), but not in the issue focusing on "medical migrations." Clearly, a new scholarly subfield of medical tourism has emerged.

46. Kangas 2011, 330.

47. Kangas 2010a, 2010b, 2011.

48. Gürtin, Inhorn, and Tremayne 2015; Inhorn and Gürtin 2012; Inhorn and Tremayne 2012.

49. Inhorn and Tremayne 2012.

50. Inhorn 2003, 2009.

51. Strathern 2000.

52. Inhorn 1994.

53. Thanks to Zeynep Gürtin for reminding me of this point.

54. Inhorn 2003.

55. Inhorn 2003, 2012.

56. Inhorn 2011a.

57. Inhorn 2012.

58. Davidson 2008; Kanna 2011, Mahdavi 2011; Vora 2013.

59. Aw 2010.

60. Inda and Rosaldo 2008, 4.

61. Inda and Rosaldo 2008.

62. Ong and Collier 2005.

63. Inhorn 2003.

64. Deleuze 1988; Ong and Collier 2005.

65. Ong 2005, 338.

66. Collier and Ong 2005, 12.
67. Collier and Ong 2005, 4.
68. Appadurai 1996.
69. Appadurai 2001, 2008.
70. Appadurai 1996, 33.
71. Appadurai 1996, 34.
72. Franklin 2012.
73. This insight comes from the famous concept of "stratified reproduction," introduced by Shelee Colen (1995) and then forwarded by Faye Ginsburg and Rayna Rapp in their seminal edited volume, *Conceiving the New World Order* (1995).
74. Gürtin, Ahuja, and Golombok 2012a, 2012b.
75. Inhorn, Patrizio, and Serour 2010; Roberts 2009.
76. I first introduced the term *reproflows* in Inhorn 2011b.
77. The importance of nonhuman actors has been emphasized in actor network theory, a theoretical approach to science (Latour and Woolgar, 1979).
78. Emily Martin has written incisively about the social constructions of women's and men's reproductive bodies, in particular the "romance" (1991) of the egg and sperm (see also 2001).
79. As noted by one of the anonymous reviewers of this book, Ong and Collier (2005) suggest that Appadurai's notion of global "flows" implies a kind of effortless mobility. In this section, I want to suggest that reproflows may be easily obstructed.
80. Arenas of constraint are the focus of my earlier work on IVF in Egypt (Inhorn 2003).
81. Blyth and Farrand 2005; Deech 2003; Hudson et al. 2011; Pennings 2002.
82. Gürtin and Inhorn 2011.
83. In the Middle East, anthropologists have mostly engaged in "separate spheres" research—that is, male ethnographers talk with men, and female ethnographers talk with women. In my 2013 Middle East Distinguished Lecture, given at the annual meeting of the American Anthropological Association, I urged Middle East anthropologists to challenge this research paradigm, partly by talking with married couples together in a new form of *marital ethnography*. (See the expanded lecture published in Inhorn 2014.)

1. Hubs

1. Pankaj Shrivastav is his real name. However, unless otherwise indicated, the names I have used for all of the patients at Conceive are pseudonyms.
2. "IVF troubadour" is a term that has been used by Robert Simpson of Durham University to describe the foreign IVF consultants who have helped to set up clinics in Sri Lanka, where he conducts his fieldwork.
3. Inhorn 2003, 2004.

4. All businesses in the Emirates must have a *kafil*, or local Emirati sponsor. Under *kafala*, or the sponsorship system, the local Emirati sponsor receives at least 51 percent of all profits, even though he or she may have very little involvement in the business. In the case of Conceive, the local sponsor receives 65 percent of the clinic's profits but pays all of its salaries and operating expenses. As a Muslim, he also occasionally pays for the IVF and ICSI cycles of very poor patients as a form of *zakat*, or charity, which is one of the five pillars of Islam.

5. Conceive was technically in the emirate of Sharjah but was strategically located only fifty meters over the Dubai border. Thus, the clinic attracted patients from both of these emirates. At the time of my study, all of the private IVF clinics serving Dubai were actually located in neighboring Sharjah. On my final trip to the Emirates in 2013, one private IVF clinic had finally opened in Dubai proper and was charging prices for IVF nearly double the going Sharjah rate.

6. Marcus 1995, 110.

7. I am grateful to my colleague P. Sean Brotherton, who helped me to trace the genealogy of the term "cosmopolitan medicine." The term is attributable to Frederick L. Dunn, who was one of my mentors in the medical anthropology program at the University of California, San Francisco. Yet I had no idea that he was the first to coin and define this term.

8. Dunn 1976. Although Charles Leslie is sometimes credited with coining the term in his edited volume, *Asian Medical Systems: A Comparative Study*, he attributes it to Dunn as follows: "While most authors in this volume follow ordinary usage [that is, 'modern,' 'scientific,' or 'Western' medicine], Fred Dunn calls attention in his essay to the biases associated with this usage and suggests the new designation 'cosmopolitan medicine,' which I have adopted" (1976, 6).

9. Dunn 1976, 135.

10. Foucault 1994. See Clarke et al. (2010) for a discussion of Foucault's influence on the terminology, as well as the addition of *bio* to *medicine* in the United States in response to the increasing importance of biotechnology and the life sciences.

11. Sassen 2001.

12. The eight medical tourism destinations most frequently identified in the literature and on the Internet are: China, India, Israel, Jordan, Singapore, Malaysia, Philippines, and the United Arab Emirates (Horowitz and Rosensweig 2007). The increase of reproductive travelers to the United Arab Emirates for fertility treatment has been reported in the local media (El Shammaa 2007; O'Driscoll 2012).

13. Ismail 2012a.

14. Ong 2005.

15. Second Biotechnology World Congress Dubai, UAE February 18–21, 2013, http://dubaiconf02.com/bwc.

16. Dajani 2011, 7.
17. Contemporary social theorists distinguish *cultural cosmopolitanism* from the normative Kantian notion of *cosmopolitanism* found in political theory—that is, good democratic governance involving a world polity with a universalistic culture—(Delanty 2006) and from the phenomenon of *transnationalism* described by globalization theorists—that is, a wide array of activities involving mobility across borders (Roudometof 2005). Cultural cosmopolitanism is about more than democracy and mobility. In the twenty-first century, it is considered to be a new moral and ethical way of living in an increasingly interconnected and heterogeneous world, characterized by geographic deterritorialization, human mobility, and cultural pluralism and hybridity.
18. Skribis, Kendall, and Woodward 2004.
19. Beck and Sznaider 2006.
20. Davidson 2008; Kanna 2011.
21. Davidson 2008.
22. Mahdavi 2011.
23. Ali 2010; DeParle 2007a. See also Makia and Koolhaas (2011) for a pictorial illustration of the ways in which the construction boom has changed Dubai over time.
24. United Nations Economic and Social Commission for Western Asia, "The Demographic Profile of the United Arab Emirates," http://www.escwa.un .org/popin/members/uae.pdf.
25. Barrett 2010.
26. Mahdavi 2011.
27. Kanna 2011; see also Asmi 2013.
28. "Most Visited Cities in the World 2012," *Forbes*, http://www.forbes.com /pictures/efik45ljkd/most-visited-cities-in-the-world-2012-8/.
29. "Most Visited Cities in the World 2012," *Forbes*, http://www.forbes.com /pictures/efik45ljkd/most-visited-cities-in-the-world-2012-8/.
30. The Gulf Cooperation Council consists of the six nations of Bahrain, Kuwait, Oman, Qatar, Saudi Arabia, and the UAE. The only Arab Gulf country missing from the council is the comparatively resource-poor Yemen.
31. "Dubai Is Most Expensive City in ME," *Gulf Business*, http://gulfbusiness .com/2012/09/Dubai-is-most-expensive-city-in-me/#.VF_EXxb4qHh.
32. "2011 Quality of Living Worldwide City Rankings—Mercer Survey," *Mercer*, http://allianceau.com/pics/advant/2011_Mercer.pdf.
33. Friedman 2005.
34. Friedman 2006.
35. Friedman 2006.
36. Davidson 2008.
37. Pheng Cheah is very critical of this type of state-sponsored cosmopolitanism in Asia: "It becomes an ideology used by a state to attract high-end expatriate workers in the high-tech, finance, and other high-end service

sectors as well as to justify its exploitation of its own citizens and the lower-end migrant workers who bear the burden of the country's successful adaptation to flexible accumulation. Cosmopolitanism is here merely a symbolic marker of a country's success at climbing the competitive hierarchy of the international division of labor and maintaining its position there. The inscription of new cosmopolitanisms (and theories about them) within the force field of uneven globalization must be broached at every turn" (2006, 495).

38. Davidson 2012b.

39. As noted above, this is the model in place at Conceive.

40. Jane Bristol-Rhys (2010) and Monica Gallant (2008) have shown that, unlike many of their male counterparts, Emirati women are pursuing higher education, and many of them have aspirations for careers in government and the private sector. I met several such highly educated Emirati career women in my study at Conceive.

41. Mahdavi 2011.

42. Ali 2010; Khalaf and Alkobaisi 1999.

43. Kanna 2011.

44. Ali 2010; Khalaf and Akobaisi 1999; DeParle 2007a.

45. Kanna 2011.

46. Kanna 2011.

47. Vora 2013.

48. DeParle 2007b.

49. This notion of disposition comes from Pierre Bourdieu's concept of *habitus*, which he defined as "a system of dispositions" (1977). Those who have propounded the notion of cosmopolitan disposition suggest that "cosmopolitanism should be understood principally as an attitude of 'openness' toward others" (Skrbis, Kendall, and Woodward 2004, 127).

50. Skribis, Kendall, and Woodward 2004, 117.

51. R. Jones 2013.

52. Inhorn and van Balen 2002.

53. In previous work, I called these IVF cycles that were combined with visits back home "IVF holidays" (Inhorn 2003) and "return reproductive tourism" (Inhorn 2011a).

54. The length of two marriages is unknown because I neglected to ask the first two couples in my study. I soon corrected this oversight.

55. In the literature, three populations are typically identified as being "archetypal cosmopolitans" (Skrbis, Kendall, and Woodward 2004). The first are global business elites, who command resources, make connections across borders and territories, and demonstrate a unique intellectual and aesthetic mind-set that characterizes them as an *uber*cosmopolitan class. The second are expatriates who choose to live abroad but maintain their transnational connections to home countries, to which they often return. The third are what Victor Roudometof calls the "ordinary folk"—ranging from migrant

workers to exiles and refugees—who do not necessarily possess the ethical imagination characteristic of cosmopolitanism but who are "capable of producing and expressing 'working-class cosmopolitanism'" through a cosmopolitanism that is "felt, imagined, consumed and fantasized" (2005, 114).

56. DeParle 2007b.
57. Mertes and Pennings 2012; Smajdor 2011.
58. Lockwood 2011; Wyndham, Marin Figueira, and Patrizio 2012.
59. Lockwood 2011.
60. Hewlett 2004.
61. Goold and Savalescu 2009.
62. Goold and Savalescu 2009, 50.
63. American Society for Reproductive Medicine, Fact Sheet, "Recurrent Pregnancy Loss," http://www.asrm.org?Recurrent_Pregnancy_Loss/.
64. Hefner 2004; Hourvitz 2009; Stoop, Nekkebroeck, and Devroey 2011; Szewczuk 2011.
65. Friese, Becker, and Nachtigall 2006, 2008.
66. The idea of "lifestyle" as a perceived cause of infertility was somewhat new to me. I had already spent years of my career studying the three main causes of infertility in the Middle East—namely, blocked fallopian tubes (as experienced by Rahnia); various ovulatory problems in women; and unusually high rates of male infertility, mostly genetic in origin. Furthermore, I had devoted considerable effort to attempting to understand infertile Middle Easterners' own answers to the question, "Why me?" In my study in Lebanon, for example, most men attributed their infertility problems to the deleterious consequences of civil war, which had led to excess stress, environmental pollution, and illicit sexuality (primarily when young men had been sent out of the country to escape the unrest, at a time when they were first experiencing their sexuality). Although some men recognized the "hereditary" nature of male infertility in close-knit, intermarrying families, the genetic nature of male infertility problems had not been made clear to most men. Thus, infertile Lebanese men in my study looked to their most obvious sources of harm—war and related stress—believing that these infertility causes were well beyond their individual control. In the peaceful Emirates, in contrast, I found a quite different set of perceived infertility factors, with lifestyle issues being the major concern. Apparently, lifestyle issues are of concern to infertile couples in the United States as well. A recent report found that American men with infertility were concerned about their use of cell phones, and women with poor egg quality were concerned about limiting their exposure to plastics (Hawkins et al. 2014). In addition, many couples considered it helpful for women to engage in rigorous exercise during the IVF cycle, avoid stress, and engage in complete bed rest after the embryo transfer.

67. One severely obese Sudanese man in the study had undergone gastric bypass surgery. One severely obese Lebanese woman—a highly paid professional who admitted that she adored food—had nearly died when she contracted a life-threatening *E. coli* infection following a premarital breast reduction surgery. Ultimately, she required a double mastectomy, and when I met her, she was anticipating undergoing breast implant surgery.

68. The genetic origins of male infertility are covered in *The New Arab Man* (Inhorn 2012). The genetics of PCOS are covered in Harris and Cheung 2006.

69. The ability to locate these microdeletions via DNA microscopy has been a major breakthrough in the understanding of so-called "idiopathic," or unexplained male infertility.

70. Hassan and Killick 2004; Marinelli et al. 2004.

71. Hassan and Killick 2004; Marinelli et al. 2004.

72. Jha et al. 2002.

73. World Health Organization, "Tobacco Facts," http://www.who.int/tobacco /mpower/tobacco_facts/en/.

74. In my study in Lebanon, many infertile men had been told to quit smoking by their physicians. However, few men had actually stopped smoking or had even attempted to quit. They pointed out that their friends and relatives who smoked had fathered children. Thus, they did not believe the physicians who told them that smoking could lead to male infertility.

75. Harris and Cheung 2006.

76. Shrivastav 2010.

77. As one authority on PCOS explains, "It has been known for some years that increases in body mass have an adverse effect on the polycystic ovary, with increasing rates of anovulation possibly linked to an increase in circulating insulin concentration. Hence, as the number of obese individuals reaching childbearing age increases, it is likely that PCOS anovulation will be seen more frequently" (Ledger 2009, S12).

78. Harris and Cheung 2006.

79. Shrivastav 2010.

80. Ismail 2012b.

81. As reported in Shrivastav 2010.

82. Shrivastav 2010.

83. The medical anthropologist Sarah Trainer (2012) has shown how college-age Emirati women struggle to manage their weight, in the midst of what they acknowledge to be an obesity epidemic among older Emirati women. Emirati women rarely exercise, and traditional family meals are becoming less common. Among the younger generation, extreme dieting strategies have led to a variety of problems, including micronutrient and protein deficiencies and underweight BMIs.

84. Schwarz 2013.

85. "Briefing," *Time*, August 18, 2014, 5.

86. "Briefing," *Time*, August 18, 2014, 1/4.

87. Fuad's story can also be found in Inhorn 2014.

88. As shown in these reprotravel stories, many cosmopolitan couples had married across ethnic, racial, religious, and national boundaries. Of the 125 couples in my study, twenty-one (16 percent) had such mixed marriages. The husbands and wives had often met through professional venues, sometimes while working in Dubai.

89. A low sperm count is defined as less than fifteen million sperm per milliliter. Furthermore, at least 50 percent of sperm should be motile, or active.

90. Fluid leaking from an infected fallopian tube into the uterus is potentially toxic to an embryo, leading to pregnancy loss.

91. Ectopic pregnancy is a potentially life-threatening condition, but if it is diagnosed early, it can often be successfully treated with a drug called methotrexate. About one-third of women who have an ectopic pregnancy are eligible for medical treatment, rather than surgery. Without more information, it is unclear whether Doina would have been eligible for methotrexate treatment. Her doctors in Abu Dhabi used the standard surgical approach, involving removal of the affected fallopian tube.

92. Embryos are "graded" on a scale of one to four (or A to D), based on an embryologist's subjective assessment of the embryo's appearance. A grade one (or grade A) embryo, for example, is one in which all of the cells are the same size and there is no sign of "fragmentation." Fragmentation means that as the embryo divides, a small portion of cytoplasm (the inside of the cell) has broken off, forming a "fragment." Embryos containing a lot of fragmentation are considered to be developmentally disadvantaged.

93. PROM involves the rupture of the membrane of the amniotic sac before the onset of labor. Min's case would be considered preterm PROM because it occurred before thirty-seven weeks of gestation. It was also prolonged, because it occurred more than eighteen hours before labor.

94. Abortion is illegal in the UAE. According to the Middle East abortion scholar Angel Foster, the UAE is famous for carrying out "sting operations" (2012), in which women feigning pregnancy are sent into doctors' offices to request abortions. The physicians who accede to these women's wishes are arrested.

95. Genetic counseling is an underdeveloped field in the Emirates and in the Arab world more generally. Thus, most men with male infertility do not receive genetic counseling of any kind. Dr. Pankaj was exceptional in that he spoke frankly to patients about the possible genetic etiology of severe male factor infertility and the potential consequences of passing on genetic defects to sons via ISCI. See Inhorn 2012 for a detailed discussion of genetic risk and male infertility.

96. Metformin is a diabetes medicine sometimes used for lowering insulin and blood sugar levels in women with PCOS. Metformin helps regulate menstrual cycles, start ovulation, and lower the risk of PCOS-related miscar-

riage. Most of the women with PCOS in my study were placed on Metformin by Dr. Pankaj.

97. Dr. Pankaj was so busy undertaking IVF and ISCI cycles that he did not have time to deliver the babies of most of his patients. Instead, he referred them for delivery to a number of trusted obstetrician colleagues in Dubai. Generally, these babies were delivered by C-section, although a minority of women with otherwise normal IVF pregnancies requested natural vaginal delivery. Nathalie was in the latter group and was exceptional in that she delivered her premature twins vaginally and without an epidural.

2. Absences

1. European Society for Human Reproduction and Embryology 2013.
2. Gallagher 2013.
3. "Interview with Geeta Nargund," BBC News, July 10, 2013.
4. Nachtigall 2006.
5. Nachtigall 2006.
6. Lunenfeld and van Steirteghem 2004, 321.
7. Jacky Boivin et al. 2007 found that slightly more couples living in developed countries (56 percent) sought infertility care than those living in less developed countries (51 percent). The authors argue that the low uptake of infertility medical services may be due to low motivation when services are known to be limited or unavailable.
8. Quoted in Sharma, Mittal, and Aggarwal 2009.
9. Ombelet 2008, Ombelet et al. 2008.
10. Dhont 2011; Lunenfeld and van Steirteghem 2004; Vayena, Rowe, and Griffin 2002; Vayena, Rowe, and Peterson 2002.
11. Ombelet 2008, 2009, 2011, 2013, 2014; Ombelet et al. 2008; Ombelet and van Balen 2010.
12. European Society for Human Reproduction and Embryology 2008, 2013; Gerrits et al. 2012.
13. Quoted in Gallagher 2013.
14. Ombelet 2014, 271.
15. A low-cost embryo culture system—developed by Jonathan Van Blerkom, a research professor at the University of Colorado, Boulder, "can fit in a shirt pocket, is designed to go anywhere, including off the grid, allowing it to be independent of the complex and costly infrastructure required by IVF programs in the developed world." According to Van Blerkom, "the system uses low-cost components, does not require complex microprocessor controlled incubators and is a closed system that generates its own unique atmospheric and culture conditions required for normal fertilization and embryogenesis using inexpensive, common chemicals" (quoted in "Low-Cost In-Vitro Fertilization Method Developed at CU May Help Couples In Developing Countries" 2013; see also Van Blerkom et al. 2014).

16. Inhorn 2012.

17. Inhorn 2012.

18. Johnson, Cohen, and Grudzinskas 2014, 266.

19. According to Ombelet, some of the most important foundations, NGOs, and international societies linked to reproductive health do not mention "infertility care in developing countries" as an issue they support (2011, 260). This includes the Cade Foundation, William J. Clinton Foundation, Compton Foundation, Ford Foundation, Bill and Melinda Gates Foundation, William and Flora Hewlett Foundation, International Planned Parenthood Federation, John D. and Catherine T. MacArthur Foundation, David and Lucile Packard Foundation, West Wind Foundation, and the United Nations. The World Health Organization is the only international organization that prioritizes infertility as a reproductive health issue.

20. Maya Mascarenhas et al. (2012) have published the most recent analysis of national, regional, and global trends in infertility prevalence in the period 1990–2010. They report the lowest numbers of infertile couples worldwide, at 48.5 million as of 2010. Jacky Boivin et al. (2007) estimated that 72.4 million women were infertile as of 2006. Shea O. Rutstein and Iqbal H. Shah (2004) found the highest number, 186 million ever-married women in developing countries (except China), based on an analysis of data from the late 1990s. This apparent drop from 186 million to 48.5 million could represent a dramatic decrease in infertility prevalence rates globally. However, the differences in estimates are more likely based on different study designs and data sources. In other words, the total number of infertile people around the world is still unknown, but the number is definitely in the many millions. Other estimates are 80 million (Nachtigall 2006) and the World Health Organization's 180 million (Ombelet 2011).

21. European Society for Human Reproduction and Embryology Task Force on Ethics and Law 2009.

22. Boivin et al. 2007.

23. Nachtigall 2006.

24. Mascarenhas et al. 2012.

25. Mascarenhas et al. 2012.

26. Mascarenhas et al. 2012.

27. Lunenfeld and van Steirteghem 2004; Rutstein and Shah 2004.

28. Lunenfeld and van Steirteghem 2004; Rutstein and Shah 2004.

29. Mascarenhas et al. 2012.

30. Mascarenhas et al. 2012; Cui 2010; Lunenfeld and van Steirteghem 2004; Nachtigall 2006.

31. Mascarenhas et al. 2012.

32. Ombelet et al. 2008.

33. Ombelet et al. 2008.

34. Inhorn and van Balen 2002; Nachtigall 2006.

35. Cui 2010; Inhorn and van Balen 2002; Nachtigall 2006.

36. Lunenfeld and van Steirteghem 2004.
37. See the many anthropological contributions in Boerma and Mgalla 2001; Gerrits et al. 2012; Inhorn and van Balen 2002; and Ombelet and van Balen 2010.
38. Lunenfeld and van Steirteghem 2004, 321.
39. Mascarenhas et al. 2012; Rutstein and Shah 2004.
40. European Society for Human Reproduction and Embryology Task Force on Ethics and Law 2009; Vayena et al. 2002, 2009.
41. Chankova 2014; Gallagher 2013.
42. Ferguson 2006.
43. Ferguson 2006, 21.
44. Ferguson 2006, 14.
45. Ferguson 2006, 8.
46. Ferguson 2006, 2.
47. Ferguson 2006, 13.
48. Colen 1995.
49. Ginsburg and Rapp 1995.
50. Inhorn 2003.
51. Ory et al. 2013.
52. Collins 2002.
53. Jones et al. 2007.
54. International Federation of Fertility Societies 2010.
55. Jones et al. 2010.
56. The history of IVF in Japan is documented in Suzuki 2014.
57. Ayo Wahlberg (2012) describes the high volume in some Chinese IVF clinics, where 20,000 annual IVF and ICSI cycles are performed, and where long lines of patients, packed body to body in winding queues, wait to be seen starting in the early hours of the morning.
58. Jones et al. 2010.
59. Adamson 2009.
60. Adamson 2009.
61. Jones et al. 2010.
62. Giwa-Osagie 2007.
63. European Society for Human Reproduction and Embryology Task Force on Ethics and Law 2009.
64. According to John Collins (2002), Kazakhstan had one clinic to serve six million Kazakhs. In the 2013 IFFS surveillance report, Kazakhstan was hailed as a new survey country, with twelve IVF clinics reported (Ory et al. 2013).
65. Mascarenhas et al. 2012.
66. Iraq's single IVF clinic in Erbil is staffed by Iraqi personnel from Baghdad, who learned their skills in neighboring Jordan. The clinic is located in Erbil because after 2003, Iraqi Kurdistan was considered the safest region of the country. The status of IVF in Iraq was described to me by

Nisreen El-Hashemite, executive director of the Royal Academy of Science International Trust, an organization founded by the former Iraqi royal family to promote science in the Middle East.

67. In my 2003 study of ICSI in Lebanon, I interviewed a significant number of infertile Syrian men who had crossed the border between the two countries (Inhorn 2012). At that time, there were only a small number of IVF clinics in Damascus and Aleppo, and the Syrian men in my study did not trust these newly opened facilities. By 2007 the number of Syrian IVF clinics had increased slightly, including a new clinic in the city of Homs, according to my informants. But with the outbreak of the civil war in 2011, infertile Syrians were fleeing their country as refugees, and were using IVF clinics in northern Jordan (Suha Alkhaldi, a Jordanian doctoral student, personal communication, July 21, 2013).

68. Inhorn 2003.

69. Jones et al. 2010. Even though these peripheral nations of the Arab Gulf were not reported in the IFFS global survey, both had started at least one IVF clinic by 2007. For example, a recent account in the *Yemen Times*, an English-language newspaper, reports that Yemen's first IVF baby was born in 2000, and since 2007, 2,000 IVF cycles have led to 800 successful pregnancies (Qaed 2013). The Arab Gulf island nation of Bahrain, also not reported in the IFFS survey, had several IVF clinics, including at least one supported by the Bahrain Defense Force and serving mostly local Bahrainis.

70. Mascarenhas et al. 2012.

71. Jones et al. 2010.

72. Nachtigall 2006.

73. Ory et al. 2014.

74. Ory et al. 2013.

75. Connolly, Hoorens, and Chambers 2010, 607.

76. Connolly, Hoorens, and Chambers 2010, 607.

77. Collins 2002, 267.

78. Collins 2002.

79. Four years after Collins undertook his global survey—and at the same time that my study was being launched at Conceive—the average cost of an American IVF cycle had increased even further, to $12,513 (Chambers et al. 2009). Yet the cost of an actual IVF live birth in the United States was $41,132, because of the need for repeated IVF cycles in many cases. The United Kingdom followed closely behind, at $40,364. Given these high costs, only about 25 percent of US demand and 40 percent of UK demand was being met. The high cost of IVF in the United States is discussed in Spar 2006.

80. This was easy for most couples to do, as the dirham had been pegged to the dollar for more than a decade ($1.00=3.67 dirhams).

81. Spar 2006.

82. Dyer and Patel 2012.

83. Dyer et al. 2013.

84. Dyer et al. 2013.

85. My first study carried out in late 1980s Egypt was devoted entirely to the plight of poor infertile urban women, who were attempting to access state-subsidized IVF services at a government maternity hospital (Inhorn 1994, 1996).

86. Inhorn 1994, 1996, 2003, 2012; Inhorn and Fakih 2006.

87. DeParle 2007a.

88. Since these labor figures were published in 2007, the population of the Emirates has reportedly grown by 3–4 million, and most of the new arrivals are imported foreign laborers. United Nations Economic and Social Commission for Western Asia, "The Demographic Profile of the United Arab Emirates," http://www.escwa.un.org/popin/members/uae.pdf.

89. Ali 2010; Aw 2010; DeParle 2007a.

90. Inhorn 2010; Mahdavi 2011.

91. Ali 2010; Khalaf and Alkobaisi 1999.

92. Barrett 2010.

93. However, there were many Indian Muslims in the Emirates. As mentioned above, during my study, I met six Muslim couples from India, most of whom preferred to undertake their IVF in the Emirates because of perceived discrimination back home in India, as well as lack of access to the technology in parts of India with high concentrations of Muslims.

94. Kanna 2011.

95. See also Vora 2013 on the generations of Indian families in Dubai.

96. Pardis Mahdavi (2011) also notes that *immigrants* and *migrants* are not the correct terms to apply to temporary laborers in the Emirates, given that they have no possibility of permanent settlement and naturalization. The term *economic refugees*, which has been used to describe poverty-stricken asylum seekers, is also not accurate. The UAE does not offer refugee status of any kind, including for those seeking protection from political violence in their own country.

97. Jones et al. 2010.

98. Berg Brigham et al. 2013.

99. Baris Ata and Emre Seli (2010) point to four historical arguments against public financing of IVF, including lack of medical necessity; low success rates; resultant low cost-effectiveness as a treatment option; and the experimental nature of some ARTs.

100. The UAE was one of several Arab Gulf countries lost to follow-up in the 2013 surveillance.

101. Al Ain is home to the Emirates' major public university, the University of the United Arab Emirates (UAEU), whose students are almost exclusively Emirati. The university hosts a medical school and government hospital, where the government IVF clinic is located.

102. Jones et al. 2010.

103. Inhorn and Gürtin 2012; Gürtin 2013.

104. Gürtin 2013.

105. Gürtin 2013.

106. Jones et al. 2010.

107. Birenbaum-Carmeli 2004, 900.

108. In her groundbreaking ethnography, *Reproducing Jews: A Cultural Account of Assisted Conception in Israel* (2000), the anthropologist Susan Martha Kahn first described how Israeli pronatalism fuels the culture of assisted conception in that country.

109. Palestinians receive these services if they live within the contemporary borders of Israel, but not if they live in the Palestinian settlements of the West Bank or Gaza Strip. See Birenbaum-Carmeli and Inhorn 2009.

110. Jones et al. 2010, 17.

111. Chambers et al. 2009.

112. One of my Australian informants told me that the Australian government "desperately wants to increase its population." A number of pronatalist measures have been put in place, including subsidies of 2,500–3,500 Australian dollars ($2,167–$3,034) to parents for the birth of every Australian baby. Infertile Australian couples also receive at least one free IVF cycle, with subsequent cycles involving negligible payments.

113. Only fourteen of the fifty US states have laws requiring minimal insurance coverage for infertility services (Katz, Nachtigall, and Showstack 2002). The most generous "mandate states"—those in which IVF cycles are largely covered for state residents—are clustered on the East Coast: Connecticut, Massachusetts, Maryland, New Jersey, New York, and Rhode Island.

114. Twenty-five European countries—almost equally divided between Eastern and Western Europe—provide some level of public financing: Austria, Belgium, Bulgaria, Croatia, the Czech Republic, Denmark, Estonia, Finland, France, Germany, Greece, Hungary, Iceland, Italy, Montenegro, the Netherlands, Norway, Portugal, Romania, Russia, Slovakia, Slovenia, Spain, Sweden, and the United Kingdom (Jones et al. 2010).

115. Estimates of UK public funding of IVF cycles range from a low of 15 percent (Culley et al. 2011) through a midlevel of 25 percent (Birenbaum-Carmeli 2004) to a high of 40 percent (Berg Brigham et al. 2013). At a minimum, 60 percent or more of IVF cycles in the United Kingdom are paid for out of pocket.

116. Birenbaum-Carmeli 2004; Culley et al. 2011.

117. Birenbaum-Carmeli 2004; Culley et al. 2011.

118. Culley et al. 2011, 11.

119. Culley et al. 2011; Hudson and Culley 2011.

120. Clomid and Metformin are the brand names of pharmaceutical medications commonly given to infertile women. Clomid stimulates ovulation, while Metformin treats insulin resistance in women with PCOS.

121. Pious Muslim women often prefer to be treated by female gynecologists who are coreligionists. This has to do with religious concerns about the "uncovering" of the female body in the presence of an unrelated male, especially one who does not understand the Islamic modesty concerns regarding "touch and gaze" by the opposite sex (Inhorn and Serour 2011).
122. Oman has experienced the world's most significant decline in total fertility rates in the past two decades. From an average of nearly eight children per woman, the number has declined by 5.3, for a current total fertility rate of 2.6 births per woman (Eberstadt and Shah 2012). Nonetheless, in more conservative regions of the country, fertility rates remain higher.
123. Sex selection is specifically prohibited in Islam, as it harkens back to early Islamic injunctions against female infanticide. Nonetheless, a thriving industry of sex selection via preimplantation genetic diagnosis is emerging in IVF clinics in Egypt, Jordan, and Dubai, with most Arab couples requesting that only male embryos be selected.
124. Masturbation is regarded as an illicit form of sexuality in most Islamic legal traditions. Masturbation thus evokes strong anxieties among some Muslim men, who have difficulty "performing" when asked to provide a semen sample in an IVF clinic (Inhorn 2010, 2012).
125. Polygyny is illegal in only three Middle Eastern countries: Israel, Tunisia, and Turkey. However, only 1–5 percent of marriages are polygynous in most Middle Eastern countries, with the highest rates of around 9 percent found in the wealthiest countries of the Arab Gulf (Omran and Roudi 1993; Tabutin 2005).
126. The celibacy trap has been a major problem in war-torn Lebanon, where, due to the loss of marriageable men through war, many women who remained in Lebanon aged out of their fertility. See Inhorn 2012 for an extended discussion.

3. Restrictions

1. I have written a great deal about hasad and infertility in the Arab world. See Inhorn 1994, 1996, 2003, 2012.
2. One of my anthropological colleagues, a Palestinian Bedouin, provided me with a beautiful hasad amulet on a key chain to protect me and my car from envy.
3. Moosa 2003, 23.
4. Inhorn 2006, 2012.
5. Shabana 2015.
6. Moosa 2003.
7. Inhorn 2003, 2005a, 2011b; Inhorn, Patrizio, and Serour 2010; Meirow and Schenker 1997; Serour 1996, 2008; Serour and Dickens 2001.
8. Most Scandinavian sperm comes from Cryos International, which is based in Denmark and is the world's largest sperm exporter.

9. Sharjah is considered the most Islamic emirate. For example, it is the only one where the sale and public consumption of alcohol is illegal. Sharjah also maintains the strictest decency laws, which require a conservative dress code and prevent the mixing of unmarried men and women.

10. Salama 2007.

11. Salama 2007.

12. Salama 2007.

13. "Federal Law No. 11 of 2008 in connection with the fertilization centers in the State" was amended through a Cabinet Resolution in 2009. The document is separated into two parts, an original 2008 draft section, followed by the 2009 amendment. The final page lists the seven rulers of the Emirates who signed the document into law.

14. The emirs were Khalifa Bin Zayed Al Nahyan, president of the UAE and ruler of Abu Dhabi; Mohamed Bin Rashid Al Maktoum, vice president and prime minister of the UAE and ruler of Dubai; Sultan Bin Mohamed Al Qasimi, member of the Supreme Council of the Federation and ruler of Sharjah; Saqr Bin Mohamed Al Qasimi, member of the Supreme Council of the Federation and ruler of Ras Al Khaima; Humaid Bin Rashid Al Naimi, member of the Supreme Council of the Federation and ruler of Ajman; Rashid Bin Ahmed Al Mualla, member of the Supreme Council of the Federation and ruler of Umm Al Quwain; and Hamad Bin Mohamed Al Sharqi, member of the Supreme Council of the Federation and ruler of Al Fujairah.

15. Jones et al. 2010.

16. Jones et al. 2010.

17. Inhorn 2005, 2012.

18. The categories in table 3.1 are adapted from Jones et al. 2010. The information in the table comes directly from the UAE's Federal Law No. 11.

19. Inhorn 2005, 2012; Serour 2008.

20. Inhorn, Patrizio, and Serour 2010.

21. This is the exact wording found in Federal Law No. 11, p. 21.

22. Federal Law No. 11, p. 21.

23. Brockopp 2003; Jones et al. 2010.

24. Jones et al. 2010.

25. "Fresh" cycles using embryos that have not been subjected to freezing have slightly higher success rates than "frozen" cycles do. Nonetheless, freezing embryos for up to five years does not significantly reduce their viability.

26. "What Is Devolution?," *Law Dictionary*, http://thelawdictionary.org /devolution.

27. I am extremely grateful to Richard Storrow and his colleagues for helping me think through an expansion of the term *legal devolution*. Professor Storrow read through this chapter carefully, making extremely insightful comments.

28. Storrow 2010.

29. Storrow 2010.
30. Storrow 2010.
31. Storrow 2010.
32. Jones et al. 2010.
33. Pennings 2009, 15.
34. Jones et al. 2010.
35. Pennings 2009.
36. For an anthropological assessment of progressive Norway's conservative assisted reproduction law, see Melhuus 2012.
37. Jones et al. 2010; Pennings 2002, 2004, 2009.
38. Inhorn, Patrizio, and Serour 2010; Jones et al. 2010; Matorras 2005; Zanini 2011.
39. Blyth 2010; Deech 2003; McKelvey et al. 2009; Pennings et al. 2008, 2009; Shenfield et al. 2010.
40. Storrow 2005–6, 307.
41. Pennings 2004.
42. Pennings 2004.
43. Mainland and Wilson 2010.
44. Shenfield 2011.
45. Pennings 2002.
46. I. Cohen 2012, 1309.
47. Pennings et al. 2008; Shenfield et al. 2010; Storrow 2011.
48. In his nearly twenty-five-year history of IVF in the Emirates, Dr. Pankaj has seen only one patient who tested positive for HIV. This patient came from sub-Saharan Africa.
49. Men who do not produce mature sperm have a genetic form of male infertility. If they use ICSI to produce offspring, then their genetic disorder will be passed onto their sons, who will also need ICSI to reproduce, like their fathers.
50. Two men in my study, one Emirati and one Sudanese, had had their sperm frozen prior to cancer treatment. Another man from South Africa underwent post-vasectomy PESA at Conceive and then had the aspirated sperm frozen.
51. The congenital absence of the vas deferens is one of the signs of cystic fibrosis, an inherited disease of the mucus glands. When absence of the vas deferens occurs alone, as in Manfred's case, it is considered to be a mild genital form of cystic fibrosis.
52. IVF clinics are found throughout Catholic countries, including Italy and most of Latin America. The fact that Catholics are avid users of IVF is revealed in Roberts 2012.
53. Inhorn 1996, 2006, 2012; Sonbol 1995; Zuhur 1992.
54. Inhorn 2006.
55. For a description of the considerable resistance to adoption among infertile Hindu couples, see Bharadwaj 2003.

56. I have written extensively about adoption versus guardianship and permanent legal fostering in the Arab world (Inhorn 1996, 2003, 2006, 2012). Although many Muslims are willing to serve as financial guardians of children in orphanages, very few Muslim couples are willing to take the next step, which would involve permanent home fostering of an orphaned child. Legal adoption—where a child is raised as if he or she belongs to the adoptive parents, taking the family name and inheriting from them—is allowed in only three Middle Eastern Muslim countries, Shia-dominant Iran and the "secular" Sunni Muslim countries of Tunisia and Turkey. A study of "secret adoption" in Morocco by the anthropologist Jamila Bargach (2002) provides the most extensive overview of the Islamic rulings and subsequent difficulties related to the legal adoption of orphaned children.
57. Inhorn and Tremayne 2012.
58. Inhorn 2012.
59. Hessini 2007.
60. Hessini 2007.
61. Hessini 2007.
62. Hessini 2007. For a study of abortion in Kuwait, see Alawadhi n.d. There, abortion is legally permitted up to four months, in cases where the pregnancy would cause harm to the mother's health or the fetus would be born with a serious physical or mental malformation.
63. Hessini 2007.
64. Hessini 2007.
65. "United Arab Emirates," United Nations Population Division, Department of Economic and Social Affairs, http:// www.un.org/esa/population /publications/abortion/doc/uae.doc.
66. Hessini 2007.
67. Jones et al. 2010, 24.
68. American College of Obstetricians and Gynecologists 2013.
69. American College of Obstetricians and Gynecologists 2013.
70. Collins 2002.
71. American College of Obstetricians and Gynecologists 2013.
72. Jones et al. 2010.
73. Serour 2008.
74. Serour 2008.
75. Interestingly, she used the term "embryo reduction" rather than "fetal reduction." Perhaps conceiving of her abortion as the loss of embryos, rather than of more developed fetuses, made it more psychologically acceptable to her.
76. Ahmed 1986; Douki et al. 2003.
77. Inhorn 2012; Kanaaneh 2002; Obermeyer 1999.
78. Inhorn 2012; Kanaaneh 2002; Obermeyer 1999.
79. Serour 2008.

80. Al-Gazali et al. 2005; Al-Gazali and Ali 2010.

81. Consanguineous unions with cousins are condoned in the Islamic scriptures and are also culturally preferred in most Middle Eastern societies for numerous reasons. These marriages are considered safer than marriages to strangers, whose backgrounds are less open to scrutiny. Furthermore, with increasing wealth in the Arab Gulf, cousin marriages solidify family ties and assets. For a fuller discussion of consanguinity in the Middle East, see Inhorn 2012, especially the chapter on "Consanguineous Connectivity," and Inhorn et al. 2009. For a fascinating study of consanguinity and state-sponsored efforts to modify marriage practices in order to eliminate "inherited blood disorders" in Oman, see Beaudevin 2014.

82. See my discussion of Muslim "local moral worlds" in Inhorn 2003.

83. As a woman under the age of thirty-five, Reem was not an ideal candidate for the transfer of four embryos. Such high numbers are appropriate only for women over forty, who are facing serious age-related infertility and are thus less likely to conceive. Reem, however, was clearly fertile, producing a large number of healthy eggs. In other words, the Greek clinic over-treated her, prescribing too much fertility medication and recommending that too many embryos be transferred.

84. An abbreviated version of Elaine's story can be found in Inhorn 2010.

85. Although I did not pry any further, I assumed that Leib was working for Mossad, the Israeli intelligence agency.

86. In fact, there were only seven children in *The Sound of Music*.

87. One of the earliest ways to detect a multiple pregnancy is through the monitoring of the level of human chorionic gonadotropin (HCG), which is a hormone secreted by the fertilized embryos. In pregnancies with multiple embryos, the level of circulating HCG in a woman's blood will therefore generally be higher than in a pregnancy with a single embryo.

88. It is interesting to note that Elaine speaks of reducing "children" rather than reducing fetuses. See note 75, above.

89. At the time of my study at Conceive, I was a professor at the University of Michigan, providing my business card and gift pens from the university to all of the couples in my study.

90. Through research in the Emirates, I soon came to realize that "fair skin" was valorized in the Indian community. Therefore, I began to notice the skin colors of husbands and wives. In these mostly middle-class professional couples, virtually all of the wives were lighter than their husbands, sometimes significantly so. To use the language that is common in the United States, I am the "white" wife of a "black," biracial husband and the mother of two "mixed-race" children. Thus, I am attuned to race and racism, and I viewed the fetishism surrounding "fair skin" in the Indian community to be a manifestation of unfortunate racial hierarchies.

91. FSH helps control the production of eggs by the ovaries. An FSH test can help to determine a woman's egg supply (the so-called ovarian reserve) and

whether a woman has gone through menopause. The more elevated the FSH level, the lower the woman's ovarian function.

92. Ramita and Karthik were also planning to apply for adoption, which was unique among the Hindu couples in my study. A small group of Christian Indian couples in my study were consistently proadoption. In contrast, both Hindu and Muslim Indian couples in my study tended to reject the possibility of adoption, thereby confirming the observation of my colleague Aditya Bharadwaj, based on his own study of IVF in India, that "adoption is not an option" for most infertile Indian couples (2003).

93. Testicular atrophy has many medical causes, including genital mumps in adolescent boys who have never been vaccinated. Steroid use in male body-builders can also cause testicular atrophy, although in that case it is often reversible. The cause of Najeeb's atrophied testicles and nonobstructive azoospermia was never identified.

94. Inhorn 2006.

95. A similar version of Ibrahim's story is also found in chapter 6 of Inhorn 2012.

96. Inhorn 2007, 2012.

97. A sperm count of less than fifteen million sperm per milliliter is the current cutoff point for a diagnosis of male infertility. Thus, Ibrahim's sperm counts of less than 0.5 million could be considered very low.

98. Ibrahim is mistaken in believing that IVF was initially rejected by Muslim religious authorities. In fact, the first fatwa condoning the use of assisted reproduction within marriage (that is, with a husband's sperm and a wife's eggs) was published only two years after the first successful case of IVF in Britain.

4. Discomforts

1. In my Lebanese study involving 220 men (120 infertile; 100 fertile but married to infertile women), the "take-home baby rate" was astonishingly low—only 4 percent (Inhorn 2012).

2. Although I had never before seen the popular American television show, *American Idol*, I was introduced to it in the Emirates and thus began to think of Dr. Pankaj in those terms. The gifted singers on *American Idol* attained a kind of celebrity status, with thousands of adoring fans. In the regional reproscape of IVF, Dr. Pankaj had achieved such idol status.

3. Maiburg et al. 2009.

4. De Mouzon et al. 2010; Mantikou et al. 2013; Nelson and Lawlor 2011.

5. Moragianni and Penzias 2010.

6. Of the 125 couples in my study, 27 were already parents of children who had been conceived naturally or with IVF, including in eleven previous marriages. Sadly, three couples in my study had lost infants, including a pair of IVF twins and two neonates who had died of acute respiratory infections.

7. Dr. Pankaj had tried offering evening clinics two nights a week, but the experiment only lasted for one and a half months. Dubai's evening traffic jams made it impossible for Conceive's staff members and patients to reach the clinic in a timely fashion. However, as a concession to working couples, Conceive was routinely open for business on Friday morning, which is the beginning of the weekend in the Emirates.

8. As South Asian couples explained to me, conception was expected early in marriage, and ideally well before the age of thirty. Grandparents hoped to meet their grandchildren before they died, in countries with relatively low life expectancies (for example, sixty-five years in both India and Pakistan).

9. Two of the female IVF physicians are Emirati, although both are of "mixed" ancestry (that is, Iranian and Palestinian). One of the female IVF physicians who has been practicing in the Emirates for many years is Iraqi.

10. Rizk et al. 2005.

11. One of the "confidential" matters in Emirati gynecology is the issue of homosexuality. Marriage is socially mandatory throughout the Arab world, including in the Emirates. This means that men and women with homosexual preferences are usually forced into heterosexual marriages. When this happens, marriages may remain unconsummated, and young brides are consequently suspected of being infertile. They may end up visiting IVF clinics, and when their homosexual husbands agree to the arrangement, intrauterine insemination (IUI) may be performed using the husband's masturbated sperm. The ensuing pregnancy thus solves the wife's purported infertility problem, while hiding her husband's sexual orientation from others. According to one of the Muslim gynecologists at Conceive, "so many young Emirati brides have been deflowered by the vaginal probe in this way," particularly at one of the IVF clinics run by a Muslim woman physician. According to Dr. Pankaj, lack of marital consummation is also found among South Asian IVF patients, sometimes due to childhood trauma and sexual abuse. I have written about sexual problems among infertility patients in Egypt (Inhorn 2005b).

12. Pennings and Ombelet 2007.

13. Van Empel et al. 2008.

14. Institute of Medicine 2001.

15. Dancet et al. 2011; Van Empel et al. 2008.

16. Van Empel 2008, 589.

17. Van Empel 2008, 589.

18. Van Empel 2008, 585.

19. Inhorn 2012.

20. Inhorn 2003, 2012.

21. I was told by Conceive staff members that Emiratis generally do not want to have their IVF children's baby photos hung on the clinic's walls.

22. Hochschild 1979.

23. Inhorn 2003, 2012.

24. This overuse of C-sections was a major problem for IVF patients who wanted to deliver their babies vaginally. One woman told me: "I don't know *anybody* who delivers naturally here." Another explained that her two friends had insisted on natural childbirth but "were left in a bit of a cupboard in the hospital." The overuse of C-sections has recently been reported by Meg Staires. She found that midwives can only legally deliver babies in hospitals in the Emirates because home birth has been made illegal. She found options for childbirth overall to be quite limited, with "incomplete services and incoherent regulations" (2013, 5).

25. Vora 2013.

26. Inhorn 2003, 2011a.

27. Inhorn 2003.

28. Inhorn 2011a.

29. Inhorn 2012.

30. The emirate of Sharjah has developed a rather remote, desert academic community called "University City." The community is the brainchild of the ruler of Sharjah, who is the only emir to have received a PhD. The city includes several colleges, technical schools, a medical school, a police academy, and a public library, the latter of which is rarely used. University City is also home to the American University of Sharjah, which was my institutional host and my family's home during our time in the Emirates.

31. Alper et al. 2002, 8.

32. Kugelman et al. 2013, 550.

33. Kugelman et al. 2013, 550.

34. One of several kinds of uterine malformations, a T-shaped uterus is also known as a DES uterus because it is usually the result of fetal exposure to diethylstilbestrol. It is unlikely that Maitha's Emirati mother was exposed to DES during her pregnancy. Thus, Maitha's uterine malformation may have been improperly diagnosed in the Emirati IVF clinic.

35. See the prologue, where Rahnia, too, underwent blastocyst transfer in the United Kingdom.

36. A blighted ovum occurs when a fertilized egg is implanted in the uterus but does not develop into an embryo. Blighted ova are the cause of nearly half of all miscarriages in the first trimester of pregnancy.

37. As of 2013 the total fertility rate in the Emirates is 2.37, or between two and three children per woman.

38. "Emiratization" is the UAE government's program to increase Emirati presence in the country's private workforce. Although many Emiratis—especially Emirati women—work for the government, foreign nationals occupy the majority of private-sector positions in the country. Since the mid-2000s, Emiratization has been in force, which means that qualified Emiratis are to be given preferential treatment in competition for private-sector employment.

39. Shorter versions of Abdullah's story can be found in Inhorn 2010 and Inhorn 2012.

40. Six couples in my study were attempting to deliver IVF "anchor babies" in either Australia, Canada, Great Britain, or the United States. Canada was the most popular country, with three couples—two Arab and one Pakistani—hoping to deliver their children there for citizenship purposes.

41. Group B streptococcus infection can lead to premature rupture of the membrane of the amniotic sac, and hence premature delivery.

42. In the Middle East, physicians and their patients are sometimes part of the same social circles. Thus, entertaining one's IVF physician was not necessarily considered unethical. Rather, it was viewed as a form of gratitude, similar to giving a physician a present.

43. As I have shown in my earlier studies of Egypt (Inhorn 1996, 2003) and Lebanon (Inhorn 2012), infertile couples rarely divorce, contrary to popular stereotypes. Instead, infertile couples often demonstrate high levels of "conjugal connectivity," including committed efforts to solve their infertility problems together. This has become much easier because of the widespread presence of IVF clinics across the Middle Eastern region since the late 1980s and early 1990s.

44. Many Arab couples seek what they call "the Canadian immigration." This is partly because Quebec is Francophone, which appeals to many Middle Easterners coming from French-speaking North Africa and Lebanon. But Canada is also "Arab friendly," especially compared to the United States. Canada makes immigration relatively easy for educated Arab professionals, who can contribute their knowledge and skill sets to the Canadian workforce.

Conclusion. Cosmopolitan Conceptions

1. Sandler 2013.
2. Yomoah 2013.
3. Franklin 1997.
4. Franklin 2013b, 753–54.
5. Franklin 2013a.
6. Franklin and Roberts 2006.
7. Franklin 2007.
8. Franklin 2013a.
9. Goold and Savulescu 2009; Lockwood 2011; Mertes and Pennings 2012; Shkedi-Rafid and Hashiloni-Dolev 2011, 2012; Stoop, Nekkebroeck, and Devroey 2010.
10. Cancer treatments involving chemotherapy often damage a woman's ovarian function, destroying her future reproductive potential. See Lockwood 2011.

11. Egg freezing is the subject of my newest research project, which is being carried out in the United States and Israel, two nations that have been front-runners in the deployment of this IVF-related technology. The Israeli portion of the study is being conducted by my colleague Daphna Birenbaum-Carmeli, of the University of Haifa.

12. Madrigal 2014.

13. Tavernise 2014.

14. Tavernise 2014.

15. "Three-Person IVF: UK Government Backs Mitochondrial Transfer," *Guardian*, June 28, 2013, http://www.theguardian.com/science/2013/jun/28/uk-government-ivf-dna-three-people.

16. "MPs Back Mitochondrial Donation Law by Majority of 254," *Guardian*, February 3, 2015, http://www.theguardian.com/politics/blog/live/2015/feb/03/william-hagues-speech-on-english-votes-for-english-laws-evel-politics-live-blog.

17. Ritter 2013.

18. Brady 2013.

19. Gallagher 2014.

20. Brady 2013.

21. Moore 2011, 9.

22. Moore 2011, chapter 6.

23. Ramirez de Arellano 2007.

24. In focusing on hope, possibility, desire, pleasure, aspiration, and satisfaction, Moore is writing against much recent "melancholic" globalization theory, with its almost exclusive focus on "the negative aspects of the impact of war, terrorism, economic reform, and new technologies" (2011, 71). The anthropologist Anna Tsing has also emphasized universal dreams and aspirations in processes of globalization, despite the inevitable zones of "friction" and "awkward engagement" (2005).

25. "Briefing," *Time*, December 16, 2013.

26. As reported on NPR Morning Edition, "Dubai Plans Airport So Big It Will Be Its Own City," October 29, 2013, http://www.npr.org/2013/10/29/241548514/last-word-in-business.

27. Forgione 2014.

28. In 2014 I was invited to give presentations at two major US children's hospitals, both of which are receiving new influxes of pediatric patients from the Arab Gulf. These patients and their families have been "medically outsourced" by their governments, which pay sizable sums to US hospitals for specialized treatment of complicated pediatric cases. See also Whittaker 2015a.

29. Whittaker 2015a.

30. Ghobari 2015.

31. Davidson 2012.

32. cooke 2013.

33. Al-Qasimi 2014.

34. Kanna 2011; Mahdavi 2011; Vora 2013.

35. Hamidi 2014.

36. Hamidi 2014.

37. Hamidi 2014; Whittaker 2015a.

38. Whittaker (2015a) uses the term "medical outsourcing" to describe the Gulf Arabs who are sent to Thailand for treatment.

39. Inhorn, Patrizio, and Serour 2010; Zanini 2011.

40. In a UAE court case reported in the *Gulf News*, an Egyptian expat husband took his New Zealander wife to court for using his frozen sperm to impregnate their Filipina maid without his knowledge or consent (Farooqui 2013).

41. Gürtin 2011.

42. Gürtin 2011.

43. For example, Guilia Zanini's "Abandoned by the State, Betrayed by the Church: Italian Experiences of Cross-Border Reproductive Care" (2011) speaks to these feelings of abandonment, anger, and exile among infertile Italians, who are forced to travel to neighboring countries because of their country's restrictive, Vatican-inspired law.

44. Vayena et al. 2009.

45. The US Affordable Care Act does not include coverage for IVF or other forms of assisted reproduction.

46. Didier Fassin (2011, 2012) and Miriam Ticktin (2011a, 2011b) have been especially concerned about citizenship and health care entitlements for undocumented immigrants.

47. Adriana Petryna (2002) has developed this concept of biological citizenship in her discussion of postsocialist Ukraine in the aftermath of the Chernobyl nuclear disease. See also Rose and Novas 2005.

48. Inhorn and Patrizio 2009; Inhorn and Serour 2011; Inhorn and Shrivastav 2010.

49. Gilmartin and White 2011; Sterling 1997.

50. These critical points have been made by Beth Kangas, who believes that the term "exile" is too political (2010b); Guido Pennings (2005), who argues that much reproductive travel is done by choice rather than by force; and Andrea Whittaker and Amy Speier (2010), who point out that unlike political exiles, reproductive travelers generally have the right to return.

51. Brody 2014.

52. Inhorn et al. 2008.

53. Inhorn 1996, 2003.

54. Nandy 2014.

55. In 2011, the Friends of Low-Cost IVF Foundation (FLCIVF), a not-for-profit organization, was created in North America by Dr. Alan Trounson and Karin Hammarberg to remedy infertility and empower women globally.

FLCIVF raises funds and works with North American IVF clinics, which are willing to donate their services pro bono, with the two main aims of: (1) providing simplified clinical IVF services for a minimal cost; and (2) delivering reproductive health education to prevent infertility and avoid transmission of HIV and other STIs. I was asked to join the board of directors as the sole anthropologist.

REFERENCES

Ackerman, Sara L. 2010. "Plastic Paradise: Transforming Bodies and Selves in Costa Rica's Cosmetic Surgery Tourism Industry." *Medical Anthropology* 29 (4): 403–23.

Adamson, G. David. 2009. "Global Cultural and Socioeconomic Factors That Influence Access to Assisted Reproductive Technologies." *Women's Health* 5 (4): 351–58.

Ahmed, Leila. 1986. "Women and the Advent of Islam." *Signs* 11 (4): 665–91.

Aizura, Aren Z. 2010. "Feminine Transformations: Gender Reassignment Surgical Tourism in Thailand." *Medical Anthropology* 29 (4): 424–43.

Alawadhi, Aseel. n.d. "Legal Background in Kuwait: How Islamic Laws Form a Legal Principle Base for Deriving New Laws, Especially in the Area of Biomedical Research." Unpublished manuscript.

Al-Gazali, Lihadh. I., et al. 2005. "United Arab Emirates: Communities and Community Genetics." *Community Genetics* 8 (3): 186–96.

Al-Gazali, Lihadh, and Bassam R. Ali. 2010. "Mutations of a Country: A Mutation of Single Gene Disorders in the United Arab Emirates (UAE)." *Human Mutation* 31 (5): 505–20.

Ali, Syed. 2010. *Dubai: Gilded Cage.* New Haven, CT: Yale University Press.

Alper, Michael M., et al. 2002. "Is Your IVF Programme Good?" *Human Reproduction* 17 (1): 8–10.

Al-Qasimi, Noor. 2014. "Post-Oil Technologies, Queer Futurities, and the Emirati Indebted Subject." Paper presented at the *Journal of Middle East Women's Studies* 2014 research workshop on Transnational Feminisms and the New Middle East Insurrections, Yale University, New Haven, CT, April 3.

American College of Obstetricians and Gynecologists. 2013. "Multifetal Pregnancy Reduction." Committee Opinion: No. 553: 1–6. Accessed on November 28, 2014. http://www.acog.org/Resources-And-Publications/Committee-Opinions/Committee-on-Ethics/Multifetal-Pregnancy-Reduction.

Appadurai, Arjun. 1996. *Modernity at Large: Cultural Dimensions of Globalization.* Minneapolis: University of Minnesota Press.

———. 2001. "Grassroots Globalization and the Research Imagination." In *Globalization*, edited by Arjun Appadurai, 1–21. Durham, NC: Duke University Press.

———. 2008. "Disjuncture and Difference in the Global Cultural Economy." In *The Anthropology of Globalization: A Reader*, edited by Jonathan Xavier Inda and Renato Rosaldo, 47–65. Malden, MA: Blackwell.

Asmi, Rehenuma. 2013. "Interview with Author Ahmed Kanna about His Recent Book, *Dubai: The City as Corporation*." *Anthropology News*, March–April: 35.

Ata, Baris, and Emre Seli. 2010. "Economics of Assisted Reproductive Technologies." *Current Opinions in Obstetrics and Gynecology* 22 (3): 183–88.

Aw, Tar-Ching. 2010. "Global Health and the United Arab Emirates." *Asia-Pacific Journal of Public Health* 22 (Supplement 3): 19S–24S.

Bargach, Jamila. 2002. *Orphans of Islam: Family, Abandonment and Secret Adoption in Morocco*. Lanham, MD: Rowman and Littlefield.

Barrett, Raymond. 2010. *Dubai Dreams: Inside the Kingdom of Bling*. London: Nicholas Brealey.

Bastos, Cristiana. 2011. "From Sulphur to Perfume: Spa and SPA at Monchique, Algarve." *Anthropology & Medicine* 18 (1): 37–53.

Beaudevin, Claire. 2014. "Old Diseases and Contemporary Crisis: Inherited Blood Disorders in the Sultanate of Oman." *Anthropology & Medicine* 29 (2): 175–89.

Beck, Ulrich, and Natan Sznaider. 2006. "Unpacking Cosmopolitanism for the Social Sciences: A Research Agenda." *British Journal of Sociology* 57 (1): 1–23.

Berg Brigham, K., B. Cadier, and K. Chevreul. 2013. "The Diversity of Regulation and Public Financing of IVF in Europe and Its Impact on Utilization." *Human Reproduction* 28 (3): 666–75.

Bergmann, Sven. 2011a. "Fertility Tourism: Circumventive Routes That Enable Access to Reproductive Technologies and Substances." *Signs* 36 (2): 280–89.

———. 2011b. "Reproductive Agency and Projects: Germans Searching for Egg Donation in Spain and the Czech Republic." *Reproductive BioMedicine Online* 23 (5): 600–608.

Bharadwaj, Aditya. 2003. "Why Adoption Is Not an Option in India: The Visibility of Infertility, the Secrecy of Donor Insemination, and Other Cultural Complexities." *Social Science & Medicine* 56 (9): 1867–80.

Bharadwaj, Aditya, and Peter Glasner. 2008. *Local Cells, Global Science: The Rise of Embryonic Stem Cell Research in India*. New York: Routledge.

Birenbaum-Carmeli, Daphna. 2004. " 'Cheaper Than a Newcomer': On the Social Production of IVF Policy in Israel." *Sociology of Health & Illness* 26 (7): 897–924.

Birenbaum-Carmeli, Daphna, and Marcia C. Inhorn. 2009. "Masculinity and Marginality: Palestinian Men's Struggles with Infertility in Israel and Lebanon." *Journal of Middle East Women's Studies* 5 (2): 23–51.

Blyth, Eric. 2010. "Fertility Patients' Experiences of Cross-Border Reproductive Care." *Fertility and Sterility* 94 (1): e11–15.

Blyth, Eric, and M. Auffrey. 2008. "International Policy on Cross Border Reproductive Services." International Federation of Social Workers Policy Statement. Accessed on November 28, 2014. http://ifsw.org/policies/cross-border -reproductive-services/.

Blyth, Eric, and Abigail Farrand. 2005. "Reproductive Tourism—A Price Worth Paying for Reproductive Autonomy?" *Critical Social Policy* 25 (1): 91–114.

Blyth, Eric, Petra Thorn, and Tewes Wischmann. 2011. "CBRC and Psychosocial Counselling: Assessing Needs and Developing an Ethical Framework for Practice." *Reproductive BioMedicine Online* 23 (5): 642–51.

Boerma, J. Ties, and Zaida Mgalla, eds. 2001. *Women and Infertility in Sub-Saharan Africa: A Multi-Disciplinary Perspective.* Amsterdam: Royal Tropical Institute.

Boivin, Jacky, et al. 2007. "International Estimates of Infertility Prevalence and Treatment-Seeking: Potential Need and Demand for Infertility Medical Care." *Human Reproduction* 22 (6): 1506–12.

Bourdieu, Pierre. 1977. *Outline of a Theory of Practice.* Cambridge: Cambridge University Press.

Brady, Tara. 2013. "Woman Who Fell Pregnant after Undergoing First Successful Womb Transplant Has Lost Her IVF Baby." May 15. Accessed on November 28, 2014. http://www.dailymail.co.uk/health/article-2324950/Woman-22 -underwent-worlds-successful-womb-transplant-loses-IVF-baby.html.

Briggs, Helen. 2006a. "Donor Crisis 'Fuels IVF Tourism.'" *BBC News,* December 22. Accessed on November 29, 2014. http://news.bbc.co.uk/2/hi/health/5317878 .stm.

———. 2006b. "IVF Tourism: An Ethical Dilemma?" *BBC News,* December 22. Accessed on November 29, 2014. http://news.bbc.co.uk/2/hi/health/5338526.stm.

Bristol-Rhys, Jane. 2010. *Emirati Women: Generations of Change.* London: Hurst.

Brockopp, Jonathan E., ed. 2003. *Islamic Ethics of Life: Abortion, War, and Euthanasia.* Columbia: University of South Carolina Press.

Brody, Jane E. 2014. "PCOS: An Infertility Issue That Is Little Understood." *New York Times,* November 24. Accessed on November 28, 2014. http://well.blogs.nytimes. com/2014/11/24/pcos-an-infertility-issue-that-is-little-understood/?_r=0.

Burkett, Levi. 2007. "Medical Tourism: Concerns, Benefits, and the American Legal Perspective." *Journal of Legal Medicine* 28 (2): 223–45.

Chambers, Georgina, et al. 2009. "The Economic Impact of Assisted Reproductive Technology: A Review of Selected Developed Countries." *Fertility and Sterility* 91 (6): 2281–94.

Chankova, Slavea. 2014. "Low-cost Fertility Treatment: Maybe Babies." *Economist,* July 19. Accessed on July 19, 2014. http://www.economist.com/news/inter national/21607881-vitro-fertilisation-once-seen-miraculous-now-mainstream -rich-countries-soon.

Cheah, Pheng. 2006. "Cosmopolitanism." *Theory, Culture & Society* 23 (2–3): 486–96.

Chopra, Anuj. 2012. "The World's Baby Factory." *Foreign Policy,* February 10. Accessed on November 28, 2014. http://www.foreignpolicy.com/articles /2012/02/10/the_worlds_baby_factory.

Clarke, Adele E., et al., eds. 2010. *Biomedicalization: Technoscience, Health, and Illness in the U.S.* Durham, NC: Duke University Press.

Cohen, I. Glenn. 2012. "Circumvention Tourism." *Cornell Law Review* 97 (6): 1309–98.

Cohen, Lawrence. 1999. "Where It Hurts: Indian Material for an Ethics of Organ Transplantation." *Daedalus* 128 (4): 135–64.

———. 2002. "The Other Kidney: Biopolitics beyond Recognition." In *Commodifying Bodies*, edited by Nancy Scheper-Hughes and Loïc Wacquant, 9–29. London: Sage.

———. 2005. "Operability, Bioavailability, and Exception." In *Global Assemblages: Technology, Politics, and Ethics as Anthropological Problems*, edited by Aihwa Ong and Stephen J. Collier, 79–90. Malden, MA: Blackwell.

———. 2011. "Migrant Supplementarity: Remaking Biological Relatedness in Chinese Military and Indian Five-Star Hospitals." *Body & Society* 17 (2–3): 31–54.

Colen, Shelee. 1995. "'Like a Mother to Them': Stratified Reproduction and West Indian Childcare Workers and Employers in New York." In *Conceiving the New World Order: The Global Politics of Reproduction*, edited by Faye D. Ginsburg and Rayna Rapp, 78–102. Berkeley: University of California Press.

Collier, Stephen, and Aihwa Ong. 2005. "Global Assemblages, Anthropological Problems." In *Global Assemblages: Technology, Politics, and Ethics as Anthropological Problems*, edited by Aihwa Ong and Stephen J. Collier, 3–21. Malden, MA: Blackwell.

Collins, John A. 2002. "An International Survey of the Health Economics of IVF and ICSI." *Human Reproduction Update* 8 (3): 265–77.

Connell, John. 2006. "Medical Tourism: Sea, Sun, Sand and . . . Surgery." *Tourism Management* 27 (6): 1093–100.

Connolly, Mark P., Stijn Hoorens, and Georgina M. Chambers. 2010. "The Costs and Consequences of Assisted Reproductive Technology: An Economic Perspective." *Human Reproduction* 16 (6): 603–13.

Connolly, Mark P., Stijn Hoorens, and William Ledger. 2008. "Money in—Babies out: Assessing the Long-Term Economic Impact of IVF-Conceived Children." *Journal of Medical Ethics* 34: 653–54.

cooke, miriam. 2013. *Tribal Modern: Branding New Nations in the Arab Gulf.* Berkeley: University of California Press.

Crooks, Valorie A., et al. 2011. "Promoting Medical Tourism to India: Messages, Images, and the Marketing of International Patient Travel." *Social Science & Medicine* 72 (5): 726–32.

Crozier, G. K. D. 2010. "Protecting Cross-Border Providers of Ova and Surrogacy Services?" *Global Social Policy* 10 (3): 299–303.

Cui, Weiyuan. 2010. "Mother or Nothing: The Agony of Infertility." *Bulletin of the World Health Organization* 88 (12): 881–82.

Culley, Lorraine, et al. 2011. "Transnational Reproduction: An Exploratory Study of UK Residents Who Travel Abroad for Fertility Treatment." Unpublished summary report for the Economic and Social Research Council.

Dajani, Rana. 2011. "The Arab Spring Offers Hope But No Quick Fix." *Nature* 477 (7362): 7.

Dancet, E. A. F., et al. 2011. "Patient-Centred Infertility Care: A Qualitative Study to Listen to the Patient's Voice." *Human Reproduction* 26 (4): 827–33.

Davidson, Christopher. 2005. *The United Arab Emirates: A Study in Survival*. Boulder, CO: Lynne Rienner.

———. 2008. *Dubai: The Vulnerability of Success*. New York: Columbia University Press.

———. 2012. "The Importance of the Unwritten Social Contract." *New York Times*, August 28.

———. 2013. *After the Sheikhs: The Coming Collapse of the Gulf Monarchies*. Oxford: Oxford University Press.

De Mouzon, J., et al. 2010. "Assisted Reproductive Technology in Europe, 2006: Results Generated from European Registers by ESHRE." *Human Reproduction* 25 (8): 1851–62.

De Sutter, Petra. 2011. "Considerations for Clinics and Practitioners Treating Foreign Patients with Assisted Reproductive Technology: Lessons from Experiences at Ghent University Hospital, Belgium." *Reproductive BioMedicine Online* 23 (5): 652–56.

Deech, Ruth. 2003. "Reproductive Tourism in Europe: Infertility and Human Rights." *Global Governance* 9 (4): 425–32.

Delanty, Gerard. 2006. "The Cosmopolitan Imagination: Critical Cosmopolitanism and Social Theory." *British Journal of Sociology* 7 (1): 25–47.

Deleuze, Gilles. 1988. *Foucault*. Translated by Sean Hand. Minneapolis: University of Minnesota Press.

DeParle, Jason. 2007a. "Fearful of Restive Foreign Labor, Dubai Eyes Reforms." *New York Times*, August 6.

———. 2007b. "Rising Breed of Migrant: Skilled and Welcome." *New York Times*, August 20.

Dhont, N. 2011. "The Walking Egg Non-Profit Organisation." *Facts, Views & Vision in ObGyn* 3 (4): 253–55.

Dolnick, Sam. 2007. "Pregnancy Becomes Latest Job Outsourced to India." *AP News*. Accessed on November 30, 2014. http://usatoday30.usatoday.com/news/health/2007-12-30-surrogacy_N.htm.

Douki, S., et al. 2003. "Violence against Women in Arab and Islamic Countries." *Archives of Women's Mental Health* 6: 165–71.

Dunn, Frederick L. 1976. "Traditional Asian Medicine and Cosmopolitan Medicine as Adaptive Systems." In *Asian Medical Systems: A Comparative Study*, edited by Charles Leslie, 133–58. Berkeley: University of California Press.

Dyer, Silke J., et al. 2013. "Catastrophic Payment for Assisted Reproductive Techniques with Conventional Ovarian Stimulation in the Public Health Sector of South Africa: Frequency and Coping Strategies." *Human Reproduction* 28 (10): 2755–64.

Dyer, Silke J., and M. Patel. 2012. "The Economic Impact of Infertility on Women in Developing Countries—A Systematic Review." *Facts, Views & Vision in ObGyn* 4 (2): 102–9.

Eberstadt, Nicholas, and Apoorva Shah. 2012. "Fertility Decline in the Muslim World: A Demographic Sea Change Goes Largely Unnoticed." *Policy Review* 173 (June–July): 29–44.

Edmonds, Alexander. 2011. "'Almost Invisible Scars': Medical Tourism in Brazil. *Signs* 36 (2): 297–302.

El Shammaa, Dina. 2007. "A Favourable Stop for Fertility Treatment." *Gulf News*, September 12. Dubai, United Arab Emirates.

European Society for Human Reproduction and Embryology. 2008. *ESHRE Special Task Force on "Developing Countries and Infertility."* Oxford: Oxford University Press.

———. 2013. "IVF for 200 Euro per Cycle: First Real-Life Proof of Principle That IVF Is Feasible and Effective for Developing Countries." Accessed on July 8, 2013. http://www.eshre.eu/Londen2013/Media/Releases/Elke-Klerckx .aspx.

European Society for Human Reproduction and Embryology Task Force on Ethics and Law. 2009. "Providing Infertility Treatment in Resource-Poor Countries." *Human Reproduction* 24 (5): 1008–11.

Farooqui, Mazhar. 2013. "'My Wife Misused My Sperm,' Says UAE Expat at Al Ain Trial." *Gulf News*, October 3. Dubai, United Arab Emirates.

Fassin, Didier. 2011. *Humanitarian Reason: A Moral History of the Present*. Berkeley: University of California Press.

———. 2012. "The Obscure Object of Global Health." In *Medical Anthropology at the Intersections: Histories, Activisms, and Futures*, edited by Marcia C. Inhorn and Emily A. Wentzell, 95–115. Durham, NC: Duke University Press.

Ferguson, James. 2006. *Global Shadows: Africa in the Neoliberal World Order*. Durham, NC: Duke University Press.

Forgione, Mary. 2014. "Dubai to Build World's Biggest Mall with 100 Hotels, Climate-Control." *Chicago Tribune*, July 24.

Foster, Angel. 2012. "Abortion." Paper presented at the Conference on Women's and Children's Health in the Middle East, Center for Middle Eastern Studies, University of Chicago, November 10.

Foucault, Michel. 1994. *The Birth of the Clinic: An Archaeology of Medical Perception*. New York: Vintage.

Franklin, Sarah. 1997. *Embodied Progress: A Cultural Account of Reproduction*. London: Routledge.

———. 2007. *Dolly Mixtures: The Remaking of Genealogy*. Durham, NC: Duke University Press.

———. 2012. "Five Million Miracle Babies Later: The Biocultural Legacies of IVF." In *Reproductive Technologies as Global Form: Ethnographies of Knowledge, Practices, and Transnational Encounters*, edited by Michi Knecht, Stefan Beck, and Maren Klotz, 27–60. Frankfurt-on-Main, Germany: Campus Verlag.

———. 2013a. *Biological Relatives: IVF, Stem Cells, and the Future of Kinship*. Durham, NC: Duke University Press.

———. 2013b. "Conception through a Looking Glass: The Paradox of IVF." *Reproductive BioMedicine Online* 27 (6): 747–55.

Franklin, Sarah, and Celia Roberts. 2006. *Born and Made: An Ethnography of Preimplantation Genetic Diagnosis*. Princeton, NJ: Princeton University Press.

Friedman, Thomas. 2005. *The World Is Flat: A Brief History of the Twenty-First Century*. New York: Farrar, Straus and Giroux.

———. 2006. "Dubai and Dunces." *New York Times*, March 15.

Friese, Carrie, Gay Becker, and Robert D. Nachtigall. 2006. "Rethinking the Biological Clock: Eleventh Hour Moms, Miracle Moms and Meanings of Age-Related Infertility." *Social Science & Medicine* 63 (6): 1550–60.

———. 2008. "Older Motherhood and the Changing Life Course in the Era of Assisted Reproductive Technologies." *Journal of Aging Studies* 22 (1): 65–73.

Gallagher, James. 2013. "IVF as Cheap as LE170, Doctors Claim." BBC News. Accessed on July 8, 2013. http://www.bbc.com/news/health-23223752.

———. 2014. "First Womb-Transplant Baby Born." BBC News. Accessed on November 30, 2014. http://www.bbc.com/news/health-29485996.

Gallant, Monica. 2008. *Emirati Women in Dubai: Navigating Cultural Change*. Frankfurt, Germany: VDM Verlag.

Gerrits, Trudie, et al. 2012. "Biomedical Infertility Care in Poor Resource Countries: Barriers, Access and Ethics." *Facts, Views & Vision in ObGyn*.

Gerrits, Trudie, and M. Shaw. 2010. "Biomedical Infertility Care in Sub-Saharan Africa: A Social Science Review of Current Practices, Experiences and View Points." *Facts, Views & Vision in ObGyn* 2 (3): 194–207.

Gender and Medical Tourism. 2011. Comparative Perspectives Symposium. *Signs* 36 (2).

Ghobari, Mohammed. 2015. "Gulf Countries, Opposition Say Houthi Takeover in Yemen a 'Coup.'" February 7. Accessed on February 9, 2015. http://news.yahoo.com/blast-hits-republican-palace-yemeni-capital-wounding-three-080403954.html;_ylt=AoLEV7.phtdUDWoA8QUnnIlQ.

Gilmartin, Mary, and Allen White. 2011. "Interrogating Medical Tourism: Ireland, Abortion, and Mobility Rights." *Signs* 36 (2): 275–80.

Ginsburg, Faye D., and Rayna Rapp, eds. 1995. *Conceiving the New World Order: The Global Politics of Reproduction*. Berkeley: University of California Press.

Giwa-Osagie, Osato F. 2007. "The Development of Assisted Conception in Sub-Saharan Africa: An Insight into the Need for Infertility Services in Developing Countries." Paper presented at the Alexandria Women's Health Forum, Egypt, March 22.

Goold, Imogen, and Julian Savulescu. 2009. "In Favour of Freezing Eggs for Non-Medical Reasons." *Bioethics* 23 (1): 47–58.

Gürtin, Zeynep B. 2011. "Banning Reproductive Travel: Turkey's ART Legislation and Third-Party Assisted Reproduction." *Reproductive BioMedicine Online* 23 (5): 555–64.

———. 2013. "The ART of Making Babies: Turkish IVF Patients' Experiences of Childlessness, Infertility and Tup Bebek." PhD Dissertation, University of Cambridge.

Gürtin, Zeynep B., Kamal K. Ahuja, and Susan Golombok. 2012a. "Egg-Sharing, Consent and Exploitation: Examining Donors' and Recipients' Circumstances and Retrospective Reflections." *Reproductive BioMedicine Online* 27 (7): 698–708.

———. 2012b. "Emotional and Relational Aspects of Egg-Sharing: Egg-Share Donors' and Recipients' Feelings about Each Other, Each Others' Treatment Outcome and Any Resulting Children." *Human Reproduction* 27 (6): 1690–701.

Gürtin, Zeynep B., and Marcia C. Inhorn. 2011. "Introduction: Travelling for Conception and the Global Assisted Reproduction Market." *Reproductive BioMedicine Online* 23 (5): 535–37.

Gürtin, Zeynep B., and Soraya Tremayne. 2015. "Islam and Assisted Reproduction in the Middle East: Comparing the Sunni Arab World, Shia Iran, and Secular Turkey." In *The Changing World Religion Map: Sacred Places, Identities, Practices and Politics*, edited by Stanley D. Brunn, 3137–53. New York: Springer.

Hamidi, Samer. 2014. "Evidence from National Health Account: The Case of Dubai." *Risk Management and Healthcare Policy* 7: 163–75.

Harris, Colette, and Theresa Cheung. 2006. *The Ultimate PCOS Handbook: Lose Weight, Boost Fertility, Clear Skin and Restore Self-Esteem*. London: Harper Thorsons.

Hassan, Mohamed A. M., and Stephen R. Killick. 2004. "Negative Lifestyle Is Associated with a Significant Reduction in Fecundity." *Fertility and Sterility* 81 (2): 384–92.

Hawkins, Leah K., et al. 2014. "Perceptions among Infertile Couples of Lifestyle Behaviors and In Vitro Fertilization (IVF) Success." *Journal of Assisted Reproduction and Genetics* 31: 255–60.

Heffner, Linda J. 2004. "Advanced Maternal Age—How Old Is Too Old?" *New England Journal of Medicine* 351: 1927–29.

Hessini, Leila. 2007. "Abortion and Islam: Policies and Practice in the Middle East and North Africa." *Reproductive Health Matters* 15 (29): 75–84.

Hewlett, Sylvia Ann. 2004. *Creating a Life: What Every Woman Needs to Know about Having a Baby and a Career*. New York: Miramax.

Hochschild, Arlie Russell. 1979. "Emotion Work, Feeling Rules, and Social Structure." *American Journal of Sociology* 85 (3): 551–75.

Horowitz, Michael D., and Jeffrey A. Rosensweig. 2007. "Medical Tourism—Health Care in the Global Economy." *Physician Executive*, 33 (6): 24–26, 28–30.

Hourvitz, Ariel, et al. 2009. "Assisted Reproduction in Women over 40 Years of Age: How Old Is Too Old?" *Reproductive BioMedicine Online* 19 (4): 599–603.

Hudson, Nicky, et al. 2011. "Cross-Border Reproductive Care: A Review of the Literature." *Reproductive BioMedicine Online* 22 (7): 673–85.

Hudson, Nicky, and Lorraine Culley. 2011. "Assisted Reproductive Travel: UK Patient Trajectories." *Reproductive BioMedicine Online* 23 (5): 573–81.

Ikemoto, Lisa C. 2009. "Reproductive Tourism: Equality Concerns in the Global Market for Fertility Services." *Law and Inequality* 27: 277–309.

Inda, Jonathan Xavier, and Renato Rosaldo. 2008. "Tracking Global Flows." In *The Anthropology of Globalization: A Reader*, edited by Jonathan Xavier Inda and Renato Rosaldo, 3–46. Malden, MA: Blackwell.

Inhorn, Marcia C. 1994. *Quest for Conception: Gender, Infertility, and Egyptian Medical Traditions*. Philadelphia: University of Pennsylvania Press.

———. 1996. *Infertility and Patriarchy: The Cultural Politics of Gender and Family Life in Egypt.* Philadelphia: University of Pennsylvania Press.

———. 2003. *Local Babies, Global Science: Gender, Religion, and In Vitro Fertilization in Egypt.* New York: Routledge.

———. 2004. "Privacy, Privatization, and the Politics of Patronage: Ethnographic Challenges to Penetrating the Secret World of Middle Eastern, Hospital-Based In Vitro Fertilization." *Social Science & Medicine* 59 (10): 2095–108.

———. 2005a. "*Fatwas* and ARTs: IVF and Gamete Donation in Sunni v. Shi'a Islam." *Journal of Gender, Race & Justice* 9 (2): 291–317.

———. 2005b. "Sexuality, Masculinity, and Infertility in Egypt: Potent Troubles in the Marital and Medical Encounters." In *African Masculinities: Men in Africa from the Late Nineteenth Century to the Present*, edited by Lahoucine Ouzgane and Robert Morrell, 289–303. New York: Palgrave.

———. 2006. "'He Won't Be My Son': Middle Eastern Muslim Men's Discourses of Adoption and Gamete Donation." *Medical Anthropology Quarterly* 20 (1): 94–120.

———. 2007. "Masculinity, Reproduction, and Male Infertility Surgeries in Egypt and Lebanon." *Journal of Middle East Women's Studies* 3 (3): 1–20.

———. 2009. "Right to Assisted Reproductive Technology: Overcoming Infertility in Low-Resource Countries." *International Journal of Gynecology & Obstetrics* 106 :172–74.

———. 2010. "'Assisted' Reproduction in Global Dubai: Reproductive Tourists and Their Helpers." In *The Globalization of Motherhood: Deconstructions and Reconstructions of Biology and Care*, edited by Wendy Chavkin and JaneMaree Maher, 180–202. New York: Routledge.

———. 2011a. "Diasporic Dreaming: Return Reproductive Tourism to the Middle East." *Reproductive BioMedicine Online* 23 (5): 582–91.

———. 2011b. "Globalization and Gametes: Reproductive Tourism, Islamic Bioethics, and Middle Eastern Modernity." *Anthropology & Medicine* 18 (1): 87–103.

———. 2012. *The New Arab Man: Emergent Masculinities, Technologies, and Islam in the Middle East.* Princeton, NJ: Princeton University Press.

———. 2014. "Middle Eastern Masculinities in the Age of Assisted Reproductive Technologies." In *Everyday Life in the Middle East*, edited by Donna Lee Bowen, Evelyn A. Early, and Becky Schulthies. 3rd ed. Bloomington: Indiana University Press.

———. 2014. "Roads Less Traveled in Middle East Anthropology—And New Paths in Gender Ethnography." *Journal of Middle East Women's Studies* 10 (3): 62–86.

Inhorn, Marcia C., et al. 2008. "Occupational and Environmental Exposures to Heavy Metals: Risk Factors for Male Infertility in Lebanon?" *Reproductive Toxicology* 25: 203–12.

Inhorn, Marcia C., et al. 2009. "Consanguinity and Family Clustering of Male Infertility in Lebanon." *Fertility and Sterility* 91 (4): 1104–9.

Inhorn, Marcia C., and Michael Hassan Fakih. 2006. "Arab Americans, African Americans, and Infertility: Barriers to Reproduction and Medical Care." *Fertility and Sterility* 85 (4): 844–52.

Inhorn, Marcia C., and Zeynep B. Gürtin. 2011. "Cross-Border Reproductive Care: A Future Research Agenda." *Reproductive BioMedicine Online* 23 (5): 665–76.

———. 2012. "Infertility and Assisted Reproduction in the Muslim Middle East: Social, Religious, and Resource Considerations." *Facts, Views & Vision in ObGyn*: 24–29.

Inhorn, Marcia C., and Pasquale Patrizio. 2009. "Rethinking Reproductive 'Tourism' as Reproductive 'Exile.'" *Fertility and Sterility* 92 (3): 904–6.

Inhorn, Marcia C., Pasquale Patrizio, and Gamal I. Servour. 2010. "Third-Party Reproductive Assistance around the Mediterranean: Comparing Sunni Egypt, Catholic Italy, and Multisectarian Lebanon." *Reproductive BioMedicine Online* 21 (7): 848–53.

Inhorn, Marcia C., and Gamal I. Serour. 2011. "Islam, Medicine, and Arab-Muslim Refugee Health in America after 9/11." *Lancet* 378 (9794): 935–43.

Inhorn, Marcia C., and Pankaj Shrivastav. 2010. "Globalization and Reproductive Tourism in the United Arab Emirates." *Asia-Pacific Journal of Public Health* 22 (Supplement 3): 68–74.

Inhorn, Marcia C., and Soraya Tremayne, eds. 2012. *Islam and Assisted Reproductive Technologies: Sunni and Shia Perspectives*. New York: Berghahn.

Inhorn, Marcia C., and Frank van Balen, eds. 2002. *Infertility around the Globe: New Thinking about Gender, Childlessness, and Reproductive Technologies*. Berkeley: University of California Press.

Institute of Medicine. 2001. *Crossing the Quality Chasm: A New Health System for the 21st Century*. Washington: National Academies Press.

International Federation of Fertility Societies. 2010. "New International Survey Shows That Your Access to Fertility Treatment Often Depends on Where You Live." Accessed on November 29, 2014. www.iffs-http://c.ymcdn.com/sites/www.iffs-reproduction.org/resource/resmgr/press_room/surveillance_final_pr.pdf.

Ismail, Manal. 2012a. "Dubai Healthcare City to Compete for Foreign Patients." *National*, Abu Dhabi, United Arab Emirates. February 18.

———. 2012b. "More Than One-third of Diabetics in the UAE Are Undiagnosed." *National*, Abu Dhabi, United Arab Emirates. November 12.

Jha, Prabhat, et al. 2002. "Estimates of Global and Regional Smoking Prevalence in 1995, by Age and Sex." *American Journal of Public Health* 92 (6): 1002–6.

Johnson, Martin H., Jacques Cohen, and Gedis Grudzinskas. 2014. "Accessible and Affordable IVF: Is Bob Edwards' Dream about to Become Reality?" *Reproductive BioMedicine Online* 28 (3): 265–66.

Johnston, Rory, et al. 2011. "An Industry Perspective on Canadian Patients' Involvement in Medical Tourism: Implications for Public Health." *BMC Public Health* 11: 416–23.

Jones, C. A., and L. G. Keith. 2006. "Medical Tourism and Reproductive Outsourcing: The Dawning of a New Paradigm for Healthcare." *International Journal of Fertility and Women's Medicine* 51 (6): 251–55.

Jones, Howard W., et al. 2007. "IFFS Surveillance 07." *Fertility and Sterility* 87 (Supplement 1): S1–67.

———. 2010. "International Federation of Fertility Societies: Surveillance 2010." Accessed on November 29, 2014. http://c.ymcdn.com/sites/www.iffs-reproduction.org/resource/resmgr/newsletters/iffs_surveillance_2010.pdf.

Jones, Radhika. 2013. "Love in the Time of Globalization." *Time*, May 13, 57.

Kahn, Susan Martha. 2000. *Reproducing Jews: A Cultural Account of Assisted Conception in Israel*. Durham, NC: Duke University Press.

Kanaaneh, Rhoda Ann. 2002. *Birthing the Nation: Strategies of Palestinian Women in Israel*. Berkeley: University of California Press.

Kangas, Beth. 2010a. "The Burden of Pursuing Treatment Abroad: Three Stories of Medical Travelers from Yemen." *Global Social Policy* 10 (3): 306–14.

———. 2010b. "Traveling for Medical Care in a Global World." *Medical Anthropology* 29 (4): 344–62.

———. 2011. "Complicating Common Ideas about Medical Tourism: Gender, Class, and Globality in Yemenis' International Medical Travel." *Signs* 36 (2): 327–32.

Kanna, Ahmed. 2011. *Dubai: The City as Corporation*. Minneapolis: University of Minnesota Press.

Katz, P., R. Nachtigall, and J. Showstack. 2002. "The Economic Impact of the Assisted Reproductive Technologies." *Nature Cell Biology* (Supplement 4): S29–32.

Khalaf, Sulayman, and Saad Alkobaisi. 1999. "Migrants' Strategies of Coping and Patterns of Accommodation in the Oil-Rich Gulf Societies: Evidence from the UAE." *British Journal of Middle Eastern Studies* 26 (2): 271–98.

Knoppers, Bartha M., and Sonia LeBris. 1991. "Recent Advances in Medically Assisted Conception: Legal, Ethical and Social Issues." *American Journal of Law and Medicine* 17:329–61.

Krane, Jim. 2009. *City of Gold: Dubai and the Dream of Capitalism*. London: St. Martin's.

Kugelman, Amir, et al. 2013. "Iatrogenesis in Neonatal Intensive Care Units: Observational and Interventional Prospective, Multicenter Study." *Pediatrics* 122 (3): 550–55.

Latour, Bruno, and Steve Woolgar. 1979. *Laboratory Life: The Construction of Scientific Facts*. Princeton, NJ: Princeton University Press.

Ledger, William. 2009. "Demographics of Infertility." *Reproductive BioMedicine Online* 18 (Supplement 2): S11–14.

Lee, Felicia R. 2005. "Fertility Tourists Go Great Lengths to Conceive." *New York Times*, January 25.

Leng, Chee Heng, and Andrea Whittaker, eds. 2010. "Why Is Medical Travel of Concern to Global Social Policy?" Special issue, *Global Social Policy* 10 (3).

Leslie, Charles. 1976. "Introduction." In *Asian Medical Systems: A Comparative Study*, edited by Charles Leslie, 1–12. Berkeley: University of California Press.

Lockwood, Gillian M. 2011. "Social Egg Freezing: The Prospect of Reproductive 'Immortality' or a Dangerous Delusion?" *Reproductive BioMedicine Online* 23(3): 334–40.

"Low-Cost In-Vitro Fertilization Method Developed at CU May Help Couples In Developing Countries." 2013. University of Colorado Boulder. Accessed September 2, 2014. http://www.colorado.edu/news/releases/2013/07/08/low-cost -vitro-fertilization-method-developed-cu-may-help-couples.

Lunenfeld, Bruno, and Andre C. van Steirteghem. 2004. "Infertility in the Third Millennium: Implications for the Individual, Family and Society: Condensed Meeting Report from the Bertarelli Foundation's Second Global Conference." *Human Reproduction Update* 10 (4): 317–26.

Madrigal, Alexis C. 2014. "Making Babies: Five Predictions about the Future of Reproduction." *Atlantic*, May 30. http://www.theatlantic.com/magazine/archive /2014/06/making-babies/361630/.

Mahdavi, Pardis. 2011. *Gridlock: Labor, Migration, and Human Trafficking in Dubai*. Stanford, CA: Stanford University Press.

Maiburg, M., et al. 2009. "Does the Genetic and Familial Background of Males Undertaking ICSI Affect the Outcome?" *Journal of Assisted Reproduction and Genetics* 26: 297–303.

Mainland, Lynn, and Elinor Wilson. 2010. "Principles of Establishment of the First International Forum on Cross-Border Reproductive Care." *Fertility and Sterility* 94 (1): e1–3.

Makia, Ahmad, and Charlie Koolhaas. 2011. *Evolving Spaces: Dubai's Emerging Cultural Districts*. Dubai: Brownbook.

Mantikou, E., et al. 2013. "Embryo Culture Media and IVF/ICSI Success Rates: A Systematic Review." *Human Reproduction Update* 19 (3): 210–20.

Marcus, George E. 1995. "Ethnography in/of the World System: The Emergence of Multi-Sited Ethnography." *Annual Review of Anthropology* 24: 95–117.

Marinelli, Daniela, et al. 2004. "Mini-Review of Studies on the Effect of Smoking and Drinking Habits on Semen Parameters." *International Journal of Hygiene and Environmental Health* 207 (3): 185–92.

Martin, Emily. 1991. "The Egg and the Sperm: How Science Has Constructed a Romance Based on Stereotypical Male-Female Roles." *Signs* 16 (3): 485–504.

———. 2001. *The Woman in the Body: A Cultural Analysis of Reproduction*. Boston: Beacon.

Martin, Lauren Jade. 2009. "Reproductive Tourism in the Age of Globalization." *Globalizations* 6 (2): 249–63.

Mascarenhas, Maya N., et al. 2012. "National, Regional, and Global Trends in Infertility Prevalence since 1990: A Systematic Analysis of 277 Health Surveys." *PLOS Medicine* 9 (12): 1–12.

Matorras, Roberto. 2005. "Reproductive Exile versus Reproductive Tourism." *Human Reproduction* 20 (12): 3571.

Mazzaschi, Andrew. 2011. "Surgeon and Safari: Producing Valuable Bodies in Johannesburg." *Signs* 36 (2): 303–12.

McKelvey A., et al. 2009. "The Impact of Cross-Border Reproductive Care or 'Fertility Tourism' on NHS Maternity Services." *BJOG: An International Journal of Obstetrics & Gynaecology* 116 (11): 1520–23.

Meirow, D., and J. G. Schenker. 1997. "The Current Status of Sperm Donation in Assisted Reproduction Technology: Ethical and Legal Considerations." *Journal of Assisted Reproduction and Genetics* 14 (3): 133–38.

Melhuus, Marit. 2012. *Problems of Conception: Issues of Law, Biotechnology, Individuals and Kinship.* New York: Berghahn.

Mertes, Heidi, and Guido Pennings. 2012. "Elective Oocyte Cryopreservation: Who Should Pay?" *Human Reproduction* 27 (1): 9–13.

Mladovsky, Philipa, and Corinna Sorenson. 2010. "Public Financing of IVF: A Review of Policy Rationales." *Health Care Analysis* 18: 113–28.

Moore, Henrietta L. 2011. *Still Life: Hopes, Desires and Satisfactions.* Cambridge, UK: Polity.

Moosa, Ebrahim. 2003. "Human Cloning in Muslim Ethics." *Voices across Boundaries*, Fall, 23–26.

Moragianni, Vasiliki A., and Alan S. Penzias. 2010. "Cumulative Live-Birth Rates after Assisted Reproductive Technology." *Current Opinions in Obstetrics and Gynecology* 22 (3): 189–92.

Nachtigall, Robert D. 2006. "International Disparities in Access to Infertility Services." *Fertility and Sterility* 85 (4): 871–75.

Nahman, Michal. 2011. "Reverse Traffic: Intersecting Inequalities in Human Egg Donation." *Reproductive BioMedicine Online* 23 (5): 626–33.

————2013. *Extractions: An Ethnography of Reproductive Tourism.* London: Palgrave Macmillan.

Nandy, Amrita. 2014. "Feminist Debates on Motherhood and Choice: A Case Study of Non-Normative Women in Delhi." PhD diss., Jawaharlal Nehru University, Delhi, India.

Naraindas, Harish. 2011. "Of Relics, Body Parts and Laser Beams: The German Heilpraktiker and His Ayurvedic Spa." *Anthropology & Medicine* 18 (1): 67–86.

Naraindas, Harish, and Cristiana Bastos, eds. 2011. "Healing Holidays? Itinerant Patients, Therapeutic Locales, and the Quest for Health." Special issue, *Anthropology & Medicine* 18 (1).

Nelson, Scott M., and Debbie A. Lawlor. 2011. "Predicting Live Birth, Preterm Delivery, and Low Birth Weight in Infants Born from In Vitro Fertilisation: A Prospective Study of 144,018 Treatment Cycles." *PLOS Medicine* 8 (1): 1–11.

Nygren, K. G., et al. 2010. "Cross-Border Fertility Care—International Committee Monitoring Assisted Reproductive Technologies Global Survey: 2006 Data and Estimates." *Fertility and Sterility* 94: e4–10.

Obermeyer, Carla Makhlouf. 1999. "Fairness and Fertility: The Meaning of Son Preference in Morocco." In *Dynamics of Values in Fertility Change*, edited by Richard Leete, 275–92. Oxford: Oxford University Press.

O'Driscoll, Sean. 2012. "Study Finds Couples are Traveling to the Emirates to Undergo Fertility Treatment." *7 Days in Dubai*, August 5.

Ombelet, Willem. 2008. "False Perceptions and Common Misunderstandings Surrounding the Subject of Infertility in Developing Countries." *ESHRE Monographs* 1: 8–11.

———. 2009. "Reproductive Healthcare Systems Should Include Accessible Infertility Diagnosis and Treatment: An Important Challenge for Resource-Poor Countries." *International Journal of Gynecology & Obstetrics* 106 (2): 168–71.

———. 2011. "Global Access to Infertility Care in Developing Countries: A Case of Human Rights, Equity and Social Justice." *Facts, Views & Vision in ObGyn* 3 (4): 257–66.

———. 2013. "The Walking Egg Project: Universal Access to Infertility Care— From Dream to Reality." *Facts, Views & Vision in ObGyn* 5 (2): 161–75.

———. 2014. "Is Global Access to Infertility Care Realistic? The Walking Egg Project." *Reproductive BioMedicine Online* 28 (3): 267–72.

Ombelet, Willem, et al. 2008. "Infertility and the Provision of Infertility Medical Services in Developing Countries." *Human Reproduction Update* 14 (6): 605–21.

Ombelet, Willem, and Frank van Balen, eds. 2010. "Social Aspects of Accessible Infertility Care in Developing Countries. *Facts, Views & Vision in ObGyn*.

Omran, Abdel Rahim, and Farzaneh Roudi. 1993. "The Middle East Population Puzzle." *Population Bulletin* 48 (1): 1–40.

Ong, Aihwa. 2005. "Economies of Expertise: Assembling Flows, Managing Citizenship." In *Global Assemblages: Technology, Politics, and Ethics as Anthropological Problems*, edited by Aihwa Ong and Stephen Collier, 337–53. Malden, MA: Blackwell.

Ong, Aihwa, and Stephen J. Collier, eds. 2005. *Global Assemblages: Technology, Politics, and Ethics as Anthropological Problems*. Malden, MA: Blackwell.

Ory, Steven J., ed. 2013. "IFFS Surveillance 2013." http://c.ymcdn.com/sites/www .iffs-reproduction.org/resource/resmgr/iffs_surveillance_09-19-13.pdf.

Ory, Steven J., et al. 2014. "International Federation of Fertility Societies Surveillance 2013: Preface and Conclusions." *Fertility and Sterility* 101 (6): 1582–83.

Pande, Amrita. 2009. "'It May Be Her Eggs but It's My Blood': Surrogates and Everyday Forms of Kinship in India." *Qualitative Sociology* 32: 379–97.

———. 2010a. "'At Least I Am Not Sleeping with Anyone': Resisting the Stigma of Commercial Surrogacy in India." *Feminist Studies* 36 (2): 292–314.

———. 2010b. "Commercial Surrogacy in India: Manufacturing a Perfect 'Mother-Worker.'" *Signs* 35 (4): 969–94.

———. 2011. "Transnational Commercial Surrogacy in India: Gifts for Global Sisters?" *Reproductive BioMedicine Online* 23 (5): 618–25.

Pennings, Guido. 2002. "Reproductive Tourism as Moral Pluralism in Motion." *Journal of Medical Ethics* 28 (6): 337–41.

———. 2004. "Legal Harmonization and Reproductive Tourism in Europe." *Human Reproduction* 19 (12): 2689–94.

———. 2005. "Reply: Reproductive Exile versus Reproductive Tourism." *Human Reproduction* 20 (12): 3571–72.

————. 2006. "International Parenthood via Procreative Tourism." In *Contemporary Ethical Dilemmas in Assisted Reproduction*, edited by F. Shenfield and C. Sureau, 43–56. Abingdon, UK: Informa Health Care.

————. 2009. "International Evolution of Legislation and Guidelines in Medically Assisted Reproduction." *Reproductive BioMedicine Online* 18 (Suppl. 2): 15–18.

————. 2010. "The Rough Guide to Insemination: Cross-Border Travelling for Donor Semen due to Different Regulations." *Facts, Views & Vision in ObGyn*: 55–60.

Pennings, Guido, et al. 2008. "ESHRE Task Force on Ethics and Law 15: Cross-Border Reproductive Care." *Human Reproduction* 23 (10): 2182–84.

————. 2009. "Cross-Border Reproductive Care in Belgium." *Human Reproduction* 24 (12): 3108–18.

Pennings, Guido, and Willem Ombelet. 2007. "Coming Soon to Your Clinic: Patient-Friendly ART." *Human Reproduction* 22 (8): 2075–79.

Petryna, Adriana. 2002. *Life Exposed: Biological Citizens after Chernobyl*. Princeton, NJ: Princeton University Press.

————. 2009. *When Experiments Travel: Clinical Trials and the Global Search for Human Subjects*. Princeton, NJ: Princeton University Press.

Pfeffer, Naomi. 2011. "Eggs-Ploiting Women: A Critical Feminist Analysis of the Different Principles in Transplant and Fertility Tourism." *Reproductive BioMedicine Online* 23 (5): 634–41.

Qadeer, Imrana. 2010. "Benefits and Threats of International Trade in Health: A Case of Surrogacy in India." *Global Social Policy* 10 (3): 303–5.

Qaed, Samar. 2013. "More Yemeni Couples Embrace In Vitro Fertilization." *Yemen Times*, Sana, Yemen, September 10. http://www.yementimes.com/en/1710/health/2867/More-Yemeni-couples-embrace-in-vitro-fertilization.htm.

Quintela, Maria Manuel. 2011. "Seeking 'Energy' vs. Pain Relief in Spas in Brazil (Caldas da Imperatriz) and Portugal (Termas da Sulfurea)." *Anthropology & Medicine* 18 (1): 23–35.

Ramirez de Arellano, Annette B. 2007. "Patients without Borders: The Emergence of Medical Tourism." *International Journal of Health Services* 37 (1): 193–98.

Ritter, Malcolm. 2013. "Once Infertile, Woman Gives Birth after Surgery." Associated Press, October 1. http://bigstory.ap.org/article/once-infertile-woman-gives-birth-after-surgery.

Rizk, Diaa E. E., et al. 2005. "Determinants of Women's Choice of Their Obstetrician and Gynecologist Provider in the UAE." *Acta Obstetrics and Gynecology Scandinavia* 84: 48–53.

Roberts, Elizabeth F. S. 2009. "The Traffic between Women: Female Alliance and Familial Egg Donation in Ecuador." In *Assisting Reproduction, Testing Genes: Global Encounters with New Biotechnologies*, edited by Daphna Birenbaum-Carmeli and Marcia C. Inhorn, 113–43. New York: Berghahn.

————. 2012. *God's Laboratory: Assisted Reproduction in the Andes*. Berkley: University of California Press.

Roberts, Elizabeth F. S., and Nancy Scheper-Hughes. 2011a. "Introduction: Medical Migrations." *Body and Society* 17 (2–3): 1–30.

———, eds. 2011b. "Medical Migrations." Special issue, *Body and Society* 17(2–3).

Rose, Nicholas, and Carlos Novas. 2005. "Biological Citizenship." In *Global Assemblages: Technology, Politics, and Ethics as Anthropological Problems*, edited by Aihwa Ong and Stephen Collier, 439–63. Malden, MA: Blackwell.

Roudometof, Victor. 2005. "Transnationalism, Cosmopolitanism and Glocalization." *Current Sociology* 53 (1): 113–35.

Rudrappa, Sharmila. 2010. "Making India the 'Mother Destination': Outsourcing Labor to Indian Surrogates." In *Research in the Sociology of Work*, edited by Christine L. Williams and Kirsten Dellinger, 253–85. London: Emerald Group.

———. 2012. "India's Reproductive Assembly Line." *Contexts* 11 (2): 22–27.

Rutstein, S. O., and I. H. Shah. 2004. "Infecundity, Infertility, and Childlessness in Developing Countries." Geneva: World Health Organization.

Salama, Samir. 2007. "FNC in Heated Debate on Bill Regulating IVF Centres." *Gulf News*, Dubai, United Arab Emirates. July 4.

Sandler, Lauren. 2013. "The Childfree Life: When Having It All Means Not Having Children." *Time*, August 12, 38–45.

Sassen, Saskia. 2001. *The Global City: New York, London, Tokyo*. Princeton, NJ: Princeton University Press.

Scheper-Hughes, Nancy. 2000. "The Global Traffic in Human Organs." *Current Anthropology* 41 (2): 191–211.

———. 2002a. "Bodies for Sale—Whole or in Parts." In *Commodifying Bodies*, edited by Nancy Scheper-Hughes and Loïc Wacquant, 1–8. London: Sage.

———. 2002b. "The Ends of the Body: Commodity Fetishism and the Global Traffic in Organs." *SAIS Review* 22 (1): 61–80.

———. 2004. "Parts Unknown: Undercover Ethnography of the Organs-Trafficking Underworld." *Ethnography* 11 (3): 16–30.

———. 2005. "The Last Commodity: Post-Human Ethics and the Global Traffic in 'Fresh' Organs." In *Global Assemblages: Technology, Politics, and Ethics as Anthropological Problems*, edited by Aihwa Ong and Stephen Collier, 145–67. Malden, MA: Blackwell.

———. 2011. "Mr. Tati's Holiday and Joao's Safari—Seeing the World through Transplant Tourism." *Body & Society* 17 (2–3): 55–92.

Schwartz, Ariel. 2013. "Dubai Is Paying Its Residents in Gold to Lose Weight." July 20. www.fastcoexist.com.

Sengupta, Amit. 2011. "Medical Tourism: Reverse Subsidy for the Elite." *Signs* 36 (2): 312–29.

Serour, Gamal I. 1996. "Bioethics in Reproductive Health: A Muslim's Perspective." *Middle East Fertility Society Journal* 1 (1): 30–35.

———. 2008. "Islamic Perspectives in Human Reproduction." *Reproductive BioMedicine Online* 17 (Supplement 3): 34–38.

———and B. M. Dickens. 2001. "Assisted Reproduction Developments in the Islamic World." *International Journal of Gynecology & Obstetrics* 74 (2): 187–93.

Shabana, Ayman. 2015. "Foundations of the Consensus against Surrogacy Arrangements in Islamic Law." *Islamic Law and Society* 22: 82–113.

Sharma, S., S. Mittal, and P. Aggarwal. 2009. "Management of Infertility in Low Resource Countries." *BJOG: An International Journal of Obstetrics and Gynecology* 116 (Supplement 1): 77–83.

Shenfield, Françoise. 2011. "Implementing a Good Practice Guide for CBRC: Perspectives from the ESHRE Cross-Border Reproductive Care Taskforce." *Reproductive BioMedicine Online* 23 (5): 657–64.

Shenfield, Françoise, et al. 2010. "Cross Border Reproductive Care in Six European Countries." *Human Reproduction* 25 (6): 1361–68.

Shkedi-Rafid, Shiri, and Yael Hashiloni-Dolev. 2011. "Egg Freezing for Age-Related Fertility Decline: Preventive Medicine or a Further Medicalization of Reproduction? Analyzing the New Israeli Policy." *Fertility and Sterility* 96 (2): 291–94.

———. 2012. "Egg Freezing for Non-Medical Uses: The Lack of a Relational Approach to Autonomy in the New Israeli Policy and in Academic Discussion." *Journal of Medical Ethics* 38: 154–57.

Shrivastav, Pankaj. 2010. "The PCOS 'Epidemic' in South Asia and the Gulf Region." Paper presented at Global Health and the United Arab Emirates: Asia-Middle East Connections, United Arab Emirates University, Al Ain, Abu Dhabi, United Arab Emirates, January 4–8.

Skrbis, Zlatko, Gavin Kendall, and Ian Woodward. 2004. "Locating Cosmopolitanism: Between Humanist Ideal and Grounded Social Category." *Theory, Culture & Society* 21 (6): 115–36.

Smajdor, Anna. 2011. "The Ethics of IVF over 40." *Maturitas* 69 (1): 37–40.

Smith, Elise, et al. 2009. "Reproductive Tourism in Argentina: Clinic Accreditation and Its Implications for Consumers, Health Professionals and Policy Makers." *Developing World Bioethics* 10 (2): 59–69.

Sobo, Elisa J., Elizabeth Herlihy, and Mary Bicker. 2011. "Selling Medical Travel to US Patient-Consumers: The Cultural Appeal of Website Marketing Messages." *Anthropology & Medicine* 18 (1): 119–36.

Solomon, Harris. 2011. "Affective Journeys: The Emotional Structuring of Medical Tourism in India." *Anthropology & Medicine* 18 (1): 105–18.

Sonbol, Amira el Azhary. 1995. "Adoption in Islamic Society: A Historical Survey." *Children in the Muslim Middle East*, edited by Elizabeth Warnock Fernea, 45–67. Austin: University of Texas Press.

Song, Priscilla. 2010. "Biotech Pilgrims and the Transnational Quest for Stem Cell Cures." *Medical Anthropology* 29 (4): 384–402.

Spar, Debora. 2006. *The Baby Business: How Money, Science, and Politics Drive the Commerce of Conception*. Boston: Harvard Business School Press.

Speier, Amy R. 2011a. "Brokers, Consumers and the Internet: How North American Consumers Navigate Their Infertility Journeys." *Reproductive BioMedicine Online* 23 (5): 592–99.

———. 2011b. "Health Tourism in a Czech Health Spa." *Anthropology & Medicine* 18 (1): 55–66.

Staires, Meg. 2013. "Observations on Reproductive Health Care in Dubai." *Issues in Middle East Studies* 35 (2): 5–6.

Stephenson, Christina. 2009. "Reproductive Outsourcing to India: WTO Obligations in the Absence of US National Legislation." *Journal of World Trade* 43 (1): 189–208.

Sterling, Abigail-Mary E. W. 1997. "The European Union and Abortion Tourism: Liberalizing Ireland's Abortion Law." *International and Comparative Law Review* 20: 385–406.

Stoop, D., J. Nekkebroeck, and P. Devroey. 2011. "A Survey on the Intentions and Attitudes towards Oocyte Cryopreservation for Non-Medical Reasons among Women of Reproductive Age." *Human Reproduction* 26 (3): 655–61.

Storrow, Richard F. 2005–6. "Quests for Conception: Fertility Tourists, Globalization, and Feminist Legal Theory." *Hastings Law Journal* 57: 295–330.

———. 2010. "The Pluralism Problem in Cross-Border Reproductive Care." *Human Reproduction* 25 (12): 2939–43.

———. 2011. "Assisted Reproduction on Treacherous Terrain: The Legal Hazards of Cross-Border Reproductive Travel." *Reproductive BioMedicine Online* 23 (5): 538–45.

Strathern, Marilyn. 2000. *Audit Cultures: Anthropological Studies in Accountability, Ethics and the Academy*. London: Routledge.

Suzuki, Masakuni. 2014. "*In Vitro* Fertilization in Japan—Early Days of *In Vitro* Fertilization and Embryo Transfer and Future Prospects for Assisted Reproductive Technology." *Proceedings of the Japan Academy of Science* 90 (5): 184–201.

Szewczuk, Elizabeth. 2011. "Age-Related Infertility: A Tale of Two Technologies." *Sociology of Health and Illness* 34(3): 429–43.

Tabutin, Dominique. 2005. "The Demography of the Arab World and the Middle East from the 1950s to the 2000s." *Population* 60 (5–6). http://www.cairn-int .info/journal-population-2005-5-page-505.htm.

Tavernise, Sabrina. 2014. "F.D.A. Weighs Fertility Method That Raises Ethical Questions." *New York Times*, February 25.

Tesoriero, Heather Won. 2008. "Infertile Couples Head Overseas for Treatments." *Wall Street Journal*, February 19.

Thompson, Charis M. 2005. *Making Parents: The Ontological Choreography of Reproductive Technologies*. Cambridge, MA: MIT Press.

Ticktin, Miriam Iris. 2011a. *Casualties of Care: Immigration and the Politics of Humanitarianism in France*. Berkeley: University of California Press.

———. 2011b. "How Biology Travels: A Humanitarian Trip." *Body & Society* 17 (2–3): 139–58.

Trainer, Sarah. 2012. "Negotiating Weight and Body Image in the UAE: Strategies among Young Emirati Women." *American Journal of Human Biology* 24 (3): 314–24.

Tsing, Anna L. 2005. *Friction: An Ethnography of Global Connection*. Princeton, NJ: Princeton University Press.

Turner, Leigh. 2007. "'First World Health Care at Third World Prices': Globalization, Bioethics and Medicine Tourism." *BioSocieties* 2: 303–25.

———. 2010. "Quality Health Care and Globalization of Health Services: Accreditations and Regulatory Oversight of Medical Tourism Companies." *International Journal for Quality in Health Care* 23 (1): 1–7.

Van Balen, Frank, and Trudie Gerrits. 2001. "Quality of Infertility Care in Poor-Resource Areas and the Introduction of New Reproductive Technologies." *Human Reproduction* 16 (2): 215–19.

Van Blerkom, Jonathan, et al. 2014. "First Births with a Simplified Culture System for Clinical IVF and Embryo Transfer." *Reproductive BioMedicine Online* 28 (3): 310–20.

Van Empel, Inge W. H., et al. 2008. "Coming Soon to Your Clinic: High-Quality ART." *Human Reproduction* 23 (6): 1242–45.

Vayena, Effy, et al. 2009. "Assisted Reproductive Technologies in Developing Countries: Are We Caring Yet?" *Fertility and Sterility* 92 (2): 413–16.

Vaynea, Effy, Patrick J. Rowe, and P. David Griffin, eds. 2002. *Current Practices and Controversies in Assisted Reproduction: Report of a World Health Organization Meeting*. Geneva: World Health Organization.

Vayena, Effy, Patrick J. Rowe, and Herbert B. Peterson. 2002. "Assisted Reproductive Technology in Developing Countries: Why Should We Care?" *Fertility and Sterility* 78 (1): 13–15.

Vora, Neha. 2013. *Impossible Citizens: Dubai's Indian Diaspora*. Durham, NC: Duke University Press.

Wahlberg, Ayo. 2012. "Selecting Donors in a Chinese Sperm Bank." Paper presented at Selective Reproductive Technologies: Routes of Routinisation and Globalisation, University of Copenhagen, Denmark, December 14.

Whittaker, Andrea M. 2008. "Pleasure and Pain: Medical Travel in Asia." *Global Public Health* 3 (3): 271–90.

———. 2009. "Global Technologies and Transnational Reproduction in Thailand." *Asian Studies Review* 33 (3): 319–32.

———. 2010. "Challenges of Medical Travel to Global Regulation: A Case Study of Reproductive Travel in Asia." *Global Social Policy* 10 (3): 396–415.

———. 2011. "Reproduction Opportunists in the New Global Sex Trade: PGD and Non-Medical Sex Selection." *Reproductive Biomedicine Online* 23 (5): 609–17.

———. 2015a. "'Outsourced' Patients and Their Companions: Stories from Forced Medical Travellers." *Global Public Health* 10(4): 485–500.

———. 2015b. *Thai In Vitro: Gender, Culture, and Assisted Reproduction*. New York: Berghahn.

Whittaker, Andrea M., Lenore Manderson, and Elizabeth Cartwright, eds. 2010. "Patients without Borders: Understanding Medical Travel." Special issue, *Medical Anthropology* 29 (4).

Whittaker, Andrea, and Amy Speier. 2010. "'Cycling Overseas': Care, Commodification, and Stratification in Cross-Border Reproductive Travel." *Medical Anthropology* 29 (4): 363–83.

World Health Organization. 2014. "Tobacco Free Initiative (TFI): Tobacco Facts." Accessed September 1, 2014. http://www.who.int/tobacco/mpower/tobacco _facts/en/.

Wyndham, Nicole, Paula Gabriela Marin Figueira, and Pasquale Patrizio. 2012. "A Persistent Misperception: Assisted Reproductive Technology Can Reverse the 'Aged Biological Clock.'" *Fertility and Sterility* 97 (5): 1044–47.

Yomoah, Doreen Akiyo. 2013. "When Being Childless Isn't a Choice." *Atlantic*, October 24. Accessed on September 9, 2014. http://www.theatlantic.com /international/archive/2013/10/when-being-childless-isn-t-a-choice/280833/.

Zanini, Giulia. 2011. "Abandoned by the State, Betrayed by the Church: Italian Experiences of Cross-Border Reproductive Care." *Reproductive BioMedicine Online* 23 (5): 565–72.

Zuhur, Sherifa. 1992. "Of Milk-Mothers and Sacred Bonds: Islam, Patriarchy, and New Reproductive Technologies." *Creighton Law Review* 25: 1725–38.

INDEX

diabetes, 70, 73–75, 148, 190, 302, 317, 332n96
diagnostic laparoscopy, 312. *See also* laparoscopy
disability: infertility as, xvii, xxvi, 289
divorce, xxiv, 60, 154
Djibouti, 118–19. *See also* East Africa
donor egg. *See* egg donation
donor insemination (DI), 25–26, 165–66, 175, 313
donor sperm. *See* sperm donation
Druze, 16
Dubai Department of Health (DOH), 165, 172
Dubai Health Authority, 33
Dubai Healthcare City, 43, 87, 294
Dubai International Airport, 19, 58, 294
Dubai, 2; abortion laws and, 87; class and, 52–53; as cosmopolitan center, 18–19, 28, 43, 51–53, 287, 292–96; as ethnocracy, 52, 127; future, 297–98; human trafficking and, 51–52; IVF in, xv, 2, 9, 33–34, 95, 132, 164–66, 191, 296; multiculturalism and, 54, 97, 101, 293; photographs of, 47–50; as techno-hub, 43–44, 115, 294; tourism and, 45–46; visitors' and tourists' visas in, 2, 9, 46, 56, 120, 140–41, 157, 252–53
Dubai: The Vulnerability of Success (Davidson), 51
Dunn, Frederick, 41–42, 327nn7–8
Dutch, 255–60
Dyer, Silke, 123–24

East Africa, 2, 9, 40, 55
ectopic pregnancy, xiii, 2, 78, 82, 132, 142, 145, 255, 262–63, 271, 313. *See also* cornual pregnancy
Edwards, Robert G., 4
egg donation, xxi, 9, 10, 69, 80, 83, 202–10, 313; as gift exchange, 24; procedure of, 25; in Spain and Eastern Europe, 23. *See also* third-party donation

egg donor. *See* egg donation
egg freezing. *See* oocyte cryopreservation
eggs, 317; "Ivy League" classification of, 24–25; quality of, 68
Egypt: IVF in, 16–18, 21, 221, 249; male fertility treatment in, 18; medical schools in, 43; reprotravel to, xii, 16
elective medicine, 13
El Rashid Hospital (Dubai), xv, 33
embodiment, 3, 13, 21, 25–26, 29, 147, 192, 298
embryo couriers, 25, 168, 219
embryo disposition, 179–80, 313
embryo donation, 168, 313. *See also* third–party donation
embryos, xiv, 216, 218, 313; frozen, 81–86
Emiratis, 15, 19, 32–34, 51–2, 55, 126, 196, 236, 298, 301; publicly funded IVF and, 131–33. *See also* United Arab Emirates
Emiratization, 346n38
Empty Quarter (Arabian Peninsula), 143, 146–47
endometrial cyst. *See* chocolate cyst
endometrioma. *See* chocolate cyst
endometriosis, 141, 176, 260, 313, 336–37. *See also* chocolate cyst
England. *See* United Kingdom
epididymis, 313
Ethiopia, xvi
Ethiopian Civil War, xi
ethnography, 18, 21; marital, 28
eugenics, 110, 178
European Society for Human Reproduction and Embryology (ESHRE), 9, 105, 174, 304
experimental medicine: and medical travel, 13

fatwa, 16, 101, 163, 168, 188, 344n98
Federal Law No. 11, 167–68, 172, 176, 179, 190, 195, 218, 340n13, 340n18. *See also* United Arab Emirates: reproductive laws in

female infertility: abortions and, 108; cultural pressures and, 153, 226–27; domestic violence and, 151, 154; infections and, 108–9, 119, 302; as "invisible disability," xvii, xxv–xxvi, 1, 3, 289; irregular menstruation and, 152; medically induced, 254–55; misdiagnosis and, 223, 243; PCOS and, 32, 71–76, 87–88, 138–39, 213, 223, 258–59, 274, 302, 317; second-hand smoke and, 72–73; work and, 67–68

Ferguson, James, 110–11

fertility postponement, 67, 302. *See also* advanced maternal age

fertility tourism. *See* reproductive tourism

fertility: rates of, 108

fetal ensoulment, 170, 189

fibroid tumor, 157–58, 314

follicle stimulating hormone (FSH), 178, 208, 258, 314

fostering, 84, 187, 303, 342n56. *See also* adoption

Foucault, Michel, 21, 42, 327n10

France: IVF in, 98–99, 134

Franklin, Sarah, 289–90

free trade zones, 43–44

Fulbright program, 18

gamete donation. *See* third-party donation

gamete intrafallopian transfer (GIFT), 272–73, 314

gamete, 314

gender, 24

Genk Institute for Fertility Technology, 106

Germany, 178

gestational surrogacy. *See* surrogacy

Ginsburg, Faye, 111

global assemblage, 21–22

global cosmopolitans, 61, 65, 77–78. *See also* medical cosmopolitanism

globalization, 9, 12, 24, 40, 348n24; characteristics of, 20–23, 292; definition of, 20; unevenness, 111

global reproductive assemblages, 20, 22

global shadows, 110, 114

glocalization, 20

Gonal F (hormonal medication), xvii, 260

gonorrhea, 109, 302, 316

Guinness Book of World Records, 83

Gulf Arabs, 15, 17, 43, 49, 293, 295

Gürtin, Zeynep, 134, 299

habitus, 329n49

halal, 162, 168–70, 187, 195, 199

haram, 144, 162–63, 166, 169–70, 185–89, 199, 207, 236

Harley Street (London), 122, 165

Harvard University, 43

hasad, 161, 339n1

health care: privatization of, 12, 14, 33–34, 106; quality of , 241–53; regulation of private sector, 2

health insurance, 106, 123, 131–35, 210

hepatitis, 168, 176–77, 324n44

hidden sperm. *See* male infertility: cryptospermia

high-order multiple pregnancy (HOMP), 166, 190–94, 201, 254, 314. *See also* multifetal pregnancy reduction

Hinduism, xxvii, 227. *See also* Hindus

Hindus: views on third-party donation, 165–66, 184

HIV/AIDS, xxiv, 109, 176

Holland. *See* the Netherlands

hormonal treatment, xii, xxii, 87; moodiness and, 225

hubs of reproductive travel. *See* reprohub

Human Reproduction (journal), 232, 254

hydrosalpinx, xv–xvi, xix, 79, 259, 314

hyperstimulation. *See* ovarian hyperstimulation syndrome

hypertension, 70, 78, 190

hysteroscopy, 157–58, 314

iatrogenesis, 254–55, 314

in vitro fertilization (IVF), xii, 4, 289–90, 315; activism and, 95–96, 103; availability of, 27; constraints on, 26–27; cost of, 2, 27, 91, 105–7, 120,

122–25, 212, 300; cultural affinity and, 226–27, 248–49; cultural barriers and, 27; debt and, xx, xxvi–xxvii, 2, 123–24; diagnosis and, 222; egg collection and, xxvii, 149, 158; in Egypt, 249; first case of, 3–4, 33; fresh cycles of, xiii–xiv; frozen cycles of, xiii–xiv; globalization of, 9, 20, 21, 33, 40, 110–12; holiday travel and, 17–18, 21; infection and, xxvii, 119, 287; Islamic law and, xxi, 2, 9, 208–11; in Lebanon, 221, 249; legal restrictions and, 2, 5–6, 22, 173–74, 292; overprescription of, 254; poverty and, 125–31; privacy and, 235–37; procedure of, 4; psychological care and, 238–39; public financing of, 98, 131–4, 137, 253; religious prohibitions on, 2, 27; salpingectomy and, 263; sex selection and, 11, 32, 145, 194–97; sperm collection and, xxvii, 149; state subsidization of, 12, 17; success rates of, 26, 27, 223–24, 254; unmet need and, 110, 114–15; work and, 64–65

India: assisted reproductive care in, 250–52; gamete donation in, 184–85; IVF in, xvii, 115, 243, 253, 263; medical travel in, xv, 13–15, 250, 257–58, 262, 292; public health in, 14; stem-cell therapy in, 12; surrogacy in, 10–11, 23, 264

Indian Medical Travel Association, 14

Indian Ministry of Tourism, 14

Indians: and reprotravel, 19, 141, 252–53, 261; views of medical care in India, 250–51. *See also* nonresident Indians (NRIs)

infertility, 315; cultural pressure to reproduce and, xx, xviii, 63, 89–93, 143–44, 153; global metrics of, 107–10; HIV risk and, 109; Internet and, 65–66, 95, 99; lifestyle factors and, 69–70, 75–76, 78; marriage and, 59; obesity and, 70, 73–76, 302; prevention of, 302; primary and secondary, 108, 135, 315; secrecy and, 235–36; as social burden, 1; stigma and, 1, 28, 93, 145–46, 163, 177, 188, 236, 264, 303;

unemployment and, 63–64. *See also* female infertility; male infertility

Institute of Medicine, 232

insulin resistance, 32, 73–76, 142, 213, 226, 237, 261, 268, 276, 290, 302, 317, 338n120

International Committee Monitoring Assisted Reproductive Technologies, 10

International Federation of Fertility Societies (IFFS), 111–12, 114, 173

Internet chat rooms, 84

interstitial pregnancy. *See* cornual pregnancy

intracytoplasmic sperm injection (ICSI), 32, 99, 130–31, 176–78, 210, 215–20, 252, 266, 269–70, 288, 315; cost of, 107; gender differences and, 24; globalization of, 18; informant views of, 92; in Lebanon, 18, 221, 249; success rates of, 223–24

intrauterine insemination (IUI), 32, 130, 252, 271, 315; Muslim views of, 185

Iran, 16, 231

Iranians: in Dubai, 44–45

Iraq War, 18

Iraq, 16, 114

ISIS, 297

Islam, xxi; male gynecologists and, 227; medical interventions and, 223; non-Muslim doctors and, 226–27; views on sex selection, 194, 197. *See also* Sunni Muslims; Shia Muslims

Israel, 112, 348n11; IVF in, 134, 203–4, 207, 283, 300, 338nn108–9

IVF absences, 16, 20, 110–15, 137

IVF clinics: in Beirut, 275; in Cairo, 21; data collection about, 16; design of, 34; government-run, 93, 132–34, 141, 159, 164–66, 215, 248; in India, 11, 142, 243, 263; marketing of, 11; referrals to, 2, 222; registration of, 10, 16; in the United Arab Emirates, 33–34, 245–47. *See also* Conceive

IVF holidays, 17–18, 21, 329n53

IVF troubadours, 33

IVF. *See* in vitro fertilization